Biomaterials and Immune Response

Complications, Mechanisms and Immunomodulation

Devices, Circuits, and Systems

Series Editor: Krzysztof Iniewski, Emerging Technologies CMOS Inc.
Vancouver, British Columbia, Canada

Edited by leading experts in the field, this series covers current and emerging technologies with a focus on applications. Authored by academics, researchers, and professionals from around the globe, the content provides an in-depth discussion and analysis of research directions in sensors, circuits, electronics, telecommunications, photonics, nanotechnology, and electronics. Graduate students, researchers, and professionals with a broad interest in various electrical engineering topics will find this series of great value.

CMOS: Front-End Electronics for Radiation Sensors
Angelo Rivetti

Laser-Based Optical Detection of Explosives
Paul M. Pellegrino, Ellen L. Holthoff, Mikella E. Farrell

Atomic Nanoscale Technology in the Nuclear Industry
Taeho Woo

Semiconductors: Integrated Circuit Design for Manufacturability
Artur Balasinski

Magnetic Sensors and Devices: Technologies and Applications
Laurent A. Francis and Kirill Poletkin

Semiconductor Radiation Detectors: Technology and Applications
Salim Reza

Nanoplasmonics: Advanced Device Applications
James W. M. Chon and Krzysztof Iniewski

Labs on Chip: Principles, Design and Technology
Eugenio Iannone

Noise Coupling in System-on-Chip
Thomas Noulis

High Frequency Communication and Sensing: Traveling-Wave Techniques
Ahmet Tekin and Ahmed Emira

3D Integration in VLSI Circuits: Implementation Technologies and Applications
Katsuyuki Sakuma

IoT and Low-Power Wireless: Circuits, Architectures, and Techniques
Christopher Siu and Krzysztof Iniewski

Biomaterials and Immune Response: Complications, Mechanisms and Immunomodulation
Nihal Engin Vrana

For more information about this series, please visit: https://www.crcpress.com/Devices-Circuits-and-Systems/book-series/CRCDEVCIRSYS

Biomaterials and Immune Response

Complications, Mechanisms and Immunomodulation

Edited by
Nihal Engin Vrana

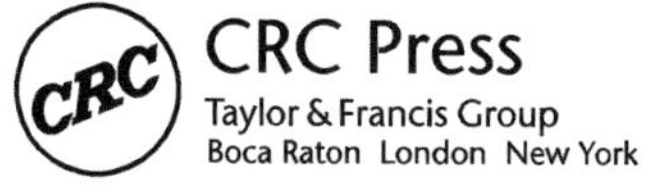
CRC Press
Taylor & Francis Group
Boca Raton London New York

CRC Press is an imprint of the
Taylor & Francis Group, an **informa** business

CRC Press
Taylor & Francis Group
6000 Broken Sound Parkway NW, Suite 300
Boca Raton, FL 33487-2742

First issued in paperback 2023

ISBN 13: 978-1-03-265302-0 (pbk)
ISBN 13: 978-1-138-50637-4 (hbk)
ISBN 13: 978-1-3151-4714-7 (ebk)

DOI: 10.1201/b22419

Publisher's Note
The publisher has gone to great lengths to ensure the quality of this reprint but points out that some imperfections in the original copies may be apparent.

Library of Congress Cataloging-in-Publication Data

Names: Vrana, Nihal Engin, author.
Title: Biomaterials and immune response : complications, mechanisms and immunomodulation / Nihal Engin Vrana.
Other titles: Devices, circuits, and systems.
Description: Boca Raton : Taylor & Francis, 2018. | Series: Devices, circuits, and systems | Includes bibliographical references and index.
Identifiers: LCCN 2018006719 | ISBN 9781138506374 (hardback : alk. paper)
Subjects: | MESH: Biocompatible Materials | Immunologic Factors | Immunity, Cellular | Prostheses and Implants | Immunomodulation
Classification: LCC QR185.35 | NLM QT 37 | DDC 616.07/9--dc23
LC record available at https://lccn.loc.gov/2018006719

Visit the Taylor & Francis Web site at
http://www.taylorandfrancis.com

and the CRC Press Web site at
http://www.crcpress.com

Contents

Preface

The advances in supramolecular chemistry, additive manufacturing and synthetic biology and related fields have been expanding the potential use of biomaterials in applications that were not even imaginable a short time ago. The transfer of 3D printing technologies for the development of artificial organs and tissues by use of cells together with biomaterial-based bioinks provide a new level of accuracy and complexity for regenerative medicine applications. The techniques developed for tissue engineering applications have been spilling over to the field of "soft robotics", and cell-laden biomaterial-based hydrogel use in biorobotics is an active field of research with exciting applications both in the biomedical field and beyond. Micro/nanoscale implantable devices, theranostic systems and biodegradable electronics benefit from the constant innovation and availability of new biomaterials. With this increase in demand, metabiomaterials of different properties will surely follow to meet the demands and needs of future engineers. However, this increasing level of complexity comes with a cost: an increasing level of complications.

Beyond mechanical or technical complications and being a potential haven for infection, the biggest roadblock for advanced implantable biomaterial-based structures is the immune system. The mammalian immune system is perplexing in its efficacy, ingenuity and level of safety in redundancy, but it is also staggering in its complexity and "no mercy" approach to its task – sometimes to the detriment of the body it is trying to protect. Allergies, chronic inflammation, granuloma formation, full-scale foreign body response or complete rejection; there are many potential bad endings for implantable biomaterials. The only way to avoid such adverse reactions is to develop a more comprehensive understanding of the immune system, its components, and its interactions with the potential insults in the context of biomaterials. In this book, we aim to provide undergraduate- and graduate-level students and researchers in the biomaterials field with a starting point for understanding the context-driven responses of the immune system by dedicated chapters to material properties, specific biomaterials, defined applications and clinical situations. We hope that the book will provide an overall appreciation of the role of the immune system in biomaterial applications and can demonstrate the need for the incorporation of immunomodulatory components in devices for better clinical outcomes.

Being implanted to a host body is a bit like starting a new job in a hostile environment. There are lots of office politics, history, mindset and interpersonal relations issues to learn to be able to tread lightly and undamaged. The immune system of the mammalian host is the "watchman" and the office bully in this context and we should send biomaterials that are able to deal with it, or at least those that can appease the immune system. One of the keys of an even bigger expansion of biomaterial use lies in this challenge. Also, in the context of auto-immune diseases, there is the standing question of "Who watches the watchmen?", which might also find its answer in advanced immunomodulation.

Acknowledgements

I dedicate this book to Dr. Yurong Liu, a great scientist who has left us at an early age. Yurong taught me how to really listen to people (which is a difficult but very important lesson). I will carry his memory with me for the rest of my career. I thank my family, my team in Protip Medical and also my colleagues in INSERM UMR 1121 for their support.

This work received funding from the European Union's Seventh Framework programme for Research, Technological Development and Demonstration under grant agreement No. 602694 (IMMODGEL) and 606624 (NanoTi). This project has received funding from the European Union's Horizon 2020 research and innovation programme under grant agreement No. 760921 (PANBioRA).

Editor

Nihal Engin Vrana is Vice President (Scientific Affairs) of Protip Medical (Strasbourg, France) and an affiliated researcher in INSERM Unit 1121 (Biomaterials and Bioengineering). He earned his PhD in 2009 (Dublin City University) as a Marie Curie ESR Fellow. He finished his post-doctoral training at INSERM Unit 977 and then in Harvard-MIT Division of Health Sciences and Technology. His research interests include tissue engineering, biomaterials, cell/material interface, materials science, and immunology.

He has been the scientific coordinator of three European projects: EuroTransBio Bimot (2012–2015), FP7 IMMODGEL (2013–2017), and Horizon 2020 PANBioRA (2018–2021). His team in Protip Medical has been involved in several national and international collaborative research projects with a total budget of more than 22 million Euros. Dr. Vrana published 62 articles in international academic journals (more than 1400 citations, h-index: 22), 6 book chapters, edited the book *Cell and Material Interface* (CRC Press, 2015) and holds 4 European patents (2 more in progress). His prizes include the Parlar Foundation's Thesis of the Year Prize (2006), European Society of Biomaterials Translational Research Award (2011), Best Patent Prize in 2nd Aegean R&D Days (2012), International Federation of Otorhinolarnygological Societies Meeting Outstanding Paper Award (2013).

Contributors

Zehra Betül Ahi
Department of Polymer Engineering
Yalova University
Yalova, Turkey

Bengü Aktaş
Institute of Biomedical Engineering
Boğaziçi University
Istanbul, Turkey

Eda Ayşe Aksoy
Department of Basic Pharmaceutical Sciences
Faculty of Pharmacy
Hacettepe University
Ankara, Turkey

Julien Barthès
Inserm UMR 1121
and
Protip Medical
Strasbourg, France

Luiz E. Bertassoni
Department of Restorative Dentistry
Oregon Health & Science University
Portland, Oregon

Eszter Bognár
IMEDIM Ltd.
Budapest, Hungary

Özge Erdemli
Department of Molecular Biology and Genetics
Başkent University
Ankara, Turkey

Emre Ergene
Department of Biomedical Engineering
Ankara University
Ankara, Turkey

Güneş Esendağlı
Department of Basic Oncology
Hacettepe University Cancer Institute
Ankara, Turkey

Praveen Gajendrareddy
Department of Periodontics
University of Illinois at Chicago
Chicago, Illinois

Bora Garipcan
Institute of Biomedical Engineering
Boğaziçi University
Istanbul, Turkey

Michael Gasik
School of Chemical Engineering
Aalto University Foundation
Espoo, Finland

Pinar Yılgör Huri
Department of Biomedical Engineering
Ankara University
Ankara, Turkey

Imre Kientzl
FERR-VÁZ Ltd.
Budapest, Hungary

Helena Knopf-Marques
Inserm UMR 1121
and
Faculté de Chirurgie Dentaire
Université de Strasbourg
Strasbourg, France

Clarence Lee
Department of Periodontology
Oregon Health & Science University
Portland, Oregon

Christopher Louie
Department of Periodontology
Oregon Health & Science University
Portland, Oregon

Kristina Nesporova
Contipro a.s.
Dolni Dobrouc
Dolni Dobrouc, Czech Republic

Hayriye Özçelik
INSERM UPR3572-Immunopathologie et Chimie Thérapeutique
Strasbourg, France

Lilian Paiva
Department of Dentistry
Federal University of Sergipe
Aracaju, Brazil

Liza Pelyhe
InDeRe
Institute for Food System Research and Innovation Nonprofit Ltd.
Budapest, Hungary

Sivaraman Prakasam
Department of Periodontology
Oregon Health & Science University
Portland, Oregon

Flavie Prévot
Ecole Supérieure de Biotechnologie de Strasbourg
Illkirch, France

Lia Rimondini
Dipartimento di Scienze della Salute Via Solaroli 17
Universitá del Piemonte Orientale
Novara, Italy

Barbora Safrankova
Contipro a.s
Dolni Dobrouc
Dolni Dobrouc, Czech Republic

Ivana Scigalkova
Contipro a.s.
Dolni Dobrouc
Dolni Dobrouc, Czech Republic

Tuğba Endoğan Tanır
Central Laboratory
Middle East Technical University
Ankara, Turkey

Ayşen Tezcaner
Department of Engineering Sciences
Middle East Technical University
and
BIOMATEN Center of Excellence in Biomaterials and Tissue Engineering
Middle East Technical University
Ankara, Turkey

Kadriye Tuzlakoğlu
Department of Polymer Engineering
Yalova University
Yalova, Turkey

Nihal Engin Vrana
Protip Medical
and
INSERM
Biomatériaux et Bioingénierie
and
Fédération de Médecine Translationnelle de Strasbourg
Fédération de Recherche Matériaux et Nanosciences Grand Est (FRMNGE)
Faculté de Chirurgie Dentaire
Université de Strasbourg
Strasbourg, France

Miklós Weszl
Department of Biophysics and Radiation Biology
Semmelweis University
and
Department of Health Economics
Corvinus University of Budapest
Budapest, Hungary

1 Editorial
Introduction to Immune Response and Biomaterials

Nihal Engin Vrana

CONTENTS

1.1 INTRODUCTION

The human immune system has evolved to be a formidable line of defence against physical and also biological insults. Both specific and non-specific immune reactions keep our bodies safe around the clock from external threats such as pathogenic microorganisms or internal threats such as tumor formation. The importance of the immune system can be easily appreciated by the debilitating and far-reaching nature of the effects of immunosuppressive and auto-immune diseases, such as AIDS, Multiple Sclerosis, Lupus etc. For example, Systemic Lupus Erythematosus is a chronic auto-immune disease that can touch many organs – including the kidney, heart and lungs – and requires life-long treatment. Although a defined etiology cannot be set, T-helper cell imbalance and high levels of pro-inflammatory cytokines are closely linked with the flares of the disease [1]. Multiple Sclerosis is a nervous system disease where an auto-immune response towards the myeline sheath (a cholesterol-rich layer surrounding some nerves which controls impulse rate by providing electrical insulation) of nerves interferes with signal transmission and leads to subsequent functional motor problems (such as loss of balance, diminished mobility etc.). This results in loss of mobility, uncontrollable muscle contractions and a wide range of other chronic problems. Again, a complete etiology has not yet been established but genetic factors involving the differentiation of T-helper cells have been strongly implicated [2]. Acquired Immune Deficiency Syndrome (AIDS) is a viral infection-driven disease (by the Human Immunodeficiency Virus) characterised by the significant depletion of a subset of T-cells ($CD4^+$) which results in an overall susceptibility to opportunistic infections of a bacterial, viral or fungal nature with fatal consequences. There is also an increased risk of tumor development, as the immune system is active in the detection and elimination of potentially cancerous cells [3]. These extreme cases clearly demonstrate the importance of a functional, efficient immune system for human health.

However, one downside of this efficacy is the unintentional barrier it creates for the application of material-based systems for improving health. Advances in biomaterials, implantology and biomedical engineering together with micro/nanotechnologies provide a wide range of potential methods where an engineered material can be used in the human body to solve a medical problem. This can be in the form of passive, material-only based structures such as dental implants, systems containing mechanically or electronically active components such as artificial heart valves and pacemakers or structures that also have cellular components such as tissue engineering scaffolds containing autologous cells. However, in all these scenarios, the materials to be used need to be accepted by the host immune system; otherwise, the potential damages might be even more drastic than the original problem. This can be appreciated in the case of transplants where host-donor match is essential for prevention of rejection of the organ. However, even in the best cases lifelong immunosuppression is required. Allografts are attacked by cytotoxic T-cells and Natural Killer (NK) cells where secretions of these cells such as perforins (which induce pores on the target cell membrane) and granzymes (serine proteases, which degrade proteins) are responsible for a significant portion of the damage of the transplanted tissue [4]. The cells of allogenic (non-self, same-species cells) origin were either eliminated or rendered dysfunctional, resulting in the rejection and failure of the transplanted organ (Figure 1.1).

The human immune system is highly complex and involves intertwined sets of reactions including a wide range of cell types, but also other bioactive molecules

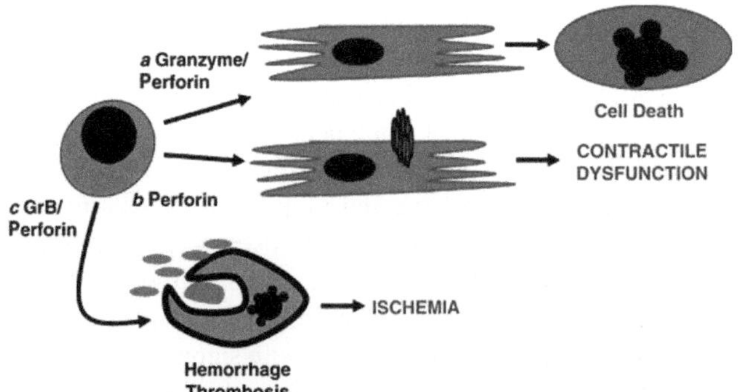

FIGURE 1.1 Modes of activity of perforins and granzymes secreted by the host immune cells on allogeneic cells in transplanted organs (the heart is given as an example). The activities of the host immune response result in transplanted cell death and dysfunction which consequently leads to organ failure and rejection in the absence of immunosuppression. (Reprinted from Choy JC, *Cell Death Differ.* 2010;17(4):567–76. With permission.)

ranging from simple, non-specific molecules to highly specific complex proteins such as cytokines, enzymes, reactive oxygen species and antibodies. In general terms, immunity is divided into cellular and humoral immunity. Humoral immunity refers to immune responses based on molecular-level activity, such as molecules involved in complement systems, antimicrobial peptides and, most importantly, antibodies (or immunoglobulins). Antibody-mediated responses are relevant for many biomaterials as the host body might already have antibodies against the biomaterial in use, particularly for those of xenogenic (from another species) origin. For example, although generally considered to have low immunogenicity, collagen (one of the main constituents of the mammalian extracellular matrix) has been shown to induce antibody responses when interspecies implantation or injection has been carried out, particularly due to the differences in aminoacid sequences and structural properties between species (at terminal, central or helical regions of the triple helix structure of collagen) [5]. Even against synthetic polymers, antibody-based reactions have been observed. (For example, Immunoglobulin Gs (IgGs) were observed against polyurethane together with cellulose acetate (a natural polysaccharide derivative) in rats when implanted as a part of a glucose sensor [6].)

In a broad sense, when an antigen (a molecule that is recognized as foreign and induces an immune response) is present, it is taken up by B-cells, processed and then presented on B-cell surface (in combination with major histocompatibility complex molecules). This leads to binding of T-helper cells and induces B-cell proliferation. The resulting B-cells can be either memory cells which will enable reaction toward the processed antigen in the future (when the antigen is detected in the body again (adaptive immunity and immunological memory)) or plasma cells which produce large quantities of the specific antibody that will interfere with the antigen and stimulate its elimination. As a system, antigen-mediated immunity is an elegant process due to its high specificity, responsiveness and efficacy. From a technological point of view, its ability to memorize antigens enabled the development of vaccine systems. B-cells, like all immune cells, have different subpopulations with differing regulatory activities. Breg (regulatory B-cells) can regulate T-cell activities and are known to be involved in the suppression of inflammation in auto-immune diseases and inflammation [7]. Even though our main focus is on adverse immune responses to biomaterials, one recent trend in the utilization of biomaterials as immunostimulators for applications such as cancer immunotherapy should be also noted [8]. In this context, the known reactions to a given biomaterial can be used to induce a local microenvironment that will enable tumor clearance.

Cellular immunity, on the other hand, refers to cell-mediated immune responses such as antigen-specific cytotoxic T-cell activity (for killing diseased cells including infected and cancerous cells via induction of apoptosis) or non-specific phagocytosis activity by macrophages, NK cells, foreign body giant cells etc. In one sense, it refers to the direct actions against infectious agents such as bacteria, fungi or protosoans. Cellular immunity is linked with humoral immunity in many ways (for example, the phagocytic activity of macrophages results in antigen presentation which triggers humoral response); moreover cell-mediated immunity also comprises the secretion of cytokines, which results in further stimulation or attenuation of immune responses.

1.2 WHY IS IMMUNE RESPONSE IMPORTANT IN BIOMATERIALS?

The presence of a biomaterial inside the body inevitably triggers an immune response. There are two aspects to the reaction: first, the presence of the biomaterial is a physical insult, but, additionally, introduction of the biomaterial in most cases also entails an injury (surgery) [9]. Thus, mobilization of the immune system due to the injury is tightly linked with the immune reaction to biomaterials. The surfaces presented by the implanted material will adsorb proteins from blood which will provide the initial signal for the immune cells to adhere to the material surface (via the adsorbed proteins). The presence of damaged capillaries and blood vessels induces clot formation on the surface of the biomaterial and accumulation of a provisional matrix rich in fibrin. From this point on, acute and chronic inflammatory responses follow as a function of the material that has been implanted, the implantation site, the patient's immune profile and the extent of injury. In an ideal implantation scenario (which practitioners are trying to implement in regenerative medicine applications), at the end of chronic inflammation, the injury site is healed, the implanted material is completely integrated with the host tissue and the inflammation is completely resolved within a timeframe of a few weeks. However, for non-degradable biomaterials or partially degradable biomaterials this would not be the case and the formation of a granulation tissue followed by a fibrous capsule formation generally takes place depending on the aforementioned parameters of the implant microenvironment and host.

One of the main activities in cellular immunity is phagocytosis, which is also highly relevant in the interaction of biomaterials and the immune system particularly for micro/nanoscale systems such as controlled drug delivery vectors. Phagocytosis is a term derived from Greek, and literally means "eating of cells". In the context of biomaterials, important phagocytes include neutrophils (in the acute phase of inflammation), monocytes/monocyte-derived macrophages (in the chronic phase) and macrophage-derived foreign body giant cells (in the end stages). Receptor-mediated phagocytosis occurs through recognition of the foreign material via surface receptors of the phagocytes, which induces stretching and invagination of the phagocyte's cell membrane to enable the intake of foreign material. The presence of a bulk or porous material in the body attracts phagocytes and their short- and long-term activities will determine the immediate microenvironment of the implanted material, as one aspect of the cell-mediated immunity is the secretion of cytokines and control over the incoming immune cells [10]. For a degradable material, the presence of phagocytes will contribute to its degradation and their activity should be taken into account while the stability of the implanted material is considered. The second question in this context is whether the degraded parts of the implanted biomaterial will be presented as antigens by macrophages or dendritic cells. If this is the case, this will induce further humoral and cell-mediated responses. In the case of non-degradable materials, the effect will be size-dependent: at nano and low microscales the material will be phagocytosed and have direct effects on the cellular pathways of immune cells or have cytotoxic effects and induce indirect immune responses. The materials at macroscale, on the other hand, will give rise to a different kind of reaction; as the size of the material compared to phagocytic cell size excludes its direct phagocytosis of the material and secretions (be it enzymes, ROS etc.) proves not enough for its removal, immune cells resort to fusion and creation of phagocytic cells with more capacity (such as foreign body giant cells) [11].

The reaction to foreign materials by the immune system "foreign body response" (the end-stage of a long sequence of events) is an integral part of the biomaterials field, as it defines the conditions that any biomaterial-based implantable, injectable, contact-with-body device needs to work in. Thus, it is essential for biomaterial scientists to develop an appreciation of the immune responses to biomaterials in order to develop innovative solutions for circumventing these reactions by design. The recent concept of Safety by Design is inherent in biomaterial development. The immune system is based on checks and balances on many levels; where a certain event (such as the presence of an antigen) can result in a cascade of events. Thus, any biomaterial-based design should take into account such events during the expected lifetime of a given implantable structure and match the desired function with host reactions spatiotemporally.

Beyond cellular and humoral immunity, another way of dividing the activities of the immune system that is regularly utilized is the distinction between innate and adaptive immunity. As the response to biomaterials has a significant innate immunity component, it is important to understand the underlying differences between these two types of immune responses. Innate immunity, a system of immediate defense particularly evolved against pathogenic agents, is based on pre-set reactions (through already-existing receptors at the birth of an individual [12]) to provide a fast and decisive response. One example of the target of recognition is bacterial lipopolysaccharide (LPS), which is highly conserved in gram-negative bacteria; thus, it can be used as a general "alarm" for the presence of unwanted organisms (other such examples would be the presence of double-stranded RNA (for viruses) or the presence of mannan on the membrane (for yeast)).

The family of receptors for such signals (such as CD-14; in general these receptors are referred to as pattern recognition receptors (PRRs)) is one of the most important components of innate immunity. For example, Toll-like receptors (TLRs) are a crucial part of innate immunity as they first recognize foreign materials and then start the immune response pathway [13]. They do this via the detection of specific pathogen-associated molecular patterns (PAMPs), indirectly. The recognition of a potential insult by the innate immune system also activates downstream activities, including adaptive immunity. Unlike innate immunity, which is a highly conserved mechanism, adaptive immunity is unique to vertebrates and evolved more recently. Instead of relying on pre-set signals, adaptive immunity relies on the detection of antigens, their presentation and the subsequent development of a memory (in the form of memory B-cells) that will enable effective defense against the same insult in a later stage of the individual's lifetime. Immunoglobulins (antibodies) are a crucial component of adaptive immune response. There are five different isotypes of antibodies, namely IgA, IgD, IgE, IgG and IgM. The isotypes differ in their function, location and also the expression during the maturation of adaptive immune cells. For example, naïve B-cells express IgM which is the first antibody to react during a first exposure and IgE which has a specific function in allergic reactions whereas IgGs are active in the clearance of pathogens [14].

In the case of biomaterials, the mechanisms of innate immunity (particularly the cellular component) are in most cases more prominent where there is potentially no or limited exposure to a given biomaterial by the host prior to implantation, thus making it highly unlikely that the implanted material will be recognized by adaptive immunity. However, the first implantation of a material will provide the necessary steps for the development of adaptive immune responses as the biomaterial has been processed before as an antigen and there is a probability that antibodies against a given biomaterial have been developed by an individual. Thus, in the future, there is room for immunodiagnostics for person-specific determination of responses to a given biomaterial for taking into account the patient's immunoprofile in biomaterial applications.

An integral part of the innate immune reaction is the secretion of cytokines. Cytokines are small, potent signaling proteins with autocrine (on the same cell), paracrine (on cells in the immediate vicinity) or endocrine (cells at a distant location) activities. They are secreted by many immune cells (such as mast cells, leucocytes and macrophages) and have important roles in immunomodulation. They can be both pro-inflammatory (such as Interferon-ɣ, Tumor Necrosis Factor α and some interleukins such as IL-1β, IL-6 or IL-12) or anti-inflammatory (such as IL-1 Receptor Antagonist, IL-4 and IL-10) [15]. Another way of dividing cytokines is functional, that is, whether they regulate cellular responses (type I) or humoral responses (type II). Cytokine nomenclature generally refers to functional activities of the given protein; for example, chemokines have distinct chemotactic features, whereas the name interleukin refers to the fact that these proteins are released by one white blood cell and act on another. The presence of a cytokine has distinct and context-dependent effects; for example, cytokines can determine the phenotype of a given immune cell; where each cytokine induces specific functional responses (IFN-ɣ, for example, induces a pro-inflammatory macrophage phenotype; on the other hand, IL-4 induces an anti-inflammatory macrophage phenotype) [16]. Over- or under-expression of cytokines are not only important actors in wound healing, chronic inflammation, cancer and infection, but can also be used as diagnostic tools and potential therapeutic targets for immunomodulation.

The complement system is another façade of innate immunity, where more than 30 soluble plasma proteins and cell surface receptors are involved in the clearance of foreign materials [9]. The complement system can be activated via three routes in the presence of foreign materials or altered self-molecules (classical pathway, alternative pathway and lectin pathway), resulting in a cascade of events that result in either enzymatic degradation of the target, lysis of the target organism (via membrane attack complex (MAC)) or decoration of the target and recruitment of cells (such as leucocytes) by complement components (for example, C3a and C5a) that results in phagocytosis or lysis of the target [17]. Finally, there is a simple but highly potent weapon in the arsenal of innate immunity: reactive oxygen species. These highly reactive oxygen components, such as superoxide ($\bullet O^{-2}$) or hydrogen peroxide (H_2O_2), are produced and released by immune cells as a part of their defence against pathogens [18]. This very efficient method of protection is highly conserved evolutionarily, as similar mechanisms are also observed in plants. However, a long-term release of ROS can have unintended collateral damage on surrounding tissues, as its activity is highly generic – unlike some other components of immunity. This is especially important in biomaterial-related situations, as frustrated phagocytosis (the inability of phagocytes to eliminate macroscopic non-degradable materials) in the presence of implants can result in high concentrations of ROS release for long periods of time.

So, in brief, the role of innate immunity, where the immune reaction is antigen-independent, is more prominent in the earlier phase of foreign body response as the initial interaction of the immune cells starts with the recruitment of neutrophils, monocytes and differentiation of monocytes into macrophages and subsequent cytokine release. Adaptive immunity – antigen-based reactions – is more material-type-dependent where the presence or absence of antigens will depend on the source of the biomaterial and its properties.

1.3 CELLS IN IMMUNE RESPONSE TO BIOMATERIALS

A confounding aspect of the immune system is the sheer number of different cell types involved in immune response. Moreover, each of these cell types have several sub-populations either defined in the form of expression or absence of a given surface marker (such as $CD14^+$ monocytes in peripheral blood mononuclear cell populations) or in more general functional terms (such as Tregs, referring to regulatory T-cells). One common way of differentiating white blood cells is through their seperation as agranulocytes (monocytes and lymphocytes) and granulocytes (such as neutrophils and mast cells). The cell types with which we are familiar from blood tests are: neutrophils (defence against bacterial and fungal infections, the first cells to arrive to implanted material surfaces in their function of bacterial clearance), basophils (release of histamine; for vasodilation, they also have roles in allergic responses), eosinophils (more specific for larger parasitic infections, such as worms), lymphocytes (T- and B-cells, adaptive immunity cells) and monocytes (phagocytes and antigen-presenting cells). Beyond these are the immune cells circulating in the lympathic system and in blood; there are tissue-residing immune cells such as resident macrophages, and mast cells, which are generally referred to as different cell types (such as osteoclasts in bone or Kuppfer cells in liver) [19].

One of the defining qualities of the immune system is its plasticity. Even though there are defined cell types with specific roles in the immune system, these cells show a significant level of phenotypic plasticity to achieve their functions. This means these cells show distinctly different phenotypes under different stimulations, which not only affects their own behaviour, but also the downstream consequences in their interactions with other cells. One of the best-defined such differences is that between Th1 and Th2 (T-helper 1 and T-helper 2, respectively) immunity related to T-lymphocytes (where helper lymphocytes are a subpopulation of T-lympocytes) [20]. This was first described in mice with CD4+ lymphocytes, and refers to two distinct secretion profiles: where the Th1 cytokine profile (IL-2/Interferon-γ, LT (lymphotoxin)) is more active in cell-mediated immunity (both inflammatory and cytotoxic functions), the Th2 cytokine profile (IL-4, IL-5, IL-10) induces more antibody-mediated responses [20,21]. Stimulation of CD4+ naïve T-cells with antigen presentation results in IL-2 secretion, which is followed by assumption of a distinct phenotype as a function of the microenvironment. In most cases, these patterns are mutually exclusive and there is a dominance of one pattern over the other in a given situation. Moreover, even though such classifications are generally useful for a better understanding of otherwise overwhelmingly complex patterns of immune response, they generally tend to fall into an n-dimensional space of potential responses and can be easily divided into several other subpopulations. However, the important distinction between these different populations remains: cytokine secretion and marker expression of immune cells is not random and is mostly predictive of the future steps of immune response.

As can be seen in the following chapters, macrophages are one of the crucial cell types when it comes to host tissue-biomaterial interactions. However, macrophages have a critical role not only in response to biomaterials but also in innate immunity in general. Macrophage polarization is implicated as an important component in normal immune responses such as bacterial clearance or remodeling after injury but also in many pathological conditions such as chronic inflammation-related diseases, cancer, atherosclerosis and auto-immune diseases. Macrophages can recognize foreign cells via receptors using Pathogen Associated Molecular Patterns (PAMPs) and they can also recognize damaged self-cells/tissue components in their function of debris clearance via Damage Associated Molecular Patterns (DAMPs). Toll-like receptors (TLRs) are important in this process. Other surface receptors also have important functions in macrophage activities, such as Mannose receptors (that recognise yeasts; CD206 is also generally used as M2 macrophage marker), Scavenger receptors (recognition of oxidized LDLs for clearance (hence the name scavenger)) and Fc receptors (for antibody-specific phagocytosis) [22]. Specific functions of macrophages are more widely covered in the next chapters, particularly in Chapter 9.

1.4 BIOMATERIAL PROPERTIES AND IMMUNE RESPONSE

Immune reaction determines the lifetime of the biomaterial inside the body, the position of the material in the body (via encapsulation, integration and in some cases actual movement of the biomaterial), its degradation and its interaction with surrounding tissues. The presence of the biomaterial is a perturbation of the tissue homeostasis, and physicochemical interactions of the material surface with the surrounding host tissue result in several inadvertent results. First, the presence of a surface in contact with blood results in adsorption of proteins where, in some cases, due to the interaction with the biomaterial surface the proteins will lose their normal conformation, which in turn results in the activation of the complement system. The activities of the complement system will bring in immune cells and their presence will, in turn, initiate further cellular and humoral responses.

The immune reaction can be something to evade through the use of biomaterials but the knowledge of immune reaction can also be used to harness it. For example, using the receptor- and phagocytosis-mediated interactions of innate immunity with nanoscale structures, it is possible to develop immune system specific delivery systems using nanobiomaterials or adjuvants to boost immune response to vaccines. On the other hand, the understanding of the innate response to scaffolds is crucial in tissue engineering for control over the remodeling and degradation of biomaterial-based tissue engineering scaffolds. Failure to take into account the potential immune response to a given structure can result in its mechanical failure due to fast degradation or fibrotic encapsulation [23]. Different properties of the biomaterial can be adjusted for achieving the desired response. For example, nano/microscale effects can be harnessed to deliver therapeutic agents into the immune cells by exploiting their phagocytic activities [24]. The aforementioned use of biomaterials as vaccine adjuvants as well as delivery systems falls into this area. Nanoscale structures are amenable to direct recognition and phagocytosis. Microscale systems can be phagocyted partially depending on their size; bulk materials – particularly non-degradable ones – can induce frustrated phagocytosis. The level and nature of immune response will be closely related to the size of the involved biomaterial; this subject is discussed in more detail in Chapter 2. For implants, the topography of biomaterial is another potential target in the form of micro/nanoscale patterns in 2D and 3D for controlling the phenotype of incoming immune cells [25]. For example, Singh et al. recently demonstrated that the presence of surface micropatterns on photocrosslinked gelatin hydrogels had a wide range of effects on the expression of genes related to protein trafficking, translation, DNA repair and cell survival (Figure 1.2), as determined by transcriptomic analysis [26]. This aspect of immune system biomaterial interactions will be covered in Chapter 3.

The physical and chemical properties of the biomaterial also have a profound effect on how the immune system will respond to it. The form of the material

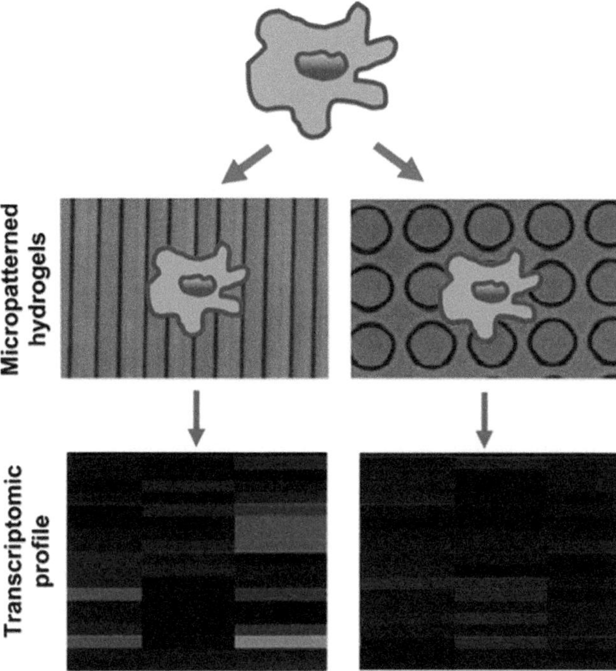

FIGURE 1.2 The effect of surface micropatterns on human macrophages. The presence of microgrooves and micropillars has distinct effects on the gene expression of primary macrophages, which can be harnessed to control their phenotype. (Reprinted from Singh S et al., *ACS Biomater Sci Eng*. 2017;3(6):969–78. With permission.)

(such as porous vs. non-porous), its bulk properties, such as mechanical properties, and its chemical nature (hydrophilic vs. hydrophilic, charge at physiological conditions, level of crosslinking etc.), together with whether it is biodegradable or not, all affect the response of immune cells. These also include treatments for reinforcing the structures. For example, McDade et al. demonstrated that glutaraldehyde crosslinking of decellularized pericardium resulted in a significant increase in pro-inflammatory cytokine release and matrix metalloproteinase release by macrophages [27]. The effects of material properties on immune cell behaviour are covered in Chapters 3, 6, 8 and 9. Another example is the effect of the molecular weight of Hyaluronic acid on the immune cell behavior, which will be covered in Chapter 7.

Beyond the bulk properties, the surface properties of the biomaterials, such as roughness and wettability, and even subtler differences such as surface crystalline phase, can have profound effects on immune reactions [28]. As the surface properties directly control protein adsorption from physiological liquids and subsequent presentation to immune cells, they can be engineered to control the behaviour of incoming immune cells (for example, surfaces causing denaturation of the proteins can induce DAMP recognition-mediated macrophage reactions, thus surfaces that cause minimal denaturation of the adsorbed proteins can have positive effects on immune reactions). Surface-related properties are covered in Chapters 5, 6 and 9.

1.5 CURRENT PARADIGMS IN IMMUNOMODULATION IN BIOMATERIALS CONTEXT

The slow but steady knowledge transfer from immunology to the field of biomaterials has led to a better appreciation of the role of the immune system on the *in vivo* performance of biomaterials. This has resulted in increased activity in the incorporation of immunomodulatory components into the design of implantable systems. In this context, the rise in the use of decellularized matrices for tissue engineering, regenerative medicine and wound healing purposes has an immunomodulatory angle, as these tissues are not only less immunogenic, due to their composition, or diminished in immunogenic components, due to decellularisation, but also have inherent immunomodulatory properties [29]. However, these properties are highly related to the source of the matrix. For example, it was recently shown that small intestinal submucosa induced an anti-inflammatory, pro-healing phenotype in macrophages, whereas dermal ECM induced a more pro-inflammatory phenotype [30]. Such fundamental research work on the immune cell biomaterial interactions will provide the necessary know-how for case- and patient-specific biomaterial selection for optimal clinical outcomes.

As mentioned above, cytokines are important mediators of immune response. Thus, there is ongoing research activity in harnessing the pro- or anti-inflammatory properties of cytokines for immunomodulation around implants and tissue engineering scaffolds. As the spatiotemporal control over the cytokine concentrations are crucial in many biological events such as wound healing and angiogenesis, sequential delivery of cytokines is a potential way of immunomodulation. Spiller et al. developed a sequential delivery system within a tissue engineering scaffold for vascularisation of tissue engineering scaffolds by exploiting the role of M1 and M2 macrophages in angiogenesis [31]. Decellularised bone scaffolds were adsorbed with IFN-ɣ to induce initial M1 polarisation of macrophages, whereas a streproavidin/biotin-based system immobilises IL-4 within the scaffold over six days, which induces M2 polarisation at a later time point (Figure 1.3). In this way, the initial capillary sprouting activity of M1 macrophages can be used first and then with the conversion of M1 macrophages to M2 macrophages by the activity of IL-4; the formed capillaries can be matured for robust vascularisation of the scaffold. Aside from sequential delivery approaches, combinatorial delivery systems for harnessing the synergistic behaviour of different cytokines, growth factors etc. are also under development [32]. For example, it was recently shown that a cytokine cocktail based on TGF-β, IL-4 and IL-10 can improve M2 macrophage polarisation fixation and help in wound healing compared to single cytokine stimulation [33]. Single or multiple cytokines can be incorporated into biomedical devices in the form of nano- or microscale coatings with anti-inflammatory properties [34]. Also, the delivery of two pro-wound healing factors (namely, a sphingosine analog (FTY720) and stromal derived factor-1 α (SDF-1α)) from a modified PEG-DA hydrogel resulted in increased vascularisation *in vivo* [35].

The direct utilization of macrophages in co-culture conditions for "immune-assisted tissue engineering" is another active area of research [36]. Macrophages with the right phenotype can help the wound healing process and vascularisation at different steps of the wound healing cascade. For example, Dohle et al. demonstrated an increase in microvessel-like structures in the presence of macrophages in the tri-culture model of osteoblasts, vascular endothelial cells and macrophages [37];

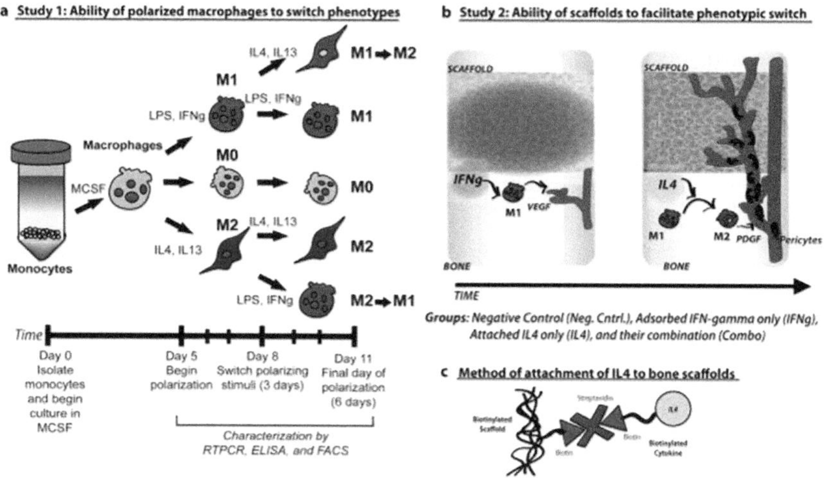

FIGURE 1.3 Sequential delivery of cytokines for control of macrophage phenotype in and around tissue engineering scaffolds. (a) Phenotypic plasticity of macrophages allows rapid assumption of a different polarisation state in the presence of proper stimuli. (b) By using sequential delivery of pro- and anti-inflammatory cytokines, the process of angiogenesis and maturation of new capillary sprouts can be tightly controlled. (c) The mode of immobilization of IL-4 into the scaffolds. (Reprinted from Spiller KL et al., *Biomaterials*. 2015;37(Supplement C):194–207. With permission.)

a similar effect was also demonstrated in tri-culture conditions where macrophages were substituted with neutrophils [38]. The co-encapsulation of macrophages with vascular endothelial cells in hydrogels resulted in macrophages assuming pericyte-like behaviour and inducing the formation of better-defined microvascular networks [39]. The encapsulation of macrophages in hydrogels also affects incoming cell behaviour and the cytokine microenvironment [40]. Such co-encapsulation systems are not only useful for potential treatments but also for development of *in vitro* models for diseases where the activities of immune cells are prominent, and in the testing of new immunomodulatory systems [41].

1.6 CHAPTER OVERVIEWS

This book aims to give the reader an overview of immune responses to biomaterials. For this end, there are chapters that are dedicated to the structure of biomaterials, whereas some other chapters focus on one type of biomaterial to emphasise the specific interactions. There are chapters that are more application-oriented and concentrate on the effect of the immune response for a given domain.

In Chapter 2, Erdemli et al. focus on biomaterials in nanoparticle form and elucidate their interactions with innate and adaptive immune systems. The interaction was covered in reference to different applications of nanoparticles, such as gene, drug and contrast agent delivery. This was followed by the elucidation of protein adsorption on nanoparticles and its potential influence on immune reactions. Finally, nanoparticle interaction with different immune cells and the role of particle properties on the outcome of the interaction was explained.

In Chapter 3, Ozcelik focuses on the effect of surface properties on immune response to biomaterials, in particular by macrophages. After an introduction to the foreign body response and the role of macrophages in this reaction, together with the definition of macrophage phenotypes, the relationship between surface properties such as roughness, wettability, chemical composition and micro/nanoscale topographies are explained. This is followed by a definition of immunological synapse and its potential role in the context of biomaterials.

In Chapter 4, Weszl et al. bring to our attention the surface properties of titanium, one of the most commonly used biomaterials, where immune responses have an important toll on clinical outcomes. Here, for a better appreciation of the complexity of a surface presented by a biomaterial, the surface crystalline phases of titanium and their potential biological effects are explained.

In Chapter 5, Gasik et al. focus on another aspect of the immune response: the biofilm formation on implants due to the failure of immune response to overcome bacterial attachment to implanted biomaterials which leads to this common biomaterial-based complication. They explain the structure and nature of biofilms on implants, the underlying causes of bacterial attachment and biofilm formation on biomaterials, biomaterial/bacteria interactions and the role of immune response in the formation of biofilms. They also give an overview of currently available methods for the potential eradication of biofilms from implant surfaces.

In Chapter 6, Tanir et al. provide a more in-depth definition of the cell types involved in immune response to biomaterials, together with elucidation of the biomaterial properties important in the determination of the extent of immune responses. This is followed by elaboration of immune responses to non-degradable, degradable and cell-grafted biomaterials, together with current immunomodulation routes, including anti-inflammatory drug treatments (steroidal or non-steroidal).

In Chapter 7, Safrankova et al. examine a widely used biomaterial, hyaluronic acid, within the context of its immunomodulatory properties. The structure, synthesis, degradation and functions of HA are described, together with industrial production and chemical modification methods of HA. This is followed by a description of the role of HA in immune system and immunomodulation, including receptors that recognise HA, specific cell interactions with HA and the role of HA in immune cell polarisation.

In Chapter 8, Aktas et al. focus on the role of immunomodulation in the context of bone regeneration with biomaterials. After describing the structure and morphology of bone and the cellular components of bone, the role of immune response in bone healing is elucidated, together with a description of the immune cells active in the process. This is followed by an introduction to osteoimmunology and recent efforts in osteoimmunomodulation in the context of orthopaedic implants and bone tissue engineering, together with immune engineering-based solutions.

In Chapter 9, Knopf-Marques et al. concentrate on macrophages and their responses to the different classes of biomaterials, namely polymers, metals and ceramics that are used in implants and as tissue engineering scaffolds. The roles of chemical and physical properties of these classes of materials from the point of view of macrophage reaction are elucidated.

In Chapter 10, Prakasam et al. focus on the clinical use of biomaterials in the field of periodontics and the role of immune response in the success and failure of currently used techniques. They describe the immune reaction to biologically sourced biomaterial systems, with the specific example of the enamel-derived matrix, together with the coverage of immune response to other tools utilised in periodontics, such as luting agents, ceramics used in crowns, metal alloys and antiseptic agents.

1.7 CONCLUSION

The human immune system is a sophisticated machine, evolved within the constraints of the mammalian body to protect and repair it – sometimes to its own detriment. Biomaterial-based solutions for healthcare problems have an indisputable place in the future of the healthcare; however, the level of impact and the share of biomaterials will be partially decided by their ability to interact with the host immune system. This chapter and the following chapters will try to provide an overview for both biologists, engineers and material scientists working in the fields of biomedical devices, implants, controlled delivery and regenerative medicine to incorporate immune components into their designs and studies for a better understanding of diseases and more potent future generations of biomaterial-based healthcare products.

ACKNOWLEDGEMENTS

This project has received funding from the European Union's FP7 research and innovation programme under grant agreement No. 602694 (IMMODGEL) and the Horizon 2020 research and innovation programme under grant agreement No. 760921 (PANBioRA).

REFERENCES

1. Wong C, Ho CY, Li E, Lam C. Elevation of proinflammatory cytokine (IL-18, IL-17, IL-12) and Th2 cytokine (IL-4) concentrations in patients with systemic lupus erythematosus. *Lupus*. 2000;9(8):589–93.
2. Consortium IMSG, 2 WTCCC. Genetic risk and a primary role for cell-mediated immune mechanisms in multiple sclerosis. *Nature*. 2011;476(7359):214–19.
3. Park LS, Tate JP, Sigel K, Rimland D, Crothers K, Gibert C et al. Time trends in cancer incidence in persons living with HIV/AIDS in the antiretroviral therapy era: 1997–2012. *AIDS*. 2016;30(11):1795–1806.
4. Choy JC. Granzymes and perforin in solid organ transplant rejection. *Cell Death Differ*. 2010;17(4):567–76.
5. Lynn AK, Yannas IV, Bonfield W. Antigenicity and immunogenicity of collagen. *J Biomed Mater Res B Appl Biomater*. 2004;71B(2):343–54.
6. Ziegler M, Schlosser M, Abel P, Ziegler B. Antibody response in rats against non-toxic glucose sensor membranes tested in cell culture. *Biomaterials*. 1994;15(10):859–64.
7. Khan AR, Hams E, Floudas A, Sparwasser T, Weaver CT, Fallon PG. PD-L1hi B cells are critical regulators of humoral immunity. *Nat Commun*. 2015;6:5997.
8. Koshy ST, Mooney DJ. Biomaterials for enhancing anti-cancer immunity. *Curr Opin Biotechnol*. 2016;40(Supplement C):1–8.
9. Anderson JM, Rodriguez A, Chang DT, eds. Foreign body reaction to biomaterials. *Semin Immunol*. 2008: Elsevier.
10. Nilsson B, Korsgren O, Lambris JD, Ekdahl KN. Can cells and biomaterials in therapeutic medicine be shielded from innate immune recognition? *Trends Immunol*. 2010;31(1):32–8.
11. Sheikh Z, Brooks PJ, Barzilay O, Fine N, Glogauer M. Macrophages, foreign body giant cells and their response to implantable biomaterials. *Materials*. 2015;8(9):5671–701.
12. Medzhitov R, Janeway CA. Innate immunity: The virtues of a nonclonal system of recognition. *Cell*. 1997;91(3):295–8.
13. Medzhitov R. Toll-like receptors and innate immunity. *Nat Rev Immunol*. 2001; 1(2):135–45.
14. Flajnik MF, Kasahara M. Origin and evolution of the adaptive immune system: Genetic events and selective pressures. *Nat Rev Genet*. 2010;11(1):47–59.
15. Zhang J-M, An J. Cytokines, inflammation and pain. *Int Anesthesiol Clin*. 2007;45(2):27.
16. Mills C. M1 and M2 macrophages: Oracles of health and disease. *Crit Rev Immunol*. 2012;32(6).
17. Ricklin D, Hajishengallis G, Yang K, Lambris JD. Complement: A key system for immune surveillance and homeostasis. *Nat Immunol*. 2010;11(9):785–97.
18. Yang Y, Bazhin AV, Werner J, Karakhanova S. Reactive oxygen species in the immune system. *Int Rev Immunol*. 2013;32(3):249–70.
19. Hashimoto D, Chow A, Noizat C, Teo P, Beasley MB, Leboeuf M et al. Tissue-resident macrophages self-maintain locally throughout adult life with minimal contribution from circulating monocytes. *Immunity*. 2013;38(4):792–804.

20. Mosmann TR, Sad S. The expanding universe of T-cell subsets: Th1, Th2 and more. *Immunol Today*. 1996;17(3):138–46.
21. Mosmann TR, Coffman R. TH1 and TH2 cells: Different patterns of lymphokine secretion lead to different functional properties. *Ann Rev Immunol*. 1989;7(1):145–73.
22. Unkeless J, Eisen HN. Binding of monomeric immunoglobulins to Fc receptors of mouse macrophages. *J Exp Med*. 1975;142(6):1520–33.
23. Anderson JM, McNally AK, eds. Biocompatibility of implants: Lymphocyte/macrophage interactions. *Semin Immunopathol*. 2011: Springer.
24. Zolnik BS, Gonzalez-Fernandez A, Sadrieh N, Dobrovolskaia MA. Minireview: Nanoparticles and the immune system. *Endocrinology*. 2010;151(2):458–65.
25. Dollinger C, Ndreu-Halili A, Uka A, Singh S, Sadam H, Neuman T et al. Controlling incoming macrophages to implants: Responsiveness of macrophages to gelatin micropatterns under M1/M2 phenotype defining biochemical stimulations. *Adv Biosyst*. 2017;1(6).
26. Singh S, Awuah D, Rostam HM, Emes RD, Kandola NK, Onion D et al. Unbiased analysis of the impact of micropatterned biomaterials on macrophage behavior provides insights beyond predefined polarization states. *ACS Biomater Sci Eng*. 2017;3(6):969–78.
27. McDade JK, Brennan-Pierce EP, Ariganello MB, Labow RS, Michael LJ. Interactions of U937 macrophage-like cells with decellularized pericardial matrix materials: Influence of crosslinking treatment. *Acta Biomaterialia*. 2013;9(7):7191–9.
28. Barthes J, Ciftci S, Ponzio F, Knopf-Marques H, Pelyhe L, Gudima A et al. the potential impact of surface crystalline states of titanium for biomedical applications. *Crit Rev Biotechnol*. 2017:1–15.
29. Dziki JL, Huleihel L, Scarritt ME, Badylak SF. Extracellular matrix bioscaffolds as immunomodulatory biomaterials. *Tissue Eng Part A*. 2017;23(19–20):1152–9.
30. Dziki JL, Wang DS, Pineda C, Sicari BM, Rausch T, Badylak SF. Solubilized extracellular matrix bioscaffolds derived from diverse source tissues differentially influence macrophage phenotype. *J Biomed Mater Res A*. 2017;105(1):138–47.
31. Spiller KL, Nassiri S, Witherel CE, Anfang RR, Ng J, Nakazawa KR et al. Sequential delivery of immunomodulatory cytokines to facilitate the M1-to-M2 transition of macrophages and enhance vascularization of bone scaffolds. *Biomaterials*. 2015;37:194–207.
32. Stewart JM, Keselowsky BG. Combinatorial drug delivery approaches for immunomodulation. *Adv Drug Deliv Rev*. 2017;114:161–74.
33. Riabov V, Salazar F, Htwe SS, Gudima A, Schmuttermaier C, Barthes J et al. Generation of anti-inflammatory macrophages for implants and regenerative medicine using self-standing release systems with a phenotype-fixing cytokine cocktail formulation. *Acta Biomaterialia*. 2017;53:389–98.
34. Knopf-Marques H, Singh S, Htwe SS, Wolfova L, Buffa R, Bacharouche J et al. Immunomodulation with self-crosslinked polyelectrolyte multilayer-based coatings. *Biomacromolecules*. 2016;17(6):2189–98.
35. Ogle ME, Krieger JR, Tellier LE, McFaline-Figueroa J, Temenoff JS, Botchwey EA. Dual affinity heparin-based hydrogels achieve pro-regenerative immunomodulation and microvascular remodeling. *ACS Biomater Sci Eng*. 2018;4(4):1241–1250.
36. Vrana NE. Immunomodulatory biomaterials and regenerative immunology. *Future Sci OA*. 2016;2(4):FSO146.
37. Dohle E, Bischoff I, Böse T, Marsano A, Banfi A, Unger R et al. Macrophage-mediated angiogenic activation of outgrowth endothelial cells in co-culture with primary osteoblasts. *Eur Cell Mater*. 2014;27:149.

38. Herath TDK, Larbi A, Teoh SH, Kirkpatrick CJ, Goh BT. Neutrophil-mediated enhancement of angiogenesis and osteogenesis in a novel triple cell co-culture model with endothelial cells and osteoblasts. *J Tissue Eng Regen Med.* 2018;12(2): e1221–36.
39. Moore EM, Ying G, West JL. Macrophages influence vessel formation in 3D bioactive hydrogels. *Adv Biosyst.* 2017;1(3).
40. Dollinger C, Ciftci S, Knopf-Marques H, Guner R, Ghaemmaghami AM, Debry C et al. Incorporation of resident macrophages in engineered tissues: Multiple cell type response to microenvironment controlled macrophageladen gelatin hydrogels. *J Tissue Eng Regen Med.* 2018;12(2):330–40.
41. Samavedi S, Diaz-Rodriguez P, Erndt-Marino JD, Hahn MS. A three-dimensional chondrocyte-macrophage coculture system to probe inflammation in experimental osteoarthritis. *Tissue Eng Part A.* 2017;23(3–4):101–14.

2 Immune Response to Nanoparticles

Özge Erdemli and Ayşen Tezcaner

CONTENTS

2.1 INTRODUCTION

The advent of nanotechnology has led to the discovery of many new approaches in the field of medicine, including drug, gene, and vaccine delivery systems and medical imaging techniques. Nanoparticles (NPs) – colloidal particles ranging from 10 to 100 nm in size – find wide applications in medicine as products of nanotechnology. NPs are increasingly studied as passive or active targeting systems for drugs, vaccine delivery systems, gene delivery systems for antimicrobial or therapeutic actions, molecular diagnostics, medical imaging and theranostic (simultaneous diagnosis and therapy with one agent) purposes, as well as for platforms capable of combining diagnostic and therapeutic agents [1,2]. In recent years, a number of NP-based therapeutic and diagnostic agents have also seen clinical use in the treatment of cancer, fungal infections, multiple sclerosis, hepatitis etc. [3].

As therapeutic delivery systems, NPs offer targeted drug delivery to the site of disease. Besides the possibility of controlled release of drugs, targeted delivery also minimizes systemic side effects. Additionally, NP-based drug delivery systems provide improved solubility of poorly soluble drugs, prolong the residence time of drugs in the systemic circulation by reducing immunogenicity, release drugs at a sustained rate and thus lower the frequency of administration and provide simultaneous delivery of two or more drugs for combination therapy [3]. From the perspective of diagnostic applications, NPs help to get information on the molecular scale for examining abnormalities such as pre-cancerous cells, disease markers and fragments of viruses that cannot be detected with traditional methods [4]. For medical imaging, NP-based imaging contrast agents have been used to improve the sensitivity and specificity of magnetic resonance imaging (MRI) compared to conventional imaging agents [5]. Besides the numerous advantages of NPs, some NPs with different physicochemical properties may cause adverse biological responses [6]. Consequently, toxicity, biocompatibility, biodistribution and biodegradation of NPs should be carefully evaluated before clinical use.

Apart from biomedical applications, NPs and other nanomaterials have been used in various industrial applications, including electronics, energy, cosmetics, agriculture and food etc. [7]. While NPs and other nanomaterials have numerous benefits, their potential dangers to human health raise much concern. NPs can enter the human body mainly through the skin, inhalation, intravenous routes or ingestion. Once they enter the body, their interactions with the biological system specify the biocompatibility, stability in the system and biological performance, as well as the side effects they cause. For these reasons, the study of the toxicity of NPs and their potential effects on the immune system has become an active area of research.

This chapter focuses on the interactions between innate and adaptive immune systems and NPs. In the first section of this chapter, current applications in biomedical imaging, diagnostics and drug, gene and vaccine delivery systems of various types of NPs are briefly reviewed. Some examples of the current trends in the field of NPs and approved NP applications in clinical use will be reviewed. These include the use of NPs as contrast agents for diagnostic imaging and theranostics and as delivery systems for drugs, genes and vaccines. The second section will address the importance of the protein adsorption on NPs for their fate *in vivo* and subsequent different interactions of NPs with cells. Finally, the interactions of NPs with the immune system and the physicochemical properties of NPs affecting immune response will be discussed.

2.2 BIOMEDICAL APPLICATIONS OF NANOPARTICLES

Many types of NPs can be used in biomedical applications, including drug, gene and vaccine delivery systems, as well as medical imaging and diagnostics, and they can be formulated from diverse materials with unique chemical and surface properties. Moreover, new formulations of NPs for biomedical applications continue to undergo extensive development. The most common types of NPs used in biomedical applications are polymeric (including nanocapsules, nanospheres, nanoconjugates, polymeric micelles or dendrimers), metallic (noble or magnetic metals), liposomal and ceramic NPs, NPs based on solid lipids, fullerenes, carbon nanotubes (CNTs), quantum dots (QDs), nanosuspensions and nanoemulsions (Figure 2.1).

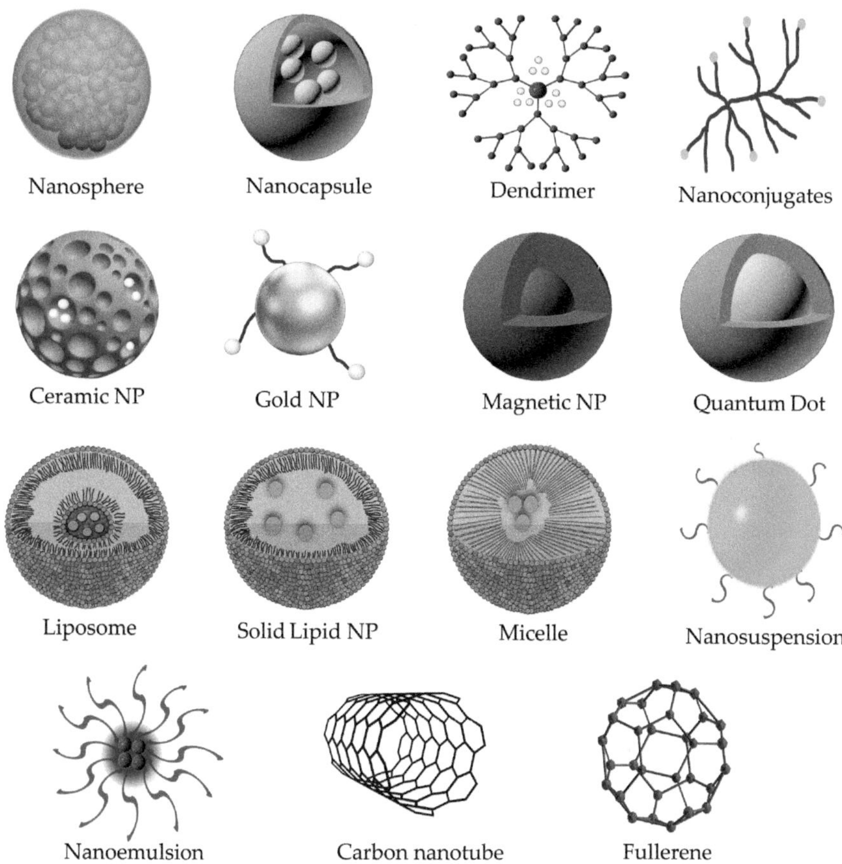

FIGURE 2.1 Types of NPs for biomedical applications.

2.2.1 Imaging and Diagnosis

Emerging NP technologies can provide improvements in molecular imaging by offering multifunctional capabilities for the targeted delivery of a large payload amount of contrast agent in a single dose to a diseased site inside the body [8,9]. Moreover, internalisation and probing of cells are facilitated by their smaller sizes, and their surfaces can be easily functionalised with a variety of molecular signaling and receptor targeting molecules.

Conventional fluorophores such as fluorescent dyes, bioluminescent proteins and fluorescent proteins are widely used in research and clinical diagnostic applications. However, these techniques have several problems, such as inadequate fluorescence intensity, photobleaching, poor circulation half-lives etc. [10]. Fluorescent NPs can provide significant improvements in traditional biological imaging with many advantages over their predecessors. For instance, fluorescent silica NPs can also allow sensitive imaging of cancer cells due to their photostability and brightness [11]. QD-based fluorophore systems also improve sensitivity, photo-stability and multiplexing capacity compared to conventional molecular fluorophores [10]. Moreover, some biorecognition molecules like peptides, antibodies, nucleic acids or small-molecule ligands can be covalently linked on QDs to improve their use as fluorescent probes [12]. In particular, cancer-specific ligands/antibodies/peptides can be conjugated on QDs to detect and image cancer cells [12].

NP-based imaging contrast agents have also been used to improve the sensitivity and specificity of magnetic resonance imaging (MRI) compared to the conventional imaging agents [5]. Magnetic NPs have been explored extensively as carriers for MRI contrast agents because of their tunable magnetism, size and easy conjugation with biologically functional units [13]. Moreover, magnetic NPs have seen wide use in multi-modal imaging applications, such as MRI-optical and MRI-positron emission tomography (PET)/single-photon emission computed tomography (SPECT) [13]. Fullerenes can be further modified to become carriers of diagnostic contrast agents for MRI [14]. For example, gadolinium endohedral fullerenes (Trimetaspheres®; Luna Innovations Incorporated, VA, USA) are being investigated for use as MRI-based contrast agents.

An interesting approach related to NPs in disease management is the use of theranostic NPs for simultaneous delivery of both contrast medium and drug, enabling detection and treatment of the disease using a single nano-construct [2,15]. In nanotheranostics, hydrophobic organic drugs, proteins, peptides and genetic materials are used as therapeutic agents, whereas diagnostic agents can be those for optical imaging (using fluorescent dyes or QDs), MRI (using superparamagnetic metals), nuclear imaging (using radionuclides) and computed tomography (using heavy elements) [15]. Some NPs such as iron oxide, gold, silica and CNTs are currently under investigation for the development of theranostic agents [2]. Additionally, the spherical configuration of the planar hexagonal rings and the conjugated double bonds in the fullerene structure offer opportunities for theranostic applications [14]. Besides, there are some preclinical studies for theranostic drug-polymer conjugates, for example, dendrimers as theranostic carriers and gold half-shell-coated drug conjugate micelles [15]. However, to date, no NP theranostics have met the clinical standards.

2.2.2 Nanoparticles in Drug Delivery

The utilization of NPs enables site-specific targeting and the controlled release of traditional pharmaceuticals, recombinant proteins, vaccines and nucleic acids for many diseases [16]. NPs can enhance the efficiency of a drug by controlling the release kinetics, regulating the biodistribution and minimizing the toxic side effects. Besides, they improve the solubility of poorly soluble drugs, prolong the residence time of drugs in the systemic circulation by reducing immunogenicity and release drugs at a sustained rate, thus lowering the frequency of administration [3]. They can also provide simultaneous delivery of two or more drugs for combination therapy [3]. Drug delivery formulations in the form of nanosuspensions can be found in the market with different application routes including oral, parenteral, pulmonary and ocular routes [17]. This approach is useful to enhance the solubility, bioavailability and physical and chemical stability of drugs and it provides passive drug targeting [17]. Nanoemulsion formulations also offer several advantages as drug delivery systems due to their high drug loading capacity, enhanced drug solubility and bioavailability, their non-toxic and non-irritant nature and variety in their formulations [18]. In recent years, nanoemulsions have been widely used for solving various difficulties in oral, topical and other routes of administration of drugs [18]. They have also had recent use in targeting to the brain [19].

Targeted drug delivery provides the delivery of a therapeutic effective dose to the diseased target area and a reduction in the associated systemic drug toxicity [20]. There are two main strategies for targeted drug delivery: active and passive. Passive targeting occurs as drug accumulation in tumours or inflamed tissues with leaky vasculature through the enhanced permeability and retention (EPR) effect and it enhances the targeted delivery of specific ligand-modified NPs into poorly accessible areas. On the other hand, active targeting is based on the specific ligand–receptor interactions between drug-loaded NPs and targeted cells. Diseased tissues in cancer or inflammation with leaky vasculature have higher expression of some specific receptors compared to normal cells that can be used as targets for nanotherapeutics with specific ligands to these receptors.

Non-specific drug delivery of conventional chemotherapeutic drugs causes major drawbacks for effective cancer treatment. To overcome the lack of specificity of these conventional drugs, NPs offer both passive and active targeting strategies to increase the intracellular concentration of drugs in cancer cells and minimize toxicity in normal cells at the same time. Various NPs, including polymeric NPs, metallic NPs, liposomes, dendrimers and CNTs, can be used as anticancer drug delivery systems [21]. Additionally, QDs have been conjugated with anticancer drugs for targeted delivery because of their ability to target specific cells [22].

The unusual behaviour of macrophages is related to a broad range of diseases, including allergic asthma, chronic ulcers, autoimmune disorders and fibrotic diseases. Certain overexpressed receptors on the infected macrophages can be used efficiently as a target for surface-engineered NPs [20]. Natural or synthetic polymer-, lipid-, dendrimer-, CNT-, liposome- and polymersome-based NP systems have been investigated for macrophage targeted drug delivery [20].

2.2.3 Vaccine and Adjuvant Delivery Systems

In the treatment and control of a broad range of infectious diseases and cancers, vaccines have been widely used for inducing cellular immunity [23]. Traditional vaccines consisting of live attenuated or whole inactivated pathogens were previously used to obtain effective and long-lasting immune responses based on antigen-specific antibody responses. However, live attenuated or inactivated/killed fatal pathogens are no longer used in new-generation vaccines because of safety issues in clinical translation. Many new-generation vaccines currently under development are based on purified subunits, recombinant protein, or DNA or synthetic peptides. Although these safe subunits with minimal toxicity can be easily produced, there are major challenges in their applications because of their lower immunogenicity compared with older-style vaccines. Thus, there is a need for improvements in the formulations of subunit vaccines with the adjuvants. Alum-based mineral salts and oil-in-water emulsions of MF59 and AS03 are the major adjuvants used in human vaccine formulations [24]. Alum adjuvants in the form of aluminum hydroxide, aluminum phosphate etc. induce Th2 immune responses and have weak capacity for inducing Th1 immune response [25]. Adjuvants can be also used in the form of delivery vehicles such as micro/nanoparticles to enhance antigen delivery and presentation by antigen-presenting cells (APCs) [26–29]. In a recent study, the immunoadjuvant potential of rod-shaped hydroxyapatite (HA), magnesium-substituted HA and zinc-substituted HA NPs with irregular nanopores was tested *in vitro* using bone marrow dendritic cells [25]. Magnesium- or zinc-substituted HA NPs induced the cellular uptake of a molecular immunopotentiator and both cell-mediated Th1 immunity and antibody-mediated Th2 immunity of bone marrow dendritic cells *in vitro*, indicating their potential as immunoadjuvants for clinical use.

In recent years, the use of NPs within vaccine formulations has been extensively investigated because they have the same dimensions as most pathogens [30]. Thus, they can provide the desired immune response. NPs can be used as either delivery systems to enhance antigen delivery and/or as an immunostimulant to activate immune response [29]. As delivery systems, NPs can be used for stimulating a short-lived, localised immune response or in the delivery of antigens, which may otherwise degrade rapidly. On the other hand, the binding of antigens on NP surfaces can allow the stimulation of immune systems in a similar way as that induced by pathogens.

Virus-like particles (VLPs) were the first NP delivery systems to be studied in vaccination due to their ease of production and ability to stimulate strong immune responses [28]. VLPs – non-infective viruses composed of viral envelope proteins without the genetic material – stimulate both cellular and humoral immunity. Several licensed recombinant hepatitis B virus (HBV9-VLP) vaccines are used in clinics [31]. Liposomes are also important carrier systems in vaccines due to their ability to induce immune responses against antigens incorporated or associated to these systems [32]. Many inorganic NPs like those based on gold, carbon, silica and calcium phosphate have been studied for vaccine developments [27]. Biodegradable polymeric NPs with entrapped antigens such as proteins, peptides or DNA have attracted much attention for their ability to control the release of vaccine antigens and optimize the desired immune response via selective targeting of the antigen to APCs [33].

2.2.4 Nanoparticle-Mediated Gene Delivery

Gene therapy is a promising method for the treatment of both acquired and inherited diseases ranging from cancer, neurodegenerative diseases and hemophilia to autoimmune diseases [34,35]. This treatment strategy aims to deliver the genetic material directly into the target pathological tissue or cells. The success of gene therapy is mostly dependent on the selective and efficient delivery of a gene to target cells with minimal toxicity. Thus, NPs can provide an effective gene delivery method due to their size-dependent ability to cross many physiological barriers and to be taken up efficiently by target cells. Several inorganic NPs such as magnetic NPs, CNTs, QDs, calcium phosphate NPs and gold NPs, and some cationic types of liposomes, solid lipids, lipids, polymeric NPs and nanoemulsions, can be used as gene delivery systems [34]. For example, mesoporous silica NPs have been widely employed for anticancer drug and gene delivery because of their easily tunable size and shape, high potential for surface functionalisation and high drug loading capacity due to their high surface area and pore volume [36]. Recently, some clinical trials of biodegradable, or natural, polymeric NPs for gene delivery have been done and a number of NP-based gene delivery systems mostly consisting of cationic polymers for binding, poly (ethylene glycol) (PEG) for stabilisation and a ligand for targeting have been developed for clinical trials [35]. However, none of these gene delivery systems has thus far been approved by the US Food and Drug Administration (FDA) for clinical applications.

2.2.5 Nanoparticles in Clinics

Adagen® (SigmaTau Pharmaceuticals, Inc., MD, USA), a polyethylene glycol (PEG) ylated bovine adenosine deaminase, was the first medical NP system to be approved (in 1990). Since then, NPs have shown great promise in emerging medical fields like medical imaging for new diagnostics and in the delivery of therapeutic agents. The main use of NPs in clinics is for anticancer applications. In recent years, various NP-based therapeutic products have been approved and are already in clinical use. Some examples of these approved NPs are given in Table 2.1. Because of the clinical success of many NPs, numerous new products are at the stage of phase II/III studies with extensive research efforts and funding worldwide.

2.3 THE INTERACTION OF NANOPARTICLES WITH THE BIOLOGICAL MICROENVIRONMENT

Research and development in the nanomaterials field has brought many advances across many sectors of industry, and these new products are already being used in many commercial applications, including electronics, energy, cosmetics, agriculture and food etc. [7]. Although they may provide huge benefits to society, there are uncertainties and concerns about the potential dangers on human health and environment imposed by nanoscale materials. NPs released from these commercial products may enter the human body and, through skin, inhalation or ingestion, depending on the type of exposure, they may adversely affect normal physiology. In addition to these unintentional exposures, intentional administration of NPs is practised as the main part of nanotechnology in medicine, including in drug, gene and vaccine delivery systems and medical imaging techniques, as mentioned in the previous sections – potentially posing even bigger risks.

Once NPs enter the biological environment, they will come into contact with various cells and extracellular proteins. These interactions of NPs are critical with respect to their potential fate and toxicity after unintentional exposure or biomedical application.

2.3.1 Protein Adsorption on NPs

In biological environments, extracellular proteins adsorb to the surface of NPs to form a protein layer or "corona" and mediate subsequent interactions with specific

TABLE 2.1
Examples of NP-Based Therapeutic Systems Approved for Clinical Use

Trade Name	Company	Therapeutic Agent	Type of NPs	Application
Adagen®	Sigma-Tau Pharmaceuticals/Enzon	Bovine adenosine deaminase	Polymer–protein conjugate	Drug delivery system for treatment of severe combined immunodeficiency disease (SCID)
Abelcet®	Sigma-Tau Pharmaceuticals	Amphotericin B	Liposome/lipid NPs	Drug delivery system for the treatment of invasive fungal infections
Doxil®	Centocor Ortho Biotech, J & J/Schering Plough, Janssen Biotech	Doxorubicin	Liposome/lipid NPs	Drug delivery system for the treatment of cancer
DaunoXome®	NeXstar Pharmaceuticals/ Gilead Sciences Ltd/ Galen Ltd	Daunorubicin citrate	Liposome/lipid NPs	Drug delivery system for the treatment of cancer

cellular receptors, which results in the cellular internalisation of these NPs and evokes an immune response [37,38]. Some proteins, like albumin, immunoglobulins, fibrinogen and apolipoproteins, can bind strongly to the iron oxide NPs, liposomes, polymeric NPs and CNTs [39]. Protein corona formation depends on the physicochemical properties of the NPs, the protein affinity towards the NPs and the nature of the physiological environment. Various parameters such as size, shape, solubility and surface properties of NPs, and the route of exposure to NPs, may affect the composition, thickness and conformation of protein corona. Therefore, the effects of these parameters have been extensively examined for biodistribution and nanosafety issues concerning NPs [38,40].

Protein adsorption on the NPs occurs as the formation of a protein–NP complex through several forces such as hydrogen bonds, solvation forces, Van der Waals interactions etc. The protein–NP complex formation alters many physicochemical properties of the NPs and, at the same time, stimulates conformational changes in the secondary structure of adsorbed proteins [41]. Due to their dynamic nature, protein adsorption on the NPs results in the formation of hard and soft corona layers. Hard corona is a tight and nearly irreversible protein binding, whereas soft corona is a quick reversible protein binding, with faster exchange rates.

The protein–NP complex formation affects the overall bioreactivity of the NPs and mediates the cellular recognition and uptake of NPs [42]. Moreover, the protein corona formation on NP surfaces regulates cellular responses including cytotoxicity and cell activation [43]. Therefore, the interaction of NPs with proteins becomes an important issue to consider for the development of better-tolerated engineered NPs with enhanced safety.

2.3.2 NP–Cell Interactions

NPs are able to enter cells and interact with subcellular structures. Due to their size and surface properties, the uptake of NPs can occur via energy-dependent intake or energy-independent insertion [42,44,45]. Endocytosis, a process in which cells internalize ions, biomolecules or particles, is an energy-dependent process that also happens for NPs [45]. NPs with very small dimensions and a positive charge can pass through cell membranes in a process called penetration [46]. During endocytosis, NPs enter the cell through endocytic vesicles but are not directly transferred into the cytosol, whereas NPs taken up by membrane penetration are directly transferred into the cytosol [46].

NPs enter cells through different endocytosis pathways, such as clathrin- and caveolae-mediated endocytosis, phagocytosis, macropinocytosis and pinocytosis [45]. NPs coated with protein corona are taken up into the cell via receptor-mediated endocytosis [47]. Phagocytosis and macropinocytosis are both actin-dependent pathways. Phagocytosis is restricted to specialized phagocytes (i.e., monocytes/macrophages, neutrophils and dendritic cells) and the interaction of receptors on the cell surface and the ligands results in the uptake of macromolecules and particles. On the other hand, almost all other cells can take up NPs by receptor-mediated endocytosis, macropinocytosis and pinocytosis pathways. Macropinocytosis and pinocytosis pathways are used by cells to take up NPs below 10 nm in size [45].

The macropinocytosis pathway is a route for non-selective endocytosis of solute macromolecules, whereas the pinocytosis pathway involves the uptake of fluids and solutes.

NPs are also able to penetrate into the cells without specific receptors on their outer surface through passive uptake or adhesive interaction. This type of uptake occurs via Van der Waals forces, electrostatic charges, steric interactions or interfacial tension effects without vesicle formation [48,49].

Following the cellular uptake of NPs, the intercellular mechanisms also decide the fate of NPs. NPs may localise in lysosomes, cytosol, nucleus, mitochondria, endosomes, golgi apparatus and endoplasmic reticulum due to their different physicochemical properties [44,50]. These up-take and intracellular pathways have been investigated in many studies and summarised in several reviews [45,50,51]. The cellular uptake of NPs is influenced by the physicochemical properties of the NPs (size [52–54] and surface properties [53,55]), the protein corona on NPs [54] and the type of interacting cell [53]. Apart from the chemistry, size and charge of the NPs, the morphology of NPs can affect the rate of cellular uptake [56]. In a previous study, hydroxyapatite NPs (HANPs) with different morphologies (long rods, dots, sheets, and fibres) were tested *in vitro* by using polymorphonuclear cells (PMNCs) [56]. They observed that fibre morphology caused higher reactive oxygen species (ROS) production compared to the other morphologies, indicating the process of phagocytosis of foreign materials.

Because of their small size, greater surface area-to-volume ratio and high surface reactivity, NPs show higher chemical reactivity and are closely associated with toxicity, including intracellular ROS generation and consequent oxidative stress, genetic damage, inflammation and carcinogenesis [57,58]. ROS, reactive species of molecular oxygen, are important molecules in cell signalling and in the defence mechanism of the immune system. Excess ROS production may result in detrimental effects on cells, alteration in biomolecule functions and the induction of cell death through apoptosis or necrosis [42]. The intracellular ROS generation by NPs is considered the primary cause of *in vivo* nanotoxicity and is dependent on the physicochemical properties of NPs, including particle size, surface charge and chemical composition [57,59]. After internalisation, NPs can interact with the mitochondria and cell nucleus, which is considered the main cause of NP-related toxicity [60]. In the nucleus, the interactions between NPs and DNA or DNA-related proteins may cause physical damage to the genetic material (nanogenotoxicity) [61]. Additionally, NPs may be involved in the other cellular responses, such as oxidative stress and inflammation [61]. Oxidative stress is a redox imbalance within cells, which is usually caused by increased intracellular ROS. This can also induce the pathways responsible for the production of redox-sensitive transcription factors (e.g., NF-κB) and mitogen-activated protein kinase (MAPK), which leads to the release of pro-inflammatory cytokines [61]. In a previous *in vivo* study, the effect of silver AgNPs (20 nm) and titanium dioxide (Aeroxide® P25 TiO2NPs, 21 nm) NPs on oxidative stress/inflammation response and components of the brain renin-angiotensin system (RAS) was examined after their intravenous injection to Wistar rats [62]. They showed that both NPs induced oxidative stress and consequent changes in the expression of brain RAS genes, which can be related to potent neurotoxic effects leading to different neurodegenerative diseases.

2.4 NANOPARTICLES AND THE IMMUNE SYSTEM

The immune system is a system of cells and intercommunicating proteins with specialized roles in the detection, recognition and elimination of infectious agents and other invaders such as dust and particles in order to protect the host. The immune system can be divided into innate and adaptive immunity. Both innate and adaptive immune responses are closely related to each other and work in a coordinated manner.

Innate immunity, an antigen-independent (non-specific) defence mechanism, represents the first line of defence against foreign agents and can immediately respond to any stimulus. The innate immune system has a primary role in early recognition and the subsequent pro-inflammatory response, and involves the recognition of pathogen-associated molecular patterns (PAMPs) [63] and damage-associated molecular patterns (DAMPs) [64] by pattern recognition receptors (PRRs) [65]. On the other hand, the adaptive immune system is an antigen-dependent and antigen-specific defence mechanism, involving the identification and elimination of pathogens by an extremely diverse repertoire of antigen-specific recognition receptors on T- and B-lymphocytes [66]. The adaptive immune system acts as a second line of defence and requires some time to attain the maximal effective response after antigen exposure. Innate immunity has no immunologic memory because of the short-lived innate immune cells. However, adaptive immunity has an immunological memory against reinfection due to the generation of long-lived, antigen-specific cells after initial exposure to an antigen or pathogen.

In some cases, defects or malfunctions in either the innate or adaptive immune response might occur, which can provoke some diseases. Immunotoxicity is an adverse or inappropriate effect on the structure or function of the immune system after exposure to a foreign agent. These adverse changes include decreases (called immunosuppression or immunodepression) or increases (called immunostimulation) in the immune response. Immunosuppression results in an increased incidence of infections and/or tumours, whereas immunostimulation results in an increased incidence of hypersensitivity reactions, inflammatory responses, or autoimmunity.

Once NPs enter the body, they can interact with immune cells and provoke immune responses. Some examples of immune responses against selected NPs are represented in Table 2.2. The initial recognition of NPs by the immune system has an important role in the fate and distribution of NPs inside the body. Interactions between NPs and the immune system may cause desirable or detrimental consequences. Avoiding immune recognition is desirable when the NPs are being used for drug delivery to the correct target site, as well as for NPs used in various industrial applications. NPs can stimulate and/or suppress immune cell responses depending on the formation of protein coronas formed in the blood [43]. However, interactions between NPs and the immune system can be beneficial for vaccine delivery or therapeutics for inflammatory and autoimmune diseases [67–69].

TABLE 2.2
Examples for Immune Responses against Selected NPs

Type of NPs	Target Cell	Experiment	Interactions with Immune System	Ref
Magnesium or zinc substituted HA NPs	Bone marrow dendritic cells	*In vitro*	Stimulation of Th1 immunity and Th2 immunity	[25]
Titania (TiO_2), silica (SiO_2), zirconia (ZrO_2) or cobalt NPs	Human macrophages (PMA-differentiated myelomonocytic U-937 cells)	*In vitro*	Changes in the expression of innate immunity receptors (TLR1-10 and the TLR4 co-receptors CD14 and MD-2), and M1 polarisation	[70]
Zinc oxide NPs	Primary mice macrophages	*In vitro*	Induce inflammatory responses in macrophages via TLR6-mediated MAPK signalling	[71]
Functionalised polystyrene NPs	Primary human macrophages and human leukaemia cell line THP-1	*In vitro*	Uptake of NPs by phagocytosis via high affinity Fc receptor for IgG antibodies and internalisation in THP-1 cells by dynamin II-dependent endocytosis	[72]

2.4.1 Nanoparticles and the Innate Immune System

The innate immune system is the first line of defence against foreign agents, where granulocytes such as basophils, neutrophils, mast cells, eosinophils and antigen-presenting cells (APCs) such as monocytes, macrophages and dendritic cells play important roles. The innate immune response is based on the phagocytosis of foreign agents. Another important part of the innate immune system is the complement system, an enzyme cascade that attacks the surfaces of pathogens or foreign materials to help antibodies and phagocytic cells to remove them.

When NPs enter the body, they may encounter innate immune responses such as opsonisation and recognition by receptors that enable phagocytosis of NPs or stimulate inflammatory responses [73,74]. In the blood stream, the binding of proteins called opsonins to the surfaces of NPs enhances recognition of these particles and leads to uptake by immune cells through various pathways [75]. Examples of key opsonins include immunoglubulins, complement proteins (C3, C4 and C5), fibronectin and apolipoproteins [76,77]. During opsonisation, unnatural protein conformations occur and these protein conformational changes promote phagocytosis and inflammatory reactions [75,78,79]. Opsonins adhere to the foreign particle by different interactions such as ionic, electrostatic, hydrophobic, hydrophilic and Van der Waals forces [76]. The binding of opsonins to NPs results in recognition by the mononuclear phagocyte system (MPS) and the clearance of particles by phagocytosis from the bloodstream [76]. Without opsonisation, phagocytic cells are not able to bind or recognise the NPs.

Phagocytosis of NPs from circulation is mediated by circulating phagocytic cells (e.g., monocytes, platelets, leukocytes and dendritic cells) and resident phagocytes such as Kupffer cells in the liver, dendritic cells in the lymph nodes and macrophages and B-cells in the spleen [78]. Macrophages are the primary phagocytic cells involved in the internalisation and clearance of NPs and in mediating host inflammatory and immunological biological responses [80]. Macrophages interact with NPs either by using phagocytic receptors or pattern recognition receptors (PRRs) [80]. NPs can be taken up by macrophages through Fc (gamma) receptor-mediated [75,81], complement receptor-mediated [75], mannose receptor-mediated [75,82] and scavenger receptor-mediated phagocytic pathways [75]. Fc (gamma) and complement receptor-mediated phagocytosis is based on the immunoglobulin G (IgG) and inactivated form of the complement fragment 3b (iC3b), respectively [83]. However, mannose- and scavenger receptor-mediated phagocytic pathways are opsonin-independent phagocytosis and they are mediated by these pattern-recognition receptors (PRRs) [84].

The innate immune system involves the recognition of pathogen-associated molecular patterns (PAMPs) [63] and DAMPs [64] by PRRs [65]. PAMPs found on pathogens are small molecular motifs including bacterial cell wall components, or viral DNA/RNA, as well as fungal glucans [85], whereas DAMPs are endogenous molecules released after tissue stress or injury. Both PAMPs and DAMPs are recognised by PRPs localised at the cell surface, in intra-cellular vesicles or in the cytosol, and thus trigger cells as part of innate immune defence, such as macrophages and epithelial cells [85].

Macrophages are capable of recognising patterns presented by foreign material; pathogens and damaged native tissues present patterns through four specific macrophage surface receptors, including Toll-like receptors (TLRs), mannose receptors, scavenger receptors and Fc receptors [80]. Different receptor-mediated pathways are involved in different types of NPs because of the specificity of the active receptors (Figure 2.2). The binding of TLRs to corresponding antigens plays a crucial role in macrophage activation and subsequently in the initiation of innate immune reactions. In a previous *in vitro* study, non-toxic concentrations of titania (TiO_2), silica (SiO_2), zirconia (ZrO_2) or cobalt NPs were tested for their ability to modulate the vital and functional parameters of human macrophages [70]. Increased expression of TLRs and the production of inflammatory cytokines were observed. In another *in vitro* study, macrophages were exposed to zinc oxide NPs and recognition of these particles by TLR6 was directly related to the activation of macrophages by the enhancement of CD11b, CDld and MHC-II to initiate immune responses [71].

Mannose receptors, expressed on the surface of macrophages, dendritic cells and some epithelial cells bind to microbial structures bearing mannose, fucose and N-acetylglucosamine on their surface [86]. Mannosylation of polymeric NPs has been used as a strategy to target macrophages such as tumour-associated macrophages (TAMs) [87,88]. In a study by Ortega et al. [87], the delivery capability of siRNA – or short, fluorescently labelled DNA strands of novel mannosylated polymer nanoparticles (MnNPs) – to the TAMs was examined in several tumour models. MnNP-DNA conjugates were directly injected into the centre of the tumour. In a murine ovarian tumour model, MnNPs improved the *in vivo* delivery of fluorescently labelled DNA to the TAMs (Figure 2.3A). The confocal images of *ex vivo* ovarian ascites TAMs showed that the MnNPs were taken up and retained by TAMs (Figure 2.3B and C) and the internal co-localisation of MnNP with the mannose

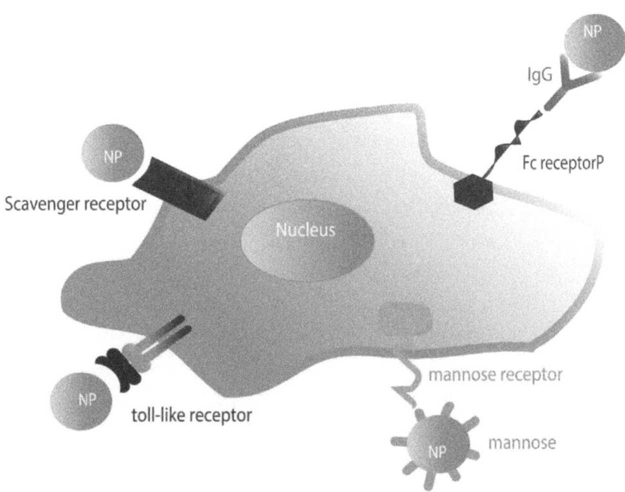

FIGURE 2.2 Phagocytic cell recognition of NPs through four specific macrophage surface receptors.

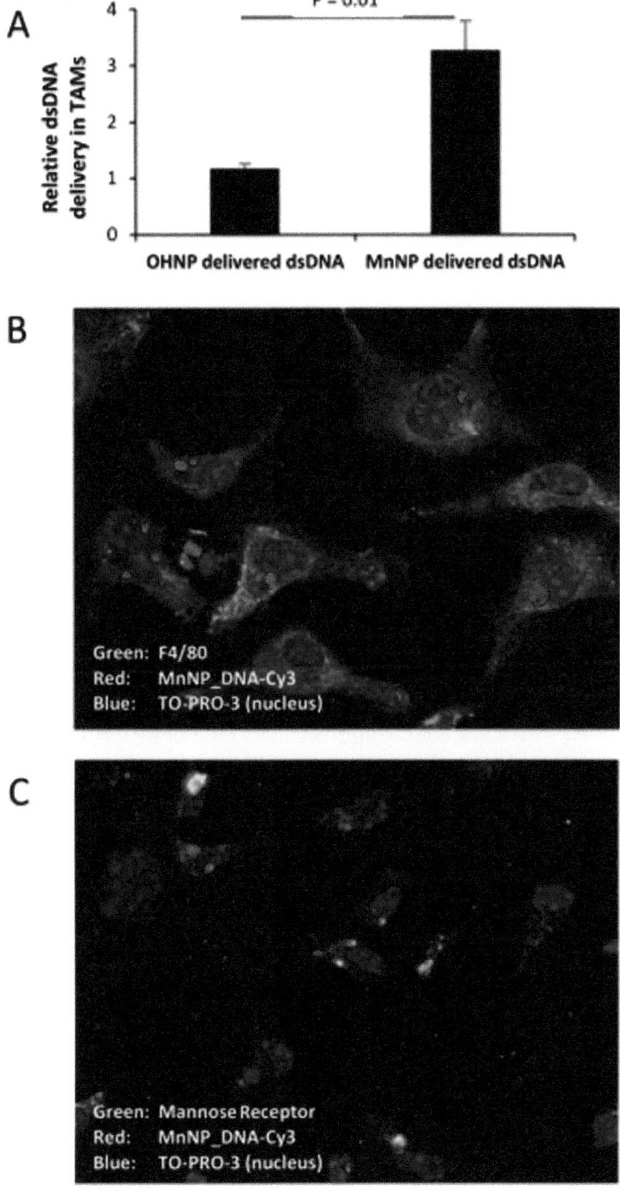

FIGURE 2.3 (A) Relative amounts of Cy5-labelled dsDNA delivered with alcohol-capped (non-targeted) endosomal escape nanoparticles (OHNP) and TAM-targeted MnNP. (B and C) *Ex vivo* murine ovarian ascites TAMs exposed to MnNP-DNA_Cy3 for 24 hours: (B) green, F4/80 labelling on the cell membrane; red, labelling of the DNA-Cy3 carrying MnNP; and blue, TO-PRO-3 staining of nucleus. (C) Green: the mannose receptor on the cell surface; red, labelling of the DNA-Cy3 carrying MnNP; and yellow, co-localisation of mannose receptor with Cy3 fluorescence of DNA carrying MnNP. (From Ortega, R.A., *Nanoscale*, 7, 500–510, 2015.)

receptor was shown by the green-red overlap (yellow) (Figure 2.3C). The endosomal uptake of MnNPs was facilitated by mannose receptors, which were transported into the cytoplasm inside the resultant endosome.

Scavenger receptors can recognise apoptotic cells, bacteria, dust particles and nanoscale objects, including engineered NPs [89]. Clathrin-mediated, scavenger receptor A-dependent endocytosis has been reported for human macrophages as a main uptake mechanism for carboxydextran-coated superparamagnetic iron oxide NPs with diameters of 20 and 60 nm [90]. In the *in vitro* and *in vivo* studies of Aldossari et al. [91], the role for scavenger receptor B1 in macrophage uptake and activation was shown by cellular recognition of silver NPs (AgNPs) and the induction of cell responses. Fc receptors for IgG (FcγRI; also known as CD64), IgM, IgA and IgE were found on the surface of most innate immune cells such as dendritic cells, macrophages and monocytes [92]. In a previous study, it was shown that carboxy and amino functionalized polystyrene NPs are internalised by human macrophages via high-affinity Fc receptors for IgG anti-bodies, CD64 in the presence of human serum [72].

2.4.2 Nanoparticles and the Adaptive Immune System

The second line of defence, the adaptive immune system, involves recognition for both self- and nonself-antigens, the formation of pathogen-specific immunologic effector pathways and the generation of immunologic memory [93]. The adaptive immune system is composed of T-cells, which are activated through APCs (cellular immunity), and B-cells, which are responsible for humoral (antibody-mediated) immunity. T-cells can participate in the elimination of pathogens by killing infected target cells and can also function as helper cells to enhance both B- and T-cell responses and to activate mononuclear phagocytes [93]. T-cells can be classified in two main groups: T-helper cells (CD4+) and CD8+ cytotoxic T-lymphocytes (CTLs). CTLs recognise and respond to foreign antigens presented by infected cells. These CTLs are crucial in defending against intracellular infections and cancer. On the other hand, T-helper cells play a major role in the suppression of immune reaction, as well as in the activation of the cells of the innate immune system, B-cells, cytotoxic T-cells and some nonimmune cells [94]. T-helper cells are subdivided into T-helper 1 (Th1), T-helper 2 (Th2), follicular helper T-cell (Tfh), induced T-regulatory cells (iTreg), the regulatory type 1 cells (Tr1), T-helper 9 (Th9) and T-helper 17 (Th17), depending on their function and cytokine profiles [94]. Th1 cells are characterised by the production of interferon-gamma (IFN-γ) [66,93,95], interleukin (IL)-2 [93,95] and tumour necrosis factor (TNF)-α [95] and they mediate B-cells for the opsonisation and neutralisation of antibodies [66]. On the other hand, Th2 cells secrete anti-inflammatory cytokines such as IL-4, IL-5, IL-10 and IL-13, and these cytokines are involved in antibody production, hypersensitivity and parasite-induced immune responses [93].

NPs can stimulate both cellular and humoral immunity. In a previous *in vivo* study with mice, the chronic pulmonary accumulation of iron oxide NPs (Fe_2O_3) induced Th1-polarised immune response stimulating the function of APCs [96]. Zhu et al. [97] showed that *in vivo* exposure to magnetic iron oxide NPs resulted in significant extracellularly secreted membrane vesicle generation involved in the triggering of Th1 immune activation in the alveolar region of Balb/C mice. Water-soluble polyhydroxylated fullerenes ($C_{60}(OH)_{20}$) showed specific immunomodulatory effects on T-cells and macrophages, both *in vivo* and *in vitro*, and they induced the production of Th1 cytokines (IL-2, IFN-γ and TNF-α) and decreased the production of Th2 cytokines (IL-4, IL-5 and IL-6) [98].

The activation of humoral immunity, the principal defence mechanism against extracellular antigens, is dependent on APCs and is mediated by antibodies (IgG, IgA, IgE, IgM and IgD) produced by B-cells [26]. Facilitating the access of antigens to APCs and subsequent antigen-specific immune responses can be used in the development of NP-based vaccine delivery systems [26,29,33]. As mentioned before, NPs can be used as either delivery systems for adjuvants and/or as immunostimulants [29]. In particular, antigens have been widely entrapped within biodegradable polymeric NPs due to their ability to control release and in order to optimise the desired immune response via selective targeting of the antigen to APCs [33]. Aluminium hydroxide NPs of ≤ 200 nm in size induced a stronger humoral response than the traditional aluminium hydroxide adjuvant with a particle size of 1–20 µm [99]. Mansoor et al. [100] reported that intranasal administration of poly (dl-lactic-co-glycolide) (PLGA) NPs loaded with bovine parainfluenza virus type-3 (BPI3V) peptide motifs and solubilised BPI3V proteins induced a stronger IgG antibody response in mice compared with solubilised BPI3V antigen alone. NP-conjugated macromolecule biomaterials (nano-mbio) also promise great potential for *in vivo* applications, although there are some safety concerns. They should therefore be investigated with caution for *in vivo* applications. For example, QDs conjugated baculovirus, a recently developed nano-mbio, which induced significantly stronger adaptive immune responses in mice compared to baculovirus alone because QDs and baculovirus facilitated each other in activating cellular immunoreaction [101].

NPs can either promote allergic reactions [102–104] or can be used as immunotherapy against allergic reactions [105–107]. The exposure of carbon nanotubes can promote pulmonary allergic responses by stimulating Th2-mediated immunity [108,109]. On the contrary, the incorporation of allergens into biodegradable and nonbiodegradable polymeric NPs has received much interest as a potential adjuvant for allergen immunotherapy [107]. Some liposomal formulations, such as Doxil® and other amphiphilic lipids, could cause a hypersensitivity syndrome known as complement activation-related pseudoallergy (CARPA) [110]. CARPA syndrome includes a consequence of activation of the complement system and is generally a mild reaction; however, it can sometimes be more severe or lethal. However, some nanoformulations consisting of neutral lipopolymers showed great potential in the minimisation of severe CARPA response [110].

2.4.3 Nanoparticle Physicochemical Properties Affecting Immune Response

The effect of NPs on the immune system varies depending on their capacity for protein binding and their unique physicochemical properties, such as size, shape, solubility, composition, charge and surface chemistry [56,75,78]. In a study by Yen et al. [111], the immunological response of macrophages against physically produced pure gold and silver NPs of varying sizes were tested *in vitro*. Depending on particle size, both types of NPs influenced macrophages negatively in various extents, but gold NPs had significant effects on macrophages compared to silver NPs of similar size, and they up-regulated the expressions of proinflammatory genes IL-1, IL-6 and TNF-α. Moreover, small gold NPs (2–4 nm) significantly increased expressions of these pro-inflammatory genes compared to medium (5–7 nm) and large (20–40 nm) NPs.

As mentioned previously, size plays a crucial role in the body's responses to NPs and subsequent distribution and elimination of the particles. Particle size also determines the pathways of endocytosis and cellular uptake [112]. NPs larger than 0.5 μm in size are internalised by macrophages, dendritic cells and neutrophils via phagocytosis pathways [45], whereas smaller NPs are internalised through macropinocytosis (0.5–5 μm) and pinocytosis pathways (20–500 nm) [80].

The size of the particles has a significant impact on their uptake by immune cells. For example, PLGA NPs were more efficiently internalised by dendritic cells *in vitro* and they were significantly more immunogenic *in vivo* compared to PLGA microparticles containing equivalent amounts of antigen and TLR ligands [113]. In a previous *in vivo* study, it was reported that large (>1 μm) industrialised particles (diesel exhaust, carbon black and silica particles) stimulated Th1-like responses, whereas smaller counterparts (<500 nm) induced Th2-like responses – an indicator of an allergic immune response [114]. On the other hand, some small engineered polymeric NPs, such as 500-nm PLGA [115], 270-nm PLGA [116] and 112-nm poly (ethylene glycol cyanoacrylate-co-hexadecylcyanoacrylate) (PEG–PHDA) [117] induced Th1-like responses. In a study by Kumar et al. [118], the interaction of immune cells with antigen-conjugated polystyrene particles of various sizes and shapes (rod or sphere) were examined both *in vitro* (e.g., antigen uptake by dendritic cells) and *in vivo* (e.g., type and strength of antibody production). They concluded that smaller spherical (193 nm) particles generated stronger Th1 and Th2 immune responses compared to other particle types.

The shape of NPs also plays an important role in modulating interactions with immune cells [119,120]. In a study by Bartneck et al. [121], the uptake capacities of human primary leukocyte populations were investigated by using rod-shaped and spherical gold NPs with diameters between 15 and 50 nm and a variety of surface chemistries. The rod-shaped NPs were taken up by macrophages more efficiently than spherical NPs, while the uptake of spherical NPs by cervical cancer cells and human lung epithelial cells was more efficient than that of rod-shaped NPs. In another study, the immunological response of primary human polymorphonuclear cells (PMNCs) and mononuclear cells (MNCs) against hydroxyapatite NPs (HANPs) with different morphologies (long rods, dots, sheets and fibres) was tested *in vitro* and the acute inflammatory response towards these NPs was examined *in vivo* in a Balb/C mice model [56]. They observed that both MNCs and PMNCs produced greater amounts of ROS when they were exposed to fibre-type NPs. Additionally, subcutaneously implanted fibre and dot-type NPs induced the highest acute inflammation as compared to the sheets.

Surface charge is another parameter that plays an important role in the uptake of NPs. Positively charged NPs are more likely to stimulate inflammatory reactions than anionic or neutral NPs [78]. Macrophage uptake increases as the surface charge (either positive or negative) of NPs increases [122,123].

Opsonisation of the NPs is also important for their uptake by immune cells. The binding of proteins onto NPs can change their bioreactivity, making them recognisable to immune cells, causing a subsequent clearance of these particles from circulation by phagocytosis [124]. The uptake by MPS phagocytes of opsonised NPs can be stimulated either in the native form of proteins [76] or after conformational changes in the protein structure [125]. However, because long circulation times are needed for these types of systems, opsonisation and non-specific clearance of NPs are undesirable for most NP-based drug delivery applications.

PEGylation of NPs is a method used to prepare NPs with stealth properties or sterically stabilised properties for preventing nonspecific protein adsorption *in vivo* and improving their biodistribution [76]. Alternatively, the functionalisation of NPs with cellular materials as a biomimetic delivery platform can provide avoidance for clearance by the immune system and prolong the circulation time of these systems [126]. In a previous study, the immunological effect of unmodified multi-stage nanovectors (MSV) and particles functionalised with a murine and human leukocyte cellular membrane, dubbed Leukolike Vectors (LLV), were tested *in vitro* and *in vivo* [127]. *In vitro* experiments examined the interactions of murine J774 macrophages with MSV and LLV coated with murine (mLLV) and human-derived cell membranes (hLLV) for 150 min by using time-lapse microscopy (Figure 2.4). The interaction of cells with MSV and hLLV resulted in cell internalisation, whereas the interaction with mLLV resulted in the release of the

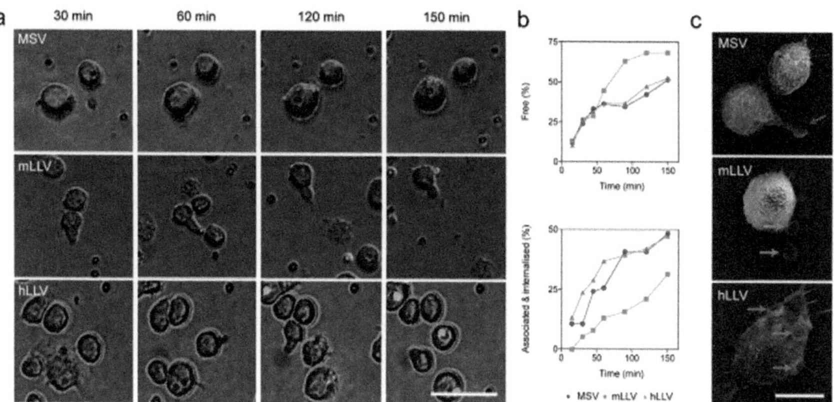

FIGURE 2.4 (a) Time-lapse microscopy images of murine J774 cells interacting with multistage nanovectors (MSV) (red) and Leukolike Vectors (LLV) coated with murine (mLLV, orange) and human-derived cell membranes (hLLV, green) after 30, 60, 120 and 150 min; scale: 20 mm. (b) Selected positions from time-lapse microscopy used for analysis for MSV, mLLV and hLLV. (c) Scanning electron micrograph images of J774 cells after 3 h incubation with MSV, mLLV and hLLV. Visible particles depicted by arrows, scale: 10 μm. (From Evangelopoulos, M., *Biomaterials*, 82, pp. 168–177, 2016.)

particles following their contact with the cell (Figure 2.4a). The group quantified free and associated/internalised particles by evaluating the representative sections of videos taken during live microscopy. They found that the percentage of free mLLV was found to be higher than MSV and hLLV at 150 min (Figure 2.4b). These results were confirmed with scanning electron microscopy (SEM) after 3 h incubation of murine J774 macrophages with MSV, hLLV and mLLV. Filopodia-like structures and subsequent particle internalisation were observed in the macrophages exposed with MSV and hLLV (Figure 2.4c). However, a simple docking of the particles on the cell surface was seen in macrophages exposed with mLLV (Figure 2.4c). The results of the *in vitro* study showed that LLV developed using a cellular coating derived from a syngeneic source (i.e., murine J774 macrophages, mLLV) can avoid uptake by macrophage cells. Additionally, the cellular membrane on systems enhanced the systemic tolerance and minimised the inflammatory response to LLV *in vivo*. The avoidance of opsonisation and phagocytosis capability of LLV functionalised with cellular membrane provides a prolonged circulation with a superior targeting of inflammation. Another biomimetic delivery platform, red blood cell membrane-coated poly (lactic-co-glycolic acid) (PLGA) NPs, also showed longer retention time in the blood due to their escape from the immune system [128].

2.5 CONCLUDING REMARKS

Apart from industrial applications, nanotechnology offers great potential for developing new treatment and diagnostic approaches in medicine. NPs with unique chemical and surface properties have been developed using different materials for drug, gene and vaccine delivery systems, medical imaging agents and in diagnostics. Some of these NP-based therapeutic and diagnostic agents are already in use in clinics for treating various diseases, and many others are currently undergoing either preclinical or clinical trials. Besides the numerous advantages of NPs, unintentional exposure or certain intentional administration of NPs with different physicochemical properties may cause adverse biological responses. The interaction of NPs with the biological system determines the biocompatibility, *in vivo* stability, biological performance and side effects caused by NPs. Due to possible health concerns, the toxicity and potential effects of NPs on the immune system should be carefully evaluated.

NPs can stimulate or suppress immune responses and their initial recognition by the immune system has an important role in the fate and distribution of NPs inside the body. Understanding how the immune system responds to NPs provides information about the development of safer NPs for biomedical and various industrial applications. However, interactions between NPs and the immune system can be beneficial for vaccine delivery or therapeutics for inflammatory and autoimmune diseases, where the avoidance of immune recognition of the NPs or targeted delivery is desired. For these purposes, further studies are required to investigate the relationship between the immunomodulatory effects of NPs and the physicochemical parameters of NPs, which define the interactions of the NPs with the immune system.

REFERENCES

1. Parveen, S. (2012). Nanoparticles: A boon to drug delivery, therapeutics, diagnostics and imaging, *Nanomedicine*, 8, pp. 147–166.
2. Xie, J. (2010). Nanoparticle-based theranostic agents, *Adv Drug Deliv Rev*, 62, pp. 1064–1079.
3. Zhang, L. (2008). Nanoparticles in medicine: Therapeutic applications and developments, *Clin Pharmacol Ther*, 83, pp. 761–769.
4. Liu, Y. (2007). Nanomedicine for drug delivery and imaging: A promising avenue for cancer therapy and diagnosis using targeted functional nanoparticles, *Int J Cancer*, 120, pp. 2527–2537.
5. Estelrich, J. (2015). Nanoparticles in magnetic resonance imaging: From simple to dual contrast agents, *Int J Nanomedicine*, 10, pp. 1727–1741.
6. Kunzmann, A. (2011). Toxicology of engineered nanomaterials: Focus on biocompatibility, biodistribution and biodegradation, *Biochim Biophys Acta*, 1810, pp. 361–373.
7. Contado, C. (2015). Nanomaterials in consumer products: A challenging analytical problem, *Front Chem*, 3(48).
8. Nune, S.K. (2009). Nanoparticles for biomedical imaging, *Expert Opin Drug Deliv*, 6, pp. 1175–1194.
9. Sivasubramanian, M. (2014). Nanoparticle-facilitated functional and molecular imaging for the early detection of cancer, *Front Mol Biosci*, 1(15).
10. Resch-Genger, U. (2008). Quantum dots versus organic dyes as fluorescent labels, *Nat Meth*, 5, pp. 763–775.
11. Santra, S. (2010). Fluorescent silica nanoparticles for cancer imaging, in R.S. Grobmyer, M.B. Moudgil (eds), *Cancer nanotechnology: Methods and protocols*, Humana Press, Totowa, NJ, pp. 151–162.
12. Shao, L. (2011). Semiconductor quantum dots for biomedicial applications, *Sensors (Basel)*, 11, pp. 11736–11751.
13. Shin, T.-H. (2015). Recent advances in magnetic nanoparticle-based multi-modal imaging, *Chem Soc Rev*, 44, pp. 4501–4516.
14. Dellinger, A. (2013). Application of fullerenes in nanomedicine: An update, *Nanomedicine (London)*, 8, pp. 1191–1208.
15. Muthu, M.S. (2014). Nanotheranostics – application and further development of nanomedicine strategies for advanced theranostics, *Theranostics*, 4, pp. 660–677.
16. Goldberg, M. (2007). Nanostructured materials for applications in drug delivery and tissue engineering, *J Biomater Sci Polym Ed*, 18, pp. 241–268.
17. Patel, V.R. (2011). Nanosuspension: An approach to enhance solubility of drugs, *J Adv Pharm Technol Res*, 2, pp. 81–87.
18. Sutradhar Kumar, B. (2013). Nanoemulsions: Increasing possibilities in drug delivery, *Eur J Nanomed*, 2013 5(2), pp. 97–110.
19. Rajshree, L.S. (2011). Microemulsions and nanoemulsions for targeted drug delivery to the brain, *Curr Nanosci*, 7, pp. 119–133.
20. Jain, N.K. (2013). Targeted drug delivery to macrophages, *Expert Opin Drug Deliv*, 10, pp. 353–367.
21. Banerjee, D. (2011). Nanotechnology-mediated targeting of tumor angiogenesis, *Vascular Cell*, 3, pp. 1–13.
22. Zhou, J. (2015). Toward biocompatible semiconductor quantum dots: From biosynthesis and bioconjugation to biomedical application, *Chem Rev*, 115, pp. 11669–11717.
23. Draper, S.J. (2010). Viruses as vaccine vectors for infectious diseases and cancer, *Nat Rev Micro*, 8, pp. 62–73.
24. Coffman, R.L. (2010). Vaccine adjuvants: Putting innate immunity to work, *Immunity*, 33, pp. 492–503.

25. Wang, X. (2016). Rod-shaped and substituted hydroxyapatite nanoparticles stimulating type 1 and 2 cytokine secretion, *Colloids Surf B Biointerfaces*, 139, pp. 10–16.
26. Sahdev, P. (2014). Biomaterials for nanoparticle vaccine delivery systems, *Pharm Res*, 31, pp. 2563–2582.
27. Zhao, L. (2014). Nanoparticle vaccines, *Vaccine*, 32, pp. 327–337.
28. Gregory, A.E. (2013). Vaccine delivery using nanoparticles, *Front Cell Infect Microbiol*, 3, pp. 13.
29. Singh, M. (2007). Nanoparticles and microparticles as vaccine-delivery systems, *Expert Rev Vaccines*, 6, pp. 797–808.
30. Xiang, S.D. (2006). Pathogen recognition and development of particulate vaccines: Does size matter?, *Methods*, 40, pp. 1–9.
31. Mohan, T. (2013). Novel adjuvants & delivery vehicles for vaccines development: A road ahead, *Indian J Med Res*, 138, pp. 779–795.
32. Schwendener, R.A. (2014). Liposomes as vaccine delivery systems: A review of the recent advances, *Ther Adv Vaccines*, 2, pp. 159–182.
33. Akagi, T. (2012). Biodegradable nanoparticles as vaccine adjuvants and delivery systems: Regulation of immune responses by nanoparticle-based vaccine, in: S. Kunugi, T. Yamaoka (eds), *Polymers in Nanomedicine*, Springer, Berlin, pp. 31–64.
34. Dizaj, S.M. (2014). A sight on the current nanoparticle-based gene delivery vectors, *Nanoscale Res Lett*, 9, pp. 252–252.
35. Chen, J. (2016). Production and clinical development of nanoparticles for gene delivery, *Mol Ther Methods Clin Dev*, 3, pp. 16023.
36. Mamaeva, V. (2013). Mesoporous silica nanoparticles in medicine—Recent advances, *Adv Drug Deliv Rev*, 65, pp. 689–702.
37. Fleischer, C.C. (2014). Nanoparticle-cell interactions: Molecular structure of the protein corona and cellular outcomes, *Acc Chem Res*, 47, pp. 2651–2659.
38. Saptarshi, S.R. (2013). Interaction of nanoparticles with proteins: Relation to bioreactivity of the nanoparticle, *J Nanobiotechnology*, 11, pp. 26.
39. Nel, A.E. (2009). Understanding biophysicochemical interactions at the nano-bio interface, *Nat Mater*, 8, pp. 543–557.
40. Lundqvist, M. (2008). Nanoparticle size and surface properties determine the protein corona with possible implications for biological impacts, *Proc Natl Acad Sci USA*, 105, pp. 14265–14270.
41. Monopoli, M.P. (2012). Biomolecular coronas provide the biological identity of nanosized materials, *Nat Nanotechnol*, 7, pp. 779–786.
42. Mu, Q. (2014). Chemical basis of interactions between engineered nanoparticles and biological systems, *Chem Rev*, 114, pp. 7740–7781.
43. Lee, Y.K. (2015). Effect of the protein corona on nanoparticles for modulating cytotoxicity and immunotoxicity, *Int J Nanomedicine*, 10, pp. 97–113.
44. Jiang, X. (2010). Endo- and exocytosis of zwitterionic quantum dot nanoparticles by live hela cells, *ACS Nano*, 4, pp. 6787–6797.
45. Oh, N. (2014). Endocytosis and exocytosis of nanoparticles in mammalian cells, *Int J Nanomedicine*, 9, pp. 51–63.
46. Wang, T. (2012). Cellular uptake of nanoparticles by membrane penetration: A study combining confocal microscopy with FTIR spectroelectrochemistry, *ACS Nano*, 6, pp. 1251–1259.
47. Lynch, I. (2007). The nanoparticle-protein complex as a biological entity; a complex fluids and surface science challenge for the 21st century, *Adv Colloid Interface Sci*, 134–135, pp. 167–174.
48. Geiser, M. (2005). Ultrafine particles cross cellular membranes by nonphagocytic mechanisms in lungs and in cultured cells, *Environ Health Perspect*, 113, pp. 1555–1560.

49. Peters, A. (2006). Translocation and potential neurological effects of fine and ultrafine particles a critical update, *Part Fibre Toxicol*, 3, pp. 13.
50. Yameen, B. (2014). Insight into nanoparticle cellular uptake and intracellular targeting, *J Control Release*, 190, pp. 485–499.
51. Iversen, T.-G. (2011). Endocytosis and intracellular transport of nanoparticles: Present knowledge and need for future studies, *Nano Today*, 6, pp. 176–185.
52. dos Santos, T. (2011). Quantitative assessment of the comparative nanoparticle-uptake efficiency of a range of cell lines, *Small*, 7, pp. 3341–3349.
53. Kettler, K. (2014). Cellular uptake of nanoparticles as determined by particle properties, experimental conditions, and cell type, *Environ Toxicol Chem*, 33, pp. 481–492.
54. Cheng, X. (2015). Protein corona influences cellular uptake of gold nanoparticles by phagocytic and nonphagocytic cells in a size-dependent manner, *ACS Appl Mater Interfaces*, 7, pp. 20568–20575.
55. Fröhlich, E. (2012). The role of surface charge in cellular uptake and cytotoxicity of medical nanoparticles, *Int J Nanomedicine*, 7, pp. 5577–5591.
56. Pujari-Palmer, S. (2016). In vivo and in vitro evaluation of hydroxyapatite nanoparticle morphology on the acute inflammatory response, *Biomaterials*, 90, pp. 1–11.
57. Manke, A. (2013). Mechanisms of nanoparticle-induced oxidative stress and toxicity, *BioMed Res Int*, 2013, pp. 15.
58. Khanna, P. (2015). Nanotoxicity: An interplay of oxidative stress, inflammation and cell death, *Nanomaterials*, 5, pp. 1163.
59. Fu, P.P. (2014). Mechanisms of nanotoxicity: Generation of reactive oxygen species, *J Food Drug Anal*, 22, pp. 64–75.
60. Aillon, K.L. (2009). Effects of nanomaterial physicochemical properties on in vivo toxicity, *Adv Drug Deliv Rev*, 61, pp. 457–466.
61. Singh, N. (2009). Nanogenotoxicology: The DNA damaging potential of engineered nanomaterials, *Biomaterials*, 30, pp. 3891–3914.
62. Krawczyńska, A. (2015). Silver and titanium dioxide nanoparticles alter oxidative/inflammatory response and renin–angiotensin system in brain, Food and Chemical *Toxicology*, 85, pp. 96–105.
63. Janeway, C.A. (2002). Innate immune recognition, *Annu Rev Immunol*, 20, pp. 197–216.
64. Matzinger, P. (1994). Tolerance, danger, and the extended family, *Annu Rev Immunol*, 12, pp. 991–1045.
65. Suresh, R. (2013). Pattern recognition receptors in innate immunity, host defense, and immunopathology, *Adv Physiol Educ*, 37, pp. 284–291.
66. Warrington, R. (2011). An introduction to immunology and immunopathology, *Allergy Asthma Clin Immunol*, 7, pp. S1.
67. Boraschi, D. (2015). From antigen delivery system to adjuvanticy: The board application of nanoparticles in vaccinology, *Vaccines*, 3, pp. 930–939.
68. Bolhassani, A. (2011). Improvement of different vaccine delivery systems for cancer therapy, *Molecular Cancer*, 10, pp. 3.
69. Dobrovolskaia, M.A. (2016). Current understanding of interactions between nanoparticles and the immune system, *Toxicol Appl Pharmacol*, 299, pp. 78–89.
70. Lucarelli, M. (2004). Innate defence functions of macrophages can be biased by nano-sized ceramic and metallic particles, *Eur Cytokine Netw*, 15, pp. 339–346.
71. Roy, R. (2014). Toll-like receptor 6 mediated inflammatory and functional responses of zinc oxide nanoparticles primed macrophages, *Immunology*, 142, pp. 453–464.
72. Lunov, O. (2011). Differential uptake of functionalized polystyrene nanoparticles by human macrophages and a monocytic cell line, *ACS Nano*, 5, pp. 1657–1669.
73. Doroud, D. (2011). Cysteine proteinase type i, encapsulated in solid lipid nanoparticles induces substantial protection against leishmania major infection in C57BL/6 mice, *Parasite Immunology*, 33, pp. 335–348.

74. Badiee, A. (2012). The role of liposome size on the type of immune response induced in BALB/c mice against leishmaniasis: Rgp63 as a model antigen, *Exp Parasitol*, 132, pp. 403–409.
75. Dobrovolskaia, M.A. (2007). Immunological properties of engineered nanomaterials, *Nat Nano*, 2, pp. 469–478.
76. Owens, D.E., 3rd (2006). Opsonization, biodistribution, and pharmacokinetics of polymeric nanoparticles, *Int J Pharm*, 307, pp. 93–102.
77. Vonarbourg, A. (2006). Parameters influencing the stealthiness of colloidal drug delivery systems, *Biomaterials*, 27, pp. 4356–4373.
78. Dobrovolskaia, M.A. (2008). Preclinical studies to understand nanoparticle interaction with the immune system and its potential effects on nanoparticle biodistribution, *Mol Pharm*, 5, pp. 487–495.
79. Aggarwal, P. (2009). Nanoparticle interaction with plasma proteins as it relates to particle biodistribution, biocompatibility and therapeutic efficacy, *Adv Drug Deliv Rev*, 61, pp. 428–437.
80. Gustafson, H.H. (2015). Nanoparticle uptake: The phagocyte problem, *Nano Today*, 10, pp. 487–510.
81. Pacheco, P. (2013). Effects of microparticle size and Fc density on macrophage phagocytosis, *PLoS One*, 8, pp. e60989.
82. Cui, Z. (2003). Physical characterization and macrophage cell uptake of mannan-coated nanoparticles, *Drug Dev Ind Pharm*, 29, pp. 689–700.
83. Mosser, D.M. (2011). Measuring opsonic phagocytosis via Fcγ receptors and complement receptors on macrophages, *Current Protocols in Immunology*, 95, pp. 14.27.1–14.27.11.
84. Su, Z. (2002). Opsonin-independent phagocytosis: An effector mechanism against acute blood-stage plasmodium chabaudi as infection, *J Infect Dis*, 186, pp. 1321–1329.
85. Farrera, C. (2015). It takes two to tango: Understanding the interactions between engineered nanomaterials and the immune system, *Eur J Pharm Biopharm*, 95, pp. 3–12.
86. Garrido, V.V. (2011). The increase in mannose receptor recycling favors arginase induction and trypanosoma cruzi survival in macrophages, *Int J Biol Sci*, 7, pp. 1257–1272.
87. Ortega, R.A. (2015). Biocompatible mannosylated endosomal-escape nanoparticles enhance selective delivery of short nucleotide sequences to tumor associated macrophages, *Nanoscale*, 7, pp. 500–510.
88. Yu, S.S. (2013). Macrophage-specific RNA targeting via 'click', mannosylated polymeric micelles, *Mol Pharm*, 10, pp. 975–987.
89. Wang, H. (2012). Scavenger receptor mediated endocytosis of silver nanoparticles into J774A.1 macrophages is heterogeneous, *ACS Nano*, 6, pp. 7122–7132.
90. Lunov, O. (2011). Modeling receptor-mediated endocytosis of polymer-functionalized iron oxide nanoparticles by human macrophages, *Biomaterials*, 32, pp. 547–555.
91. Aldossari, A.A. (2015). Scavenger receptor B1 facilitates macrophage uptake of silver nanoparticles and cellular activation, *J Nanopart Res*, 17, pp. 1–14.
92. Guilliams, M. (2014). The function of Fcγ receptors in dendritic cells and macrophages, *Nat Rev Immunol*, 14, pp. 94–108.
93. Bonilla, F.A. (2010). Adaptive immunity, *J Allergy Clin Immunol*, 125, pp. S33–S40.
94. Luckheeram, R.V. (2012). $CD4^+$ T cells: Differentiation and functions, *Clin Dev Immunol*, 2012, pp. 12.
95. Ganesh, B.B. (2011). Role of cytokines in the pathogenesis and suppression of thyroid autoimmunity, *Journal Interferon Cytokine Res*, 31, pp. 721–731.
96. Park, E.J. (2015). Chronic pulmonary accumulation of iron oxide nanoparticles induced Th1-type immune response stimulating the function of antigen-presenting cells, *Environ Res*, 143, pp. 138–147.
97. Zhu, M. (2012). Nanoparticle-induced exosomes target antigen-presenting cells to initiate Th1-type immune activation, Small, 8, pp. 2841–2848.

98. Li, X. (2014). Aluminum hydroxide nanoparticles show a stronger vaccine adjuvant activity than traditional aluminum hydroxide microparticles, *J Control Release*, 173, pp. 148–157.
99. Ying, L. (2009). Immunostimulatory properties and enhanced tnf-α mediated cellular immunity for tumor therapy by C60(OH)20 nanoparticles, *Nanotechnology*, 20, pp. 415102.
100. Mansoor, F. (2014). Intranasal delivery of nanoparticles encapsulating BPI3V proteins induces an early humoral immune response in mice, *Res Vet Sci*, 96, pp. 551–557.
101. Wang, M. (2015). In vivo study of immunogenicity and kinetic characteristics of a quantum dot-labelled baculovirus, *Biomaterials*, 64, pp. 78–87.
102. Nygaard, U.C. (2009). Single-walled and multi-walled carbon nanotubes promote allergic immune responses in mice, *Toxicological Sciences*, 109, pp. 113–123.
103. Larsen, S.T. (2010). Nano titanium dioxide particles promote allergic sensitization and lung inflammation in mice, *Basic Clin Pharmacol Toxicol*, 106, pp. 114–117.
104. Yoshida, T. (2011). Promotion of allergic immune responses by intranasally-administrated nanosilica particles in mice, *Nanoscale Res Letters*, 6, pp. 195.
105. Gamazo, C. (2014). Nanoparticle based-immunotherapy against allergy, *Immunotherapy*, 6, pp. 885–897.
106. Ballester, M. (2015). Nanoparticle conjugation enhances the immunomodulatory effects of intranasally delivered CPG in house dust mite-allergic mice, *Sci Rep*, 5, pp. 14274.
107. De Souza Reboucas, J. (2012). Nanoparticulate adjuvants and delivery systems for allergen immunotherapy, *J Biomed Biotechnol*, 2012, pp. 13.
108. Rydman, E.M. (2014). Inhalation of rod-like carbon nanotubes causes unconventional allergic airway inflammation, *Part Fibre Toxicol*, 11, pp. 1–17.
109. Inoue, K.-I. (2010). Repeated pulmonary exposure to single-walled carbon nanotubes exacerbates allergic inflammation of the airway: Possible role of oxidative stress, *Free Radic Biol Med*, 48, pp. 924–934.
110. Zhang, X.Q. (2012). Interactions of nanomaterials and biological systems: Implications to personalized nanomedicine, *Adv Drug Deliv Rev*, 64, pp. 1363–1384.
111. Yen, H.-J. (2009). Cytotoxicity and immunological response of gold and silver nanoparticles of different sizes, *Small*, 5, pp. 1553–1561.
112. Shang, L. (2014). Engineered nanoparticles interacting with cells: Size matters, *J Nanobiotechnology*, 12, pp. 1–11.
113. Silva, A.L. (2015). Poly-(lactic-co-glycolic-acid)-based particulate vaccines: Particle uptake by dendritic cells is a key parameter for immune activation, *Vaccine*, 33, pp. 847–854.
114. van Zijverden, M. (2000). Adjuvant activity of particulate pollutants in different mouse models, *Toxicology*, 152, pp. 69–77.
115. Lutsiak, M.E.C. (2006). Biodegradable nanoparticle delivery of a Th2-biased peptide for induction of Th1 immune responses, *J Pharm Pharmacol*, 58, pp. 739–747.
116. Chong, C.S.W. (2005). Enhancement of T helper type 1 immune responses against hepatitis B virus core antigen by PLGA nanoparticle vaccine delivery, *J Control Release*, 102, pp. 85–99.
117. de Kozak, Y. (2004). Intraocular injection of tamoxifen-loaded nanoparticles: A new treatment of experimental autoimmune uveoretinitis, *Eur J Immunol*, 34, pp. 3702–3712.
118. Kumar, S. (2015). Shape and size-dependent immune response to antigen-carrying nanoparticles, *J Control Release*, 220, Part A, pp. 141–148.
119. Sharma, G. (2010). Polymer particle shape independently influences binding and internalization by macrophages, *J Control Release*, 147, pp. 408–412.
120. Doshi, N. (2010). Macrophages recognize size and shape of their targets, *PLoS One*, 5, pp. e10051.

121. Bartneck, M. (2010). Rapid uptake of gold nanorods by primary human blood phagocytes and immunomodulatory effects of surface chemistry, *ACS Nano*, 4, pp. 3073–3086.
122. He, C. (2010). Effects of particle size and surface charge on cellular uptake and biodistribution of polymeric nanoparticles, *Biomaterials*, 31, pp. 3657–3666.
123. Roser, M. (1998). Surface-modified biodegradable albumin nano- and microspheres. II: Effect of surface charges on in vitro phagocytosis and biodistribution in rats, *Eur J Pharm Biopharm*, 46, pp. 255-263.
124. Patel, H.M. (1998). Serum-mediated recognition of liposomes by phagocytic cells of the reticuloendothelial system—The concept of tissue specificity, *Adv Drug Deliv Rev*, 32, pp. 45–60.
125. Deng, Z.J. (2011). Nanoparticle-induced unfolding of fibrinogen promotes Mac-1 receptor activation and inflammation, *Nat Nano*, 6, pp. 39–44.
126. Sawdon, A. (2013). Engineering antiphagocytic biomimetic drug carriers, *Ther Deliv*, 4, pp. 825–839.
127. Evangelopoulos, M. (2016). Cell source determines the immunological impact of biomimetic nanoparticles, *Biomaterials*, 82, pp. 168–177.
128. Hu, C.-M.J. (2011). Erythrocyte membrane-camouflaged polymeric nanoparticles as a biomimetic delivery platform, *Proc Natl Acad Sci USA*, 108, pp. 10980–10985.

3 The Effects of Biomaterials with Micro/Nanotopographies on Immune Cells *In Vitro* and *In Vivo*

Hayriye Özçelik

CONTENTS

3.1 INTRODUCTION

The biochemical and biophysical microenvironments of cells play a significant part in their phenotype and behaviour. The presence of a biomaterial surface in the vicinity of the cells can change their behaviour through its physicochemical characteristics, such as its wettability, roughness, porosity etc. One such property that has been widely used for biomedical purposes is surface topography. The advances in surface patterning technologies spearheaded by the requirements of stereolithography in the field of electronics have been slowly applied to biomaterials, resulting in the creation of high-fidelity micro/nanosurface topographies. As structural anisotropy is an important functional feature of several tissues, such as muscle, cornea, ligament etc., in many cases the functional advantages of such topographical cues have been widely demonstrated. So far, much progress has been made in understanding these effects on both somatic cells and stem cells. Recently, the effects of such biophysical and biochemical cues on immune cells, specifically macrophages, has started to draw the attention of researchers.

In the field of immunology, one of the main tools used to control immune cell behaviour is cytokines. In terms of biomaterial biocompatibility, cytokines are described based on their role in influencing foreign body response to the implanted material, promoting either inflammation or wound healing. One of the most active cells in this context is the macrophage, where cytokine induction is one of the main determinants of macrophage plasticity. For example, interferon gamma (IFN-gamma) is widely used to induce M1 macrophages, whereas interleukin-4 (IL-4) is a known M2 macrophage inducer. However, cells receive various signals from their surroundings, not only through biochemical cues, but also through biophysical cues such as inherent material properties and externally applied forces, which collectively direct the future behaviour of the cells. Therefore, the complexity of the microenvironments in which macrophages are often present underlines the necessity to consider other factors that may influence macrophage polarisation. This chapter reviews a range of cues presented by biomaterials, such as roughness, stiffness, mechanical loading, surface topography and chemistry. These sections are followed by the concept of immunological synapse and the use of a model method of supported lipid bilayers (SLBs) to investigate it.

3.2 POLARISATION OF MACROPHAGES AND FOREIGN BODY RESPONSE

Macrophages are immune cells that reside in tissue and are the first to respond to invading pathogens. The microenvironment of macrophages directly affects their polarisation and can give rise to distinct functional phenotypes in a spectrum defined by M1 and M2 macrophages in two extremes. In the case of implantable or injectable structures, these varying microenvironmental cues may be biomaterial-based. Macrophages are generally classified in two groups by their way of activation: classic (M1) or alternative (M2) [1]. The M2 subpopulation can be further subdivided into M2a–d. *In vivo* and *in vitro* macrophage subpopulations exist simultaneously and generate a specific response in their microenvironment as a function of their role in that specific tissue.

The "classically activated" or M1 phenotype polarises as a result of macrophage interaction with pro-inflammatory signals such as Interferon-γ (IFN-γ) and microbial products such as lipopolysaccharide (LPS). TNFα, IL-8 and IL-6 are considered pro-inflammatory cytokines due to their collective ability to promote inflammation by cellular activation and chemotaxis. M1 macrophages are capable of high antigen presentation, as well as promoting Th1 differentiation of lymphocytes that produce pro-inflammatory cytokines (such as IFN-γ and IL-2) in response to intracellular pathogens. Pro-inflammatory M1 cells are predominantly involved in antimicrobial reactions and are capable of degrading the extracellular matrix (ECM) with specific enzymes [1,2]. In the context of biomaterial implantation, while the initial presence of M1 macrophages promotes a necessary initial inflammatory response, a prolonged M1 presence leads to a severe foreign body response, granuloma and fibrous encapsulation, resulting in chronic inflammatory events and failure of biomaterial integration.

Anti-inflammatory M2 cells promote angiogenesis, cell proliferation and ECM remodelling; hence, they are found in the resolution phase of inflammation. Cytokines that inhibit the inflammatory response and promote wound healing, such as IL-1RA, are considered anti-inflammatory or pro-wound healing. IL-1β is considered a pro-inflammatory/pro-wound healing cytokine due to its ability to activate both inflammatory cells (lymphocytes and monocytes) and wound healing cells (fibroblasts). IL-10 acts in the opposite fashion by down-regulating the activity of these cell types and suppressing further cytokine production, leading to an anti-inflammatory/anti-wound healing effect. The M2 phenotype of macrophages, which is referred to as "alternatively activated", is the result of activation by signals (e.g., IL-4, IL-13) from basophils, mast cells and other granulocytes. M2 macrophages consistently express scavenger and mannose receptors (CD206), release anti-inflammatory cytokines such as IL-10, display a high level of iron export aiding in tissue remodelling and encompass a range of different subsets (i.e., M2a, M2b, M2c), including "wound healing" and "regulatory macrophages". Within the M2 subsets, the M2a (induced by IL-4 and IL-13) and M2b (induced by immune complexes and Toll-like receptor (TLR) agonists) subsets perform immune regulatory functions by initiating Th2 lymphocyte anti-inflammatory responses (through the secretion of IL-10, IL-1ra and IL-6). Alternatively, the M2c subset is induced by IL-10 and plays a major role in tissue remodelling and the suppression of inflammatory immune reactions by secreting transforming growth factor β (TGF-β) and IL-10. Moreover, M1 and M2 can be identified by associated antigens. M1 macrophages express the S100A8–S100A9 heterodimer on the cell surface [3,4], while the CD163 receptor is a typical surface antigen of M2 cells [4].

Foreign body response of the host to the implanted material determines the biocompatibility of implanted medical devices and prostheses. Monocyte and macrophages are key players in the host tissue reaction to implants [5–7]. The biocompatibility of a material is partially determined by the inflammatory response of macrophages, which makes up the first line of defence by migrating to the site of implantation long before other cell types arrive. Moreover, in later stages they are also involved in integration of the implant and wound healing and tissue repair [8–10].

Following implantation, the surface of the material is coated with plasma proteins. Monocytes migrate to the tissue/material interface and adhere to the protein-coated surface of the implant. They then differentiate into adherent macrophage cells. The activated macrophages in contact with the biomaterial will start to secrete cytokines, which recruit other immune cells, including leukocytes. If the inflammation remains unresolved within a time frame of a few weeks, a significant level of macrophage fusion leads to multi-nucleated foreign body giant cells (FBGCs) in the biomaterial microenvironment. This is particularly the case for non-degradable biomaterials, which are generally covered by a fibrotic capsule. The FBGCs, with the aim of degrading the foreign material, secrete enzymes and abrasive chemicals such as oxygen radicals, which might deteriorate the mechanical properties of the implants and also cause collateral damage to the tissues in the immediate vicinity of the implants and create further complications.

The available strategies to avoid excessive foreign body response include: (i) protein adsorption (reduction via coatings); (ii) controlling immune cell adhesion; (iii) decreasing the levels of inflammatory cytokines in the implant vicinity; and (iv) preventing FBGC formation on the implant surface. Different ways of modulating the presence and activity of biomaterial-adherent macrophages and FBGCs and their overall response to the surface of implanted medical devices and are currently being sought and comprise an active area of research in surface modification. Simultaneously, understanding the control of the M2:M1 ratio by controlling biomaterial and microenvironmental cues will therefore be a key strategy in the design of next-generation immuno-informed biomaterials to enhance the positive healing period, which includes tissue remodelling, integration and regeneration.

3.3 MACROPHAGE ADHESION

Macrophages are derived from nonadherent monocytes and become adherent when activated. They then migrate through tissue to reach the site of injury or inflammation. Macrophages adhere to the extracellular matrix by different types of integrins and scavenger receptors. Interestingly, modes of adhesion of macrophages to collagen type I may be dependent on species, the underlying adhesion conditions and cell source. β1 integrin is generally the main mediator of adhesion of macrophages to collagen type I [11]. However, in rats, CD18 (β2 integrin subunit) is involved in adhesion to collagen [12]. Whereas in mice (in the most widely used macrophage cell line RAW264.7) the adhesion is modulated mostly by class A scavenger receptors (SR-A) [13].

For most cell types, adhesion to a surface induces the formation of focal adhesions (FA), which are protein structures that are directly linked to the cell cytoskeleton and can transduce the physical and mechanical cues from the adhered surface. In macrophages, podosomes replace FAs. Unlike FAs, podosomes are less-stable, dynamic complexes with a dot-like shape and a size of up to 1 µm [14–16]. Most of the cytoskeletal components of FAs (for example, talin, paxillin, talin, vinculin etc.) are also present in podosomes; however, there are also podosome-specifc molecules such as dynamin2 and Tks4/5 [17–19]. Podosomes have been observed in activated endothelial cells, smooth muscle cells and cells of myeloid origin, including osteoclasts, monocytes, macrophages and dendritic cells (DCs) [20,21]. Podosomes are perpendicular to the membrane (whereas FAs are tangential to the cell membrane) and have a cylindrical structure. Their unstable nature is accounted to be important for macrophage migration [22]. The stable adhesion of macrophages results in larger podosomes [23]. Another distinguishing property of podosomes is the presence of CD44 in their cores with known affinity to hyaluronic acid (whose role in immune reaction is covered in a later chapter). Moreover, podosomes are generally considered as mechanosensors as the traction force exerted on the substrate is directly related to the rigidity of the substrate [24]. As with other cells, adhesion to a surface activates focal adhesion kinase (FAK) in macrophages [25,26]. The downstream signalling proteins that are activated after FAK phosphorylation are important for actin cytoskeletal dynamics and can affect macrophage spreading and lateral movement [27–30]. It has been shown that by mediating the attachment of macrophages via the

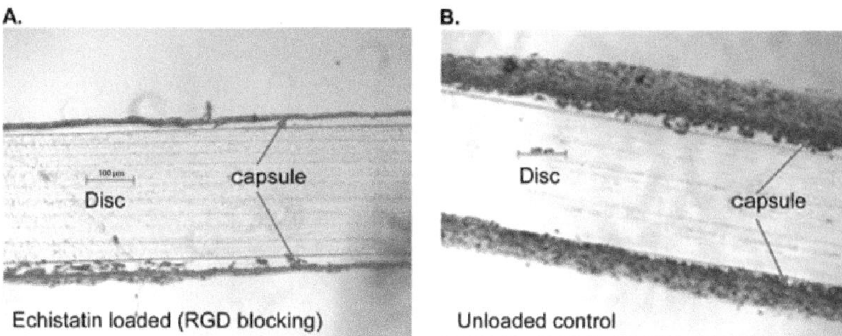

FIGURE 3.1 The blocking of integrin-mediated macrophage adhesion to PET implants via echistatin loading (an integrin blocker) significantly decreases the thickness of the fibrous capsule in formation after 14 days. (Reprinted from Zaveri, T.D. et al., *Biomaterials*, 35, 3504–3515, 2014. With permission.)

blocking of integrin, the thickness of the fibrous capsule towards non-degradable biomaterials can be controlled (Figure 3.1).

3.4 CUES PRESENTED BY A BIOMATERIAL

3.4.1 Surface Roughness, Stiffness and Mechanical Stimulation

Roughness is one of the parameters extensively studied for the cell implant interface. Thus, it is necessary to assess the effects of changes in roughness on immune cells. In fact, it has long been observed that macrophages adhere more to rough surfaces than to flat surfaces [31]. A study by Salthouse [32] examined the effect of surface shape and roughness on macrophages and showed a strong correlation between smooth implanted surfaces without physical acute angles and enhanced tissue compatibility. It has been suggested that the level of roughness is important for polarisation of macrophages. Without LPS stimulation, sandblasted and acid-etched titanium implant surfaces were demonstrated to increase TNF-α secretion while decreasing the production of chemoattractants monocyte chemotactic protein 1 (MCP-1) and macrophage inflammatory protein-1a (MIP-1a) in RAW264.7 macrophages. In the presence of LPS, surface roughness synergistically upregulates inflammatory cytokine secretion, such as TNF-α, IL-1β, IL-6, MCP1 and MIP-1a.

However, pro-inflammatory activation might not mean less wound repair in the long run. For example, Barth et al. [33] tested the effect of polished and sandblasted acid-etched epoxy surfaces (roughness of 0.06 and 4.33 μm, respectively) on RAW 264.7 macrophages. A rough SLA surface was shown to reduce M1 chemokine IFN-γ-induced protein 10 (IP-10), but increase monocyte chemotactic protein-1 (MCP-1) and macrophage inflammatory protein-1α (MIP-1α). Rough SLA surfaces did not affect Arg-1 (M2 marker) and NOS2 (M1 marker) expression.

Similarly, Mao et al. [34] have shown that while TiO_2 surfaces with greater roughness led to inflammatory activation, moderately roughened surfaces induced polarisation toward a prohealing phenotype. Contrarily, in murine J744A.1 macrophages, SLA surfaces did not have an effect on pro-inflammatory cytokine production

(IL-1b, IL-6, IL-10) [35], whereas nanorough titanium surfaces attenuated secretion of NO, TNFa, IL-1b and NO. However, as the induction of roughness also changes other properties simultaneously on titanium surfaces, a definitive conclusion on the effect of roughness on macrophage behaviour on metallic surfaces has not yet been established. Currently, there are no canonical relationships established with surface roughness and macrophage activities, which requires further studies.

Not only the mechanical properties of the substrate but also the mechanical properties of macrophages are determinant in their activation. Colloidal force microscopy studies demonstrated that LPS stimulation decreases the Young's modulus of macrophages nearly three times, while also increasing the strength of adhesion to the substrate [36]. However, as in the case of roughness, there are species-related effects; as in murine RAW264.7 cells, LPS treatment increased Young's modulus, with similar observations made as a function of substrate rigidity. The increase in elasticity in turn resulted in higher ROS secretion and improved phagocytosis. Depending on the cell source, the change in elasticity is correlated with actin polymerisation [37,38]. Thus, beyond the control of surface stiffness, methods to control the mechanical properties of macrophages can also have application potential.

Tissue stiffness changes dramatically during aging and the development of diseases. One of the earliest studies, by Beningo and Wang [39], used mouse bone marrow-derived macrophages to investigate the effects of substrate stiffness on macrophage function. It has been reported that stiff polyacrylamide particles were phagocytised preferentially over soft particles of identical chemistry through a Rac-1-mediated mechanosensory pathway. It has been shown that RAW264.7 cells on elasticity gradients established using PEG hydrogels adhere more to the stiffer regions without having any distinct effect on polarisation [40]. However, on stiffer substrates, LPS stimulation increases the secretion of pro-inflammatory cytokines (TNF-α, IL-6, IL-1β). In line with *in vitro* observations, stiffer hydrogels implanted in mice resulted in a more pronounced inflammation compared to the softer hydrogels *in vivo.*

Patel et al. [38] tested murine and differentiated human macrophages side by side on polyacrylamide gels with elastic moduli ranging from 0.3 to 76.8 kPa. Without LPS activation, substrate rigidity showed little effect on TNF-α secretion in both RAW264.7 and human U937 macrophages. Under LPS stimulation, for both cell types, less TNF-α was secreted in more rigid hydrogels with more phagocytosis.

Blakney et al. [41] showed that increasing the stiffness of 3D polyethylene glycol–RGD (PEG–RGD) hydrogels (130, 240 and 840 kPa) increased the FBR and the thickness of the fibrous capsule formed (~30 μm for 130 kPa and ~208 μm for 840 kPa). *In vitro* studies with the same gels revealed that the cells retained a round morphology on 130 kPa substrates, with localised and dense F-actin and localised αV integrin stainings, whereas on stiffer substrates cell spreading was more pronounced and the cells had a more defined F-actin and greater αV integrin staining. An increase in production of both pro-inflammatory (IL-1b, IL-6, TNF-a) and anti-inflammatory (IL-10) cytokines with increasing stiffness of gels has also been noted.

Macrophages express Toll-like receptor 4 (TLR4) in numerous diseases where tissue stiffness is altered, including cancer, atherosclerosis and cardiovascular disease. Previreta et al. [42] mimicked a wide range of tissue stiffnesses by using polyacrylamide gels to test the proinflammatory response of bone marrow-derived macrophages. The TLR4 signalling pathway was examined by evaluating TLR4, p–NF–κB p65, MyD88 and p–IκBα expression as well as p–NF–κB p65 translocation. They reported that the expression of the various signalling molecules were higher in macrophages grown on stiff substrates than on soft substrates. Furthermore, TLR4 knockout experiments showed that TLR4 activity increased pro-inflammatory effects on stiff substrates.

Using substrates of varying stiffness, Adlerz et al. [43] showed that macrophage migration rate, spreading and proliferation can be controlled as a function of substrate stiffness. On substrates with stiffnesses ranging from 1 to 5 kPa, macrophage area only slightly changed after 18 hours, whereas on substrates with higher stiffnesses (280 kPa–70 GPa) the macrophage area increased eightfold with prominent F-actin stress fibres. Macrophages travelled fastest on the 280-kPa substrate (12.0 ± 0.5 μm/h) and slowest on the 3-kPa substrate (5.0 ± 0.4 μm/h). Cells grown on the 280-kPa gel had a shorter doubling time than those grown on the softer substrate. As can be seen in the previous paragraphs, the effect of stiffness on macrophage behaviour is better defined and the control of stiffness of implanted biomaterials is a viable method of controlling the initial immune response to them.

Mechanical stimulation is also another important parameter for the growth and maturation of cells in several tissues. For example, resident macrophages in bone, lungs etc. are under the constant mechanical stimuli to which they have been known to respond. The effect of stress on macrophage activation has been linked to mechanically sensitive potassium channels [44], NF-κB [45] and NLRP3 inflammasome [46] activation. Osteoclasts, resident macrophages in bone, resorb more bone under cyclic stretch [47]. In another study, the effect of cyclical pressure on cytokine production in cultured human macrophages was quantified where an increase in pro-inflammatory cytokines (TNF-a, IL-6, IL-1b) was observed compared to controls for all levels of cyclical pressures tested (17–138 kPa). The introduction of polyethylene particles to represent wear debris from implants resulted in a further hike in pro-inflammatory cytokine release. It was proposed that this pattern of effects in response to cyclical pressure and the presence of wear debris contributes towards the aseptic loosening of implants [48]. When primary rat peritoneal macrophages were subjected to static stretch, inflammatory genes including inducible nitric oxide synthase (iNOS), cyclooxygenase-2 (COX-2), IL-1b, IL-6, MIP-1a and MIP-2 were up-regulated [49]. Cyclic stretch applied to THP-1 cells and human alveolar macrophages increased secretion of IL-8. When LPS stimulation and stretch were applied sequentially, stretch enhanced LPS-mediated secretion of TNF-a, IL-6 and IL-83 [50].

Cyclic stretch has also been shown to affect the polarisation of macrophages, along with other biophysical cues such as the presence of biomaterials. For Human Peripheral Mononuclear Cells (PBMCs) on electrospun fibers, 12% cyclic strain negatively affected the M2:M1 macrophage ratio, whereas at 7% cyclic strain the ratio increased after seven days compared to no strain conditions [51]. This is a good demonstration of the induction of inflammatory reactions under non-physiological mechanical stimuli. Moreover, resident macrophages in different tissues have different biomechanical microenvironments, which should be taken into account during the study of their responses to mechanical stimuli.

3.4.2 Effects of Surface Micro-Nanotopography

Tissue architecture has a crucial role in directing cell behaviour and cell movement. The architecture of the local tissue might have strong influences on the accumulation of macrophages in the inflammation sites. It has also been shown that the architecture of the substrate may enhance the chemotactic response of human neutrophils and leukocytes if the directional cues of the substrate conform with direction of the gradient of chemoattractant [52]. Therefore, surface modification of the substrate provides a starting point to direct adherent monocyte/macrophage cytokine production. The most commonly used surface topographical properties to achieve desired effects are surface roughness and engineered regular surface patterns. The use of different patterns and geometry, such as micropillars, microgrooves or micropits, have been beneficial for understanding their functional reactions to topography.

Biomaterial surface microtopography has extensively been explored as a physical cue to control immune response and offers the advantage of long-term stability and cost-effective fabrication methods. Studies have generally suggested that surfaces that contain microscale features appear to enhance the adhesion of macrophages and their secretion of inflammatory cytokines, including IL-1β, IL-6 and nitric oxide, when compared to macrophages on smooth surfaces [35,53–55]. It can also be hypothesised that topography close to biological scale, in the micron and nanometric range, can provide enough cues to modulate macrophage behaviour, obviating the need for biochemical stimuli.

In an early study, Wojciak et al. [56] grew murine P388D1 macrophages on poly(methyl methacrylate), smooth or micro-grooved substrates with varying depths (0.5 μm and 5 μm) and widths (10 μm). For stimulation, LPS was added to the culture medium (1 μg/mL). It was found that a patterned substrate activated cell spreading and elongation and significantly increased the persistence and speed of cell movement. On patterns with 10 μm-wide and 0.5 μm-deep grooves, murine P388D1 macrophages aligned parallel to the grooves and ridges and the patterns enhanced macrophage migration in terms of speed, distance and persistence (shallow grooves being more effective than deep ones). LPS-activated macrophages appeared to be more sensitive to topography than nonstimulated ones. Moreover, phagocytic activity of macrophages was more prominent on microgrooved surfaces where the dominant factor effecting the phagocytosed polystyrene microbeads was the depth of microgrooves. The contact of the cells with microgrooves increased the F-actin content in cells. It is possible that the mechanical interaction of groove/ridge edges with the cell membrane triggers F-actin polymerisation, which in turn influences cell orientation and movement.

Chen et al. [57] examined topography-induced changes in macrophage behaviour by using parallel gratings (250 nm–2 μm line width) imprinted on poly(e-caprolactone) (PCL), poly(lactic acid) (PLA) and poly(dimethyl siloxane) (PDMS). RAW 264.7 macrophages adhered and elongated along the gratings, irrespective of the substrate, in a grating size-dependent way; the most significant spreading was observed for 2-μm gratings (Figure 3.2). However, macrophages were less sensitive to nanoscale gratings in this study.

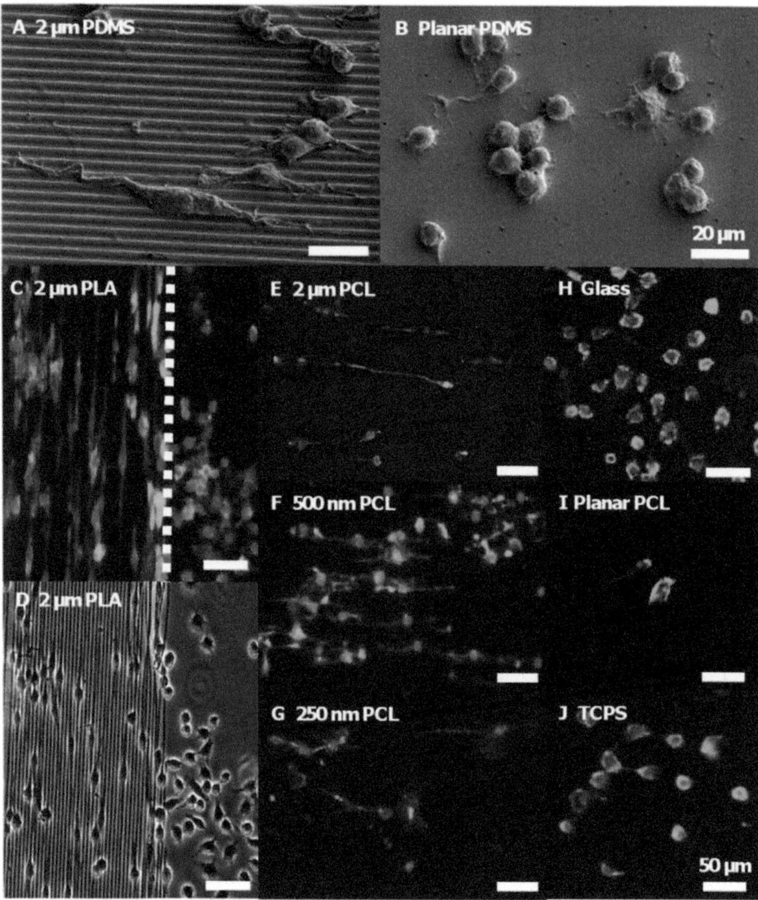

FIGURE 3.2 RAW 264.7 macrophages on planar or micropatterned PDMS, PCL and PLA substrates. The presence of 2-μm gratings induced cellular elongation parallel to the gratings for all substrates. *In vivo*, these gratings also decreased cell fusion. (Reprinted from Chen, S. et al., *Biomaterials*, 31, 3479–3491, 2010. With permission.)

The relative insensitivity of macrophages to nanotopography on polymeric surfaces can be compared to the differences in phagocytosis of nano and microparticles. This can be related with surface area, shape and size dependence of nanoparticles in determining inflammatory response and internalisation kinetics. The sensivity of macrophages is consonant with that of phagocytosis; where phagocytosis peak for macrophages was around 2 μm and smaller, nanoscale polymeric particles are internalised less [58,59]. The reaction is not completely absent as the presence of nanogratings affected the secretion of TNF-α and VEGF secreted by RAW 264.7 cells. Nanotopographies can provide stimuli in other contexts, such as in motility and movement into different tissue types, to perform specific functional roles that differ widely, such as MHC (major histocompatibility complex) presentation in the innate immune response, phagocytosis and wound healing [60,61].

The dimensions of surface features are another parameter controlling macrophage responses. For example, Bartneck et al. [62] investigated the influence of different perfluoropolyether (PFPE) cylindrical post micropatterns prepared by radical cross-linking with different sizes and centre-to-centre distances and line micropatterns on macrophages.

Substrates made out of a novel PFPE-based biomaterial have been prepared by UV-initiated radical cross-linking via methacrylate end groups, which resulted in a densely cross-linked bulk material. Photo-curable polymers are one of the most commonly used substrates for micropatterning studies [62,63].

Each micropattern induces a distinct morphology of the cells, together with specific polarisation and chemokine secretion profiles. The line-like structure induced a pro-inflammatory phenotype (27E10high, CD163low) similar to LPS stimulation. On the other hand, large posts led to an anti-inflammatory phenotype (27E10low, CD163high), whereas small posts at the smaller distance induced M1 phenotype marker expression (27E10high) without affecting CD163 (M2 marker) expression.

The micropatterns stimulated the expression of inflammatory chemokines. CCL2, CXCL10 and IL8 demonstrated the most influence of micropattern presence. IL-8 is known as a pro-inflammatory cytokine that attracts neutrophils [64] and has pro-angiogenic effects [65,66]. CXCL10 is involved in endothelial cells to leukocytes [67] and inhibits angiogenesis [68,69]. CCL2 has chemotactic activity for monocytes and basophils [70].

In accordance with the pro-inflammatory phenotype observed with surface markers, small posts induced CCL2 expression. In contrast, the same posts more widely separated did not stimulate CCL2 production. Upregulation of IL8 expression was seen in all the cylindrical structures, similar to the profiles previously induced by PVDF micropatterns [71]. CXCL10 gene expression is inversely proportional to increasing post separation [72].

In the work of Luu et al. [73], they investigate how surface topology alters macrophage cell morphology and polarisation states. To this end, by using a deep etching technique they fabricated titanium surfaces containing micro- and nanopatterned grooves whose widths varied from 0.15 to 50 μm, and whose pitch was twice that of the groove width. Groove depth ranged between 0.8 and 1.3 μm. Unlike in some polymeric substrates, here nanoscale topography induced morphological changes where the macrophages elongated the most on 500 μm nanopatterns, whereas groove width did not have an effect on cell area (Figure 3.3). The elongation level correlated with the expression of M2 marker Arginase 1 (Argl) and IL-10 secretion (an anti-inflammatory cytokine). Thus, the presence of nanogrooves on titanium substrates induced a more M2-like phenotype.

Alterations in cell shape have been associated with changes in cell function. Macrophages also change their morphologies in response to physical and soluble factors. For example, LPS-stimulated BMDMs are more flattened. In order to harness the effect of cell shape on macrophage activation, Mc Whorter et al. [74] demonstrated that elongation induced by micropatterns results in M2-like phenotype markers with significant reduction in pro-inflammatory cytokine secretion. Upon identifying that

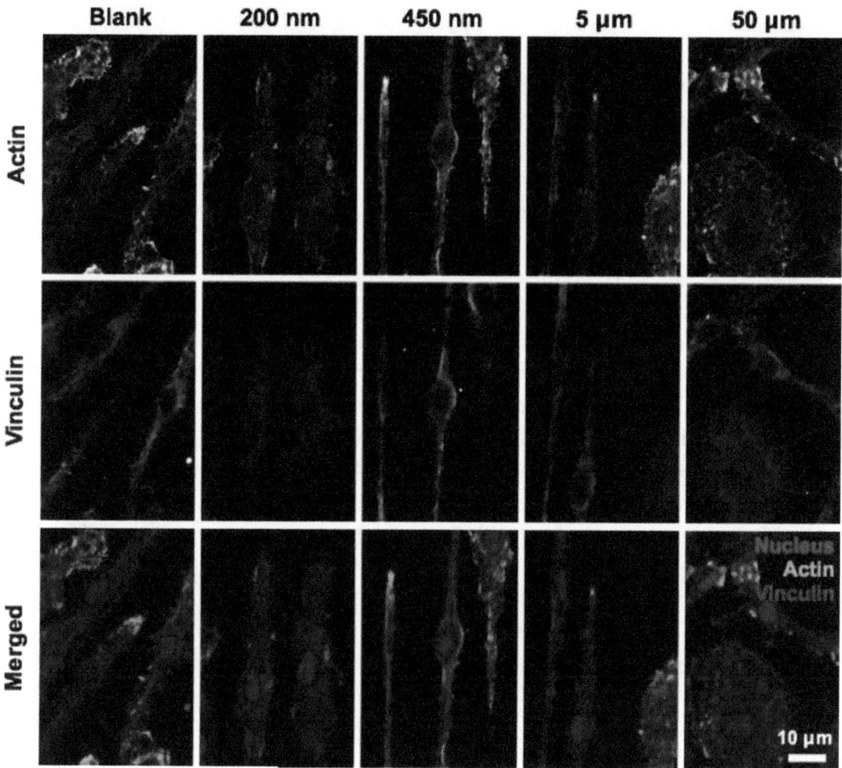

FIGURE 3.3 The effect of surface nano-/microgrooves on macrophage elongation (groove sizes ranging from 200 nm to 50 μm). Fluorescence microscope images of cell cytoskeleton (F-actin, green) and focal adhesions (represented by vinculin (a protein involved in focal adhesion complexes), red). (Reprinted from Luu, L.U. et al., *ACS Appl Mater Interfaces*, 7, 28665–28672, 2015. With permission.)

M1-polarised cells assume a rounded shape and M2-polarised cells assume an elongated shape, the authors used engineered cell culture substrates with 20- and 50-μm grooves to control cell shape and consequently direct polarisation. Moreover, elongation protects cells from M1-inducing stimuli (LPS and IFN-γ). As a result, the effects of M2-inducing cytokines IL-4 and IL-13 were enhanced and the cells exhibited much more elongated morphologies, suggesting that, in addition to directing polarisation, biophysical cues directly presented by biomaterials may be used as complimentary factors. Interestingly, while cytoskeletal inhibitors inhibited shape-induced polarisation, their presence did not affect the cells' ability to respond to cytokine stimulation, pointing out that shape-induced and cytokine-induced polarisation occur through distinct pathways. However, it should be noted that the morphological changes are not fully generalisable – although there are studies that demonstrate marked differences in M1/M2 macrophage actin organisations [74,75]. Altogether, these findings highlight the possibility of using micro-/nanotopography to control macrophage phenotype, even though the dimensions of the patterns need to be optimised in a cell type- and substrate type-dependent manner.

Understanding and having the capacity to regulate the inflammatory response elicited by 3D scaffolds aimed at tissue regeneration is crucial. Porous structures promote faster healing and form a thinner fibrous capsule than dense solid implants [76,77], suggesting that implant architecture can play a role in foreign body reaction. Thus, not only the intrinsic material properties but also the geometry/architecture and surface cues of the 3D scaffolds may be of importance in the design of new surfaces and scaffolds that can tailor macrophage activation towards a regenerative pathway.

Sussman et al. [78] compared macrophage polarity on poly-hydroxy-ethyl-methacrylate (p-HEMA) scaffolds with: (i) no-pores; (ii) 34-μm pores; and (iii) 160-μm pores implanted in mice subcutaneously and explanted after three weeks. With the porous materials they observed reduced fibrosis and increased vascularisation. Interestingly, an increased presence of M1 phenotype and greater remodelling in the small pore size scaffold was observed, suggesting that M1 cells are not always detrimental to the tissue remodelling process (where they are known to be highly active in angiogenesis). The authors were also the first to report specific locations of polarised cells. Macrophages in implant pores displayed a shift towards an M1 phenotype compared to externalised cells. In contrast, a significant enrichment in M2 phenotypic cells was localised immediately outside the porous structure. This study also indicated that macrophages may gain a "functionally active" phenotype, with simultaneous upregulation of both M1 and M2 markers instead of terminally polarised M1 or M2 phenotypes. This is expected, since macrophages are plastic cells that can assume a wide spectrum of activation states and respond to subtle microenvironmental changes. Therefore, determination of macrophage activation, instead of concentrating on a single marker or a very narrow set of markers, and complementing phenotypical analyses with functional analyses is relevant to the intended application of the biomaterials.

Rapid prototyping (RP) is a perfect tool to fabricate 3D structures with well-defined and reproducible geometries and architectures. It is possible to build 3D scaffolds with different characteristics and well-distinguished geometric and physico-chemical features, allowing the study of the effect of these factors on inflammatory cell responses.

In a recent report, Almeida et al. [79] analysed the cytokine secretion profile of human monocytes/macrophages in contact with biodegradable 3D-printed scaffolds of different architecture and pore size (based on PLA, PLA/calcium phosphate glass or chitosan). PLA-based scaffolds induced higher production of IL-6, IL-12/23 and IL-10, while chitosan led to increased secretion of TNF-α, with the scaffold geometry impacting on the amounts of TNF-α and IL-12/23 secreted. Chitosan scaffolds with large pores led to the secretion of more pro-inflammatory cytokines.

Another important antigen-presenting cell type is dendritic cells (DCs). Immature DCs (iDCs) reside in tissues as a surveillance system for pathogenic insults. Once they come into contact with an antigen, they differentiate into mature DCs (mDCs), which leads to the presentation of the antigen by mDCs to T-cells in lymph nodes [80,81]. The maturation process of DCs is highly related to podosomes, where iDCs are highly adhesive with a significant number of podosomes that dissolve during the maturation process to enable the fast migration of mDCs to lymph nodes [82,83].

For iDCs seeded on flat surfaces, it has been shown that the binding of prostaglandin E2 (PGE2) to the prostaglandin receptors EP2 and EP4 results in rapid podosome dissolution in iDCs – one of the first steps towards a fully mature DC phenotype [84,85].

To demonstrate the effect of topography on DC signalling, van den Dries et al. [86] stimulated iDCs, either on 2D or 3D micropatterned substrates, with PGE2. To investigate how 2D surface geometry dictates the formation and spatial organisation of podosomes in DCs, 2D micropatterning of fibronectin spots on the hydrogels has been used (spots of 5–20 μm). It was observed that the constraints exerted by the fibronectin spots had a significant effect on podosome density. Once micropatterned surfaces with varying widths between 2 and 20 μm were utilised, it was noted that DCs were able to align parallel to the micropatterns. Finally, whereas on a 2D surface PGE2 causes a rapid increase in activated RhoA levels leading to fast podosome dissolution, 3D geometric cues prevent PGE2-mediated RhoA activation, thus keeping podosomes intact. These results demonstrate that the presence of biophysical cues can have significant effects on DC attachment and mobility under stimulation.

Cell migration is an important cellular behaviour in many physiological and pathological events. Geometrical and physical properties of the ECM must also be important in regulating cell migration. Based primarily on studies of cells migrating on flat surfaces, the physical events that produce cell migration have been described as a series of steps: (1) cell membrane extension to form lamellipodia; (2) cell adhesion to substratum; (3) cytoskeletal contraction; and (4) detachment of cell membrane at rear. The speed of cell migration depends on the integration of the rates of all these processes, although one step can be rate-determining under certain conditions.

Surface topography also has effects on macrophage/DC migration; for example, surface-presenting nanoscale features (or nanoroughness) decrease the rate of migration [87]. The rate of migration is also related to the polarisation state of macrophages, where it has been shown in mice that M2 macrophages are more mobile compared to M1 macrophages [75]. Similar to DCs, 3D matrix properties together with matrix stiffness have also been shown to affect the migratory properties of macrophages (mostly due to differential RhoA and Rac activation) [88].

T-cells travel through several tissues and organs, such as lymph nodes and blood vessels, to perform their functions for immune detection and response. Within tissues, T-cells migrate with a peak velocity of 25 μm/min [89]. It has been shown that the migration of T-cells is guided by stromal cells/extracellular matrix (ECM) exhibiting unique fibrous structures such as stromal cell networks, reticular fibre structures in the brain induced by infection and collagen fibers. Thus, nanostructured surfaces can be an ideal platform for the study of topography-guided migration of T-cells [90,91]. The motility of T-cells was studied on the surfaces containing various complex nanoscale zigzag structures, which were fabricated by UV-assisted capillary force lithography. Motility of the T-cells was not affected by the side length, but, rather, influenced by the turning angle on the zigzag patterns. T cells on zigzag patterns with an acute turning angle exhibited significantly reduced migration speed and altered migration direction with respect to T cells on zigzag patterns with right or wider angles. When lamellipodia formation at the leading edges of migrating cells inhibited by CK-636 treatment, a pharmacological inhibitor (ARP 2/3) targeting a key regulator for lamellipodia formation, a substantial fraction of treated T cells on zigzag patterns with an acute turning angle were trapped near the interfaces formed by the turning points. These findings suggested that lamellipodia play essential roles in rapid migration of T cells under complex topographical microenvironments. In a later study the same research group investigated mechanisms of T-cell migration on nanotopographies. When the nanopatterns were present, lamellipodia leading edges were guided towards the nanogrooves.

Although most of the current work has been focused on 2D biomaterial surfaces, controlling the immune response to 3D architecture may be useful for the management of immune-mediated healing in tissue engineering and regenerative medicine. It is likely that 3D structures that present topographical cues, including fibrous tissue architectures, may simulate an immunological niche and hence macrophage function and the wound healing response.

These results emphasize the importance of selecting biomaterials based on the right chemistry, surface properties and geometry. However, the ideal response and cytokine environment still remain uncertain, and more complex studies (e.g., with co-cultures with other cell types, testing more surface features) are required.

3.4.3 Electrospun Fibre as a 3D Substrate

As an alternative to surface patterned materials, 3D electrospun micro- or nanoscale fibre meshes have been employed by several groups [92–94]. Recent studies show that macrophage activation and FBGC formation respond to differing polymer fibre diameter [92,95]. It has been observed that nanofibers elicit significantly less macrophage adhesion and inflammatory activation, and minimise the host response, when compared to microfibers randomly aligned or flat PLLA substrates. Under LPS stimulation, less inflammatory cytokines were secreted on fibrous PLLA by macrophages compared to flat PLLA films after 24 h; however, the effect was temporary and was not observed after seven days.

Using RAW264.7 cells, Saino et al. [93] have shown on electrospun poly(L-lactic acid) (PLLA) fibrous substrates that both fibre alignment and also fiber diameter had significant effects on macrophage activation and adhesion compared to flat films. In another study, electrospun polydioxanone (PDO) scaffolds decreased M1 activation and increased M2 macrophage polarisation, with increased expressions of Arginase-1, VEGF, TGF-β1 and bFGF [94]. When Cao et al. [92] implanted random and aligned polycaprolactone (PCL) nanofibres, they observed thinner fibrous capsules and reduced inflammation, together with faster wound healing with fibrillar scaffolds. When the size of the fibres was compared [95], it was shown that fibres in the range of 1–5 μm in diameter resulted in thinner fibrous capsules compared to fibres in the range of 10–15 μm in diameter.

3.4.4 Surface Chemistry and Chemical Patterning

Macrophages respond to chemotactic factors that induce phagocytosis and stimulate cell movement causing their accumulation in the inflammatory sites. It has conventionally been considered that the chemistry of biomaterials dictates the behaviour of immune cells by altering cell adhesive interactions. Therefore, controlling biomaterial-adherent monocyte/macrophage cytokine expression through the modification of surface/substrate chemistry is a possible method. To this end, Brodbeck et al. [96] tested surfaces consisting of hydrophobic, hydrophilic, anionic and cationic surface chemistries. It was found that hydrophilic and anionic surfaces promote an anti-inflammatory response by promoting increased IL-10 production and decreased IL-8 production by macrophages. In experiments, where IL-4 was added to promote macrophage fusion, cells adherent to the cationic surface expressed decreased levels of IL-1RA and IL-10 (anti-inflammatory cytokines). Therefore, biomaterial surface chemistry can dictate the levels of cytokines produced by macrophages, having strong implications for the determination of biomaterial biocompatibility.

Expression levels of cytokines among the different substrate surface chemistries, IL-8 and IL-10 expressions, were significantly influenced by hydrophilic and anionic surface chemistries. IL-8 is well known for its chemoattractant capabilities. A decrease in monocyte/macrophage IL-8 production would lead to a decrease in the chemotaxis of leukocytes to the site of the implant. IL-10 is responsible for decreasing cellular activity by inhibiting cytokine expression by a variety of cell types. Therefore, an increase of IL-10 production would indicate an overall suppression in the response to the implanted device.

However, there are conflicting results in the literature regarding the extent of dependence of the FBR on biomaterial surface chemistry. For example, Schutte et al. and Castner et al. [97,98] argued that there are no differences between inert, non-degradable materials with different surface chemistries one month post-implantation and hence any short-term effect observed is inconsequential. This was also highlighted by Chen et al. [57], who demonstrated that subtle changes in topography override the effects of surface chemistry.

Recent studies have progressed towards a possible explanation for the conflicting reports on the surface chemistry dependence of the FBR. Dadsetan et al. [99] showed a significant effect of hydrophobic (contact angle –120°) PDMS films on protein adsorption and a reduction in human macrophage adhesion. On the contrary, Jones et al. [100] found that the number of adherent cells on polyacrylamide-based hydrophilic and neutrally charged surfaces was decreased in comparison with hydrophobic surfaces. Moreover, the adherent cells switched from pro-inflammatory (IL-1β and IL-6) to anti-inflammatory (IL-10) cytokine production over time. Similarly, McBane et al. [101] observed that a degradable polar hydrophobic ionic polyurethane (D-PHI) surface affected human monocyte-derived macrophages (MDM) by decreasing the secretion level of pro-inflammatory cytokines (TNF-α, IL-1β and HMGB1) and increasing IL-10 in comparison to tissue culture polystyrene (TCPS).

Alfarsi et al. [102] tested surface chemistry and topography simultaneously using titanium surfaces (polished (SMO), microrough (SLA) and hydrophilic-modified microrough (modSLA) and used trascriptomics analysis to show that the macrophages behaved differently on these surfaces. Interaction with a modSLA surface resulted in down-regulation of ten pro-inflammatory genes (such as TNF, IL-1β, CCL3 etc.), whereas on the other surfaces up-regulation of 16 pro-inflammatory genes was observed. It can be said that changes in surface chemistry and topography have overlapping effects and must be validated for each biomaterial.

Higher-resolution patterning, down to single ligands (i.e., less than 10 nm) may be an ideal platform for regulation of the number and nanoscale arrangement of ligands. Deeg et al. [103] have employed well-established nanolithography techniques to present T-cell ligands with nanometer-scale accuracy by introducing nanopatterned antigen arrays that mimic the antigen presentation. They demonstrated that the overall number of presented major histocompatibility class II proteins (pMHCs) dominates over local pMHC density.

During inflammation, the degradation of glycocalyx (the surface layer of the vascular endothelium) has been shown to facilitate leukocyte recruitment. Conversely, an undamaged layer, and thus, mimicking undamaged/intact the endothelial glycocalyx surface can be a method of inhibiting a cascade of inflammatory events [104]. Since the glycocalyx is heterogeneous structure in terms of composition and roughness, it can be speculated that the spatial organisation of its polysaccharide content and the topography play an important role in the adhesion of macrophages and inflammatory response of the surface. To this end, Tsai et al. [105] reported two methods: microcontact printing and photodegradation by UV exposure for patternining dextran and hyaluronic acid. Two geometries (90 μm × 90-μm squares and 22-μm stripes) were tested with human macrophages. The presence of hyaluronic acid-modified surfaces significantly decreased macrophage adhesion relative to other studied surfaces, showing polysaccharide patterning as a potential method to control innate immune responses.

Another key event of inflammation is the release of small molecules such as reactive oxygen species (ROS), including superoxide anion (O_2-), hydrogen peroxide (H_2O_2) and hydroxyl radicals (-OH). Therefore, ROS can be used as a diagnostic marker of inflammation using electrochemical biosensors (such as the detection of nitric oxide secreted from cells [106,107] and a recent report describing H_2O_2 release from leukocytes [108]). For such studies, Yan et al. [109] developed a biomaterial micropatterning strategy and a microdevice to enable macrophages to be in close contact with H_2O_2 biosensors (with a limit of detection of 2 μM), enabling on-chip, real-time monitoring of H_2O_2 levels. Such microdevices can be used for ROS release by immune cells in clinical settings. Moreover, such devices that integrate electrochemical biosensors into micropatterned co-cultures can be employed to simultaneously define and detect endocrine signalling between two distinct cell types.

Central nervous system recording electrodes have been used in clinics for the treatment of deafness, for symptoms associated with Parkinson's disease and to control limb prostheses. However, a foreign body response develops over time around electrodes implanted in the brain. Braden et al. [110] used silicon microelectrodes to determine the nature of the immune response to their presence. There was a persistent macrophage presence around the implanted electrodes over a 12-week period. CD68/ED1-expressing cells remained at the interface over the indwelling period. Many of the cells were also CD11b (a marker of activated microglia). They then checked several potential coatings prepared via spin coating. A general trend of increased cytokine release per adherent cell was observed on the more hydrophobic materials for MCP-1, IL-1β, TNF-α and TGF-β1. The results suggested that low protein-binding coatings may be useful in reducing activated microglial attachment to the electrode after implantation in brain tissue; hence, for improving the biocompatibility of the electrodes.

Although there are various studies that have shown the effect of surface chemistry on immune cells, as described above, some investigators have also reported that surface chemistry does not have any significant influence on macrophage polarisation. Thus, the diversity of the results points out the requirement of systematic studies in this area involving multiple materials and chemical modifications.

3.4.4.1 Co-Culturing by (Chemical) Patterning

Patterning of co-cultures of cells is a promising technique to investigate cell–cell communication. In the most common methods for co-culturing adherent cells with nonadherent cells, the nonadherent cells are placed on top of the adherent cells either directly or on a porous filter insert. Recently, novel co-culturing techniques have been developed, enabling nonadherent cells to be immobilised on the substrate just as adherent cells attach to the substrate by using a cell membrane anchoring reagent (CMAR) [111,112]. These studies are especially valuable since the interactions between adherent and nonadherent cells are important in many physiological events. For example, cancer cells release chemotactic factors and recruit monocytes and lymphocytes to their surrounding environments. Thus, such systems might be useful for recreating the cancer microenvironment to investigate the influence of immune cells in the tumour stroma on cancer drug sensitivity. In a recent study, a patterned co-culture composed of micropatterned neuroblastoma cells surrounded by immobilised myeloid cells was successfully prepared. For the immobilisation of nonadherent cells on the substrate, the CMAR and serum albumin conjugate was prepared by reacting CMAR with albumin. They observed that monocytes enhanced the drug sensitivity of cancer cells and this influence was limited to cancer cells located near the monocytes [113].

Co-culture models are particularly useful for investigating heterotypic interactions and have previously been used extensively for the investigation of mucosal barrier and cell function. Stybayeva et al. [114] has created a co-culture system/model by capturing T-cells on printed arrays of anti-CD3 Ab spots and then cultivating mucosal epithelial cells (human HT-29) alongside the surface-bound HIV-infected or uninfected T-cells (Jurkats). Gene expression analysis of the epithelial cells pointed to increases in inflammation-associated gene transcription, juxtaposed by marked decreases in genes mediating epithelial cell adhesion (E-cadherin), growth and development (homeobox5, VEGF) and Wnt signalling (catenin beta 1, transcription factor 7-like2).

3.4.5 Immunological Synapse: Another Approach for Patterning

T-cells are a subset of lymphocytes with a central role in the adaptive immune response. "T" stands for thymus, the organ in which the final stage of their development occurs. T-cells are especially important in cell-mediated immunity, which is the defence against tumour cells and pathogenic organisms. There are several different kinds of T-cells, which can be divided into two different general classifications: killer T-cells and helper T-cells.

T-cell activation occurs after engagement of the T-cell antigen-specific receptor (TCR) by the antigen-major histocompatibility complex (MHC) at the surface of antigen-presenting cells (APCs) and by subsequent engagement of co-stimulatory molecules such as CD28. These signals result in the clonal expansion of T-cells, upregulation of activation markers on the cell surface, differentiation into effector cells, induction of cytotoxicity or cytokine secretion and apoptosis.

The binding of T-cell receptors (TCRs) to peptide-MHC (pMHC) triggers nucleation of clusters of signalling and cytoskeletal molecules, which assemble into a central supramolecular activation cluster (cSMAC). This junction is called an "immunological synapse" (IS) because of its similarity to a neural synapse. These two synapses share a common feature: information is transferred through a tight cell-cell interface. Although, while the neural synapse is permanent, the immunological synapse lasts for only minutes or at most hours [115].

Monks et al. [116] observed the pattern of the mature IS by confocal microscopy of 3D interactions between T-cells and APCs. This study was followed by a key study utilising a model of glass-supported lipid bilayers (SLBs) bearing mobile peptide–MHC (pMHC) complexes and adhesion protein functions as live APC substitutes, where the dynamics of receptor clustering following T-cell engagement with these molecules could be analysed in detail. As the synapse evolves, certain important components migrate either inward or outward, suggesting that spatiotemporal organisation may regulate signalling [117,118]. SLBs may be formed by several methods, including Langmuir-Blodgett/Schäfer deposition, spin coating, microcontact printing, solvent-exchange deposition, lipid-surfactant micelles, evaporation-induced assembly, bubble collapse deposition, lipid dip-pen nanolithography and vesicle fusion. However, mostly two methods have successfully been applied to immune cell studies: polymer liftoff and diffusion barriers.

Arrays of SLB regions can be produced by liftoff of a polymer such as parylene. The polymer is patterned by photolithography on a SiO_2 substrate; then the lipid membrane is deposited; then the polymer is peeled off, to leave fluid lipid islands that hold their shape. The resolution of this technique has improved to the micron level [119]. The diffusion barrier approach is amenable to both photolithography and electron-beam lithography [120]. SLBs are deposited on a hydrophilic substrate on which lithographically defined patterns have been fabricated. By this method, micron-scale arrays of membrane corrals may be defined, which are spatially addressable. Barriers may be fabricated from protein, photoresist, or many inorganic materials, especially metals [121]. Electrostatic or chemical properties, and not topography, are responsible for the barrier action, since fluid membranes will spread over and conform to SiO_2 barriers, while barriers of similar dimensions fabricated from metal will block diffusion. The most significant advantage of barrier-partitioned SLBs is that the barriers may be defined by electron-beam lithography, and therefore made extremely small (~100 nm), so that their width is negligible compared with the diameter of a large cell such as a T-lymphocyte.

Several other papers have reported the results concerning the dynamic nature of the synapse such as dependence of pattern clustering in immunological synapse on the density and quality of antigen [122–125], the identity and activation state of the APC [126,127] and the maturity and activation state of the T-cell [128–130].

Moreover, several 3D-SLBs have been constructed, including lipid bilayers on a core of hydrogel, PLGA or silica [131–133]. Cell-sized silica beads with an SLB coating were more effective in cytotoxic T-cell induction compared to liposomes; however, they could not induce T-cell expansion (most probably due to the absence of necessary cytokines such as IL-2) [134]. Another approach was to extract antigen-bearing LBs and transfer them onto microspheres to mimic APCs [135].

The researchers were able to extract information about both the physical mechanism of IS formation and the relationship between spatial organization and the signalling which leads to T-cell activation. T-cells interacting with a membrane partitioned by a 1-μm grid formed TCR clusters of uniform size. Each of these TCR clusters was oriented in the corner of its grid square, which strongly suggests a centralised, cytoskeletal mechanism of TCR organisation, as opposed to a passive process driven by binding, bending and stretching energies, which Qi et al. put forward as a possibility [136].

For studying the IS, researchers used electron-beam lithography to constrain the freedom of motion of lipids and GPI-linked pMHC and ICAM in a SLB [137]. T-cells interacting with this membrane initiated synapse formation, but barrier constraints on membrane ligands were transferred to the receptors on the T-cell membrane, and the mature distribution of ligands and receptors was dictated by substrate geometry. ICAM and TCR/pMHC distributions were mutually exclusive, as in the wild-type synapse.

Recently, Hsu et al. [138] formed stimulatory lipid bilayers on glass surfaces from binary lipid mixtures with varied composition to investigate the effects of the mobility of the ligands on formation of IS and T-cell activation. On less mobile SLBs, formation of cSMAC was delayed. Zheng et al. [139] have combined the glass-supported planar lipid bilayer system with stimulated emission depletion (STED) technique and demonstrated the feasibility and application of this combined technique for examining immunological synapses with super-resolution.

Shen et al. [140] tested whether the increased IL-2 level in T-cell–APC pairs is driven by the pattern itself or by upstream events that precipitate the patterns. For this purpose, features of It was demonstrated that presenting anti-CD28 in the cell periphery, instead of having these signals combined in the centre of the IS, enhances IL-2 secretion by naïve CD4+ T-cells. The incorporation of protein patterns onto SLBs provides a new level of control over T-cell proliferation [141]. In spite of small differences between ISs of CD4+ and CD8+ T-cells, there is a high level of similarity in IS structure in T-cell subsets [142]. There are other potential uses of SLBs such as studying TCR-containing vesicles excreted within the IS [143] or differences in activation of CD4+ and CD8+ T-cells [144] and high-resolution microscopy-based observations of IS [145]. "Artificial APC"-type synthetic surfaces play a significant role in dissecting the structure and function of the immunological synapse (IS) since its discovery [146,147]. Synthetic surface models provide several advantages, such as investigation of ligand density, composition of the APCs, spatio-temporal resolution of receptor binding events between the T-cell and model surface by optical and total interference microscopy. Recent surface micro/nanofabrication techniques have been successful in addressing a number of key problems to control the spatial distribution and mobility of ligands displayed from synthetic substrates [137,148].

3.5 CONCLUSION

The new approach in biomaterials and tissue engineering is to communicate with the immune system, rather than trying to avoid it. With the many advances in our knowledge about macrophage biology and engineering, we can now integrate this information into design options for novel multipurposed/immuno-informed biomaterials, which leads to a favourable immune response upon implantation. Ongoing research is unveiling more details of inherent biomaterial cues as well as their effects on the polarisation of macrophages and immune-modulation, of which many examples have been provided in recent research [145,149–151]. Alternatively, under the light of newly considered regulation pathways of macrophage activation such as epigenetic regulations [152] and post-translational modifications and improved understanding of other components of the immune system such as neutrophil and dendritic cell modulation will ultimately lead to the design of a new generation of biomaterials that can actively direct the innate immune system. In the case of adaptive immunity, the study of IS using biomaterial-based techniques provides new insights into adaptive immunity and can also pave the way for the utilisation of IS as a potential target for controlling adaptive immunity-based reactions to biomaterials.

REFERENCES

1. Martinez, F.O., Sica, A., Mantovani, A., Locati M. (2008). Macrophage activation and polarization, *Front Biosci*, 13, pp. 453–61.
2. Katsuda, S. and Kaji, T. (2003). Atherosclerosis and extracellular matrix, *J Atheroscler Thromb*, 10(5), pp. 267–274.
3. Odink, K., Cerletti, N., Bruggen, J., Clerc, R.G., Tarcsay, L., Zwadlo, G., Gerhards, G., Schlegel, R., Sorg, C. (1987). Two calcium-binding proteins in infiltrate macrophages of rheumatoid arthritis, *Nature*, 330(6143), pp. 80–82.
4. Zwadlo, G., Bruggen, J., Gerhards, G., Schlegel, R., Sorg, C. (1988). Two calcium-binding proteins associated with specific stages of myeloid cell differentiation are expressed by subsets of macrophages in inflammatory tissues, *Clin Exp Immunol*, 72(3), pp. 510–515.
5. Ratner, B.D. and Bryant, S.J. (2004). Biomaterials: Where we have been and where we are going, *Annu Rev Biomed Eng*, 6, pp. 41–75.
6. Williams, D.F. (2008). On the mechanisms of biocompatibility, *Biomaterials*, 29, pp. 2941–2953.
7. Anderson, J.M., Rodriguez, A., Chang, D.T. (2008). Foreign body reaction to biomaterials, *Semin Immunol*, 20, pp. 86–100.
8. Cromack, D.T., Porras-Reyes, B., Mustoe, T.A. (1990). Current concepts in wound healing: Growth factor and macrophage interaction, *J Trauma*, 30(12Suppl), pp. 129–133.
9. Park, J.E. and Barbul, A. (2004). Understanding the role of immune regulation in wound healing, *Am J Surg*, 187, pp.11S–16S.
10. Ingham, E. and Fisher, J. (2005). The role of macrophages in osteolysis of total joint replacement, *Biomaterials*, 26(11), pp. 1271–1286.
11. Friedl, P., Weigelin, B. (2008). Interstitial leukocyte migration and immune function, *Nat Immunol*, 9, pp. 960–969.
12. Féréol, S., Fodil, R., Labat, B., Galiacy, S., Laurent, V.M., Louis, B., Isabey, D., Planus, E. (2006). Sensitivity of alveolar macrophages to substrate mechanical and adhesive properties, *Cell Motil Cytoskeleton*, 63, pp. 321–340.

13. Gowen, B.B., Borg, T.K., Ghaffar, A., Mayer, E.P. (2000). Selective adhesion of macrophages to denatured forms of type I collagen is mediated by scavenger receptors, *Matrix Biol*, 19, pp. 61–71.
14. David-Pfeuty, T., Singer, S.J. (1980). Altered distributions of the cytoskeletal proteins vinculin and alpha-actinin in cultured fibroblasts transformed by Rous sarcoma virus, *Proc Natl Acad Sci USA*, 77(11), pp. 6687–6691.
15. Marchisio, P.C., Cirillo, D., Naldini, L., Primavera, M.V., Teti, A., Zambonin-Zallone, A. (1984). Cell-substratum interaction of cultured avian osteoclasts is mediated by specific adhesion structures, *J Cell Biol*, 99(5), pp. 1696–1705.
16. Tarone, G., Cirillo, D., Giancotti, F.G., Comoglio, P.M., Marchisio, P.C. (1985). Rous sarcoma virus-transformed fibroblasts adhere primarily at discrete protrusions of the ventral membrane called podosomes, *Exp Cell Res*, 159(1), pp. 141–157.
17. Ochoa, G.C., Neff, L., Ringstad, N., Takei, K., Daniell, L., Kim, W., Cao, H., McNiven, M., Baron, R., De Camilli, P. (2000). A functional link between dynamin and the actin cytoskeleton at podosomes, *J Cell Biol*, 150(2), pp. 377–389.
18. Seals, D.F., Azucena, E.F., Jr., Pass I., Tesfay, L., Gordon, R., Woodrow, M., Resau, J.H., Courtneidge, S.A. (2005). The adaptor protein Tks5/Fish is required for podosome formation and function, and for the protease-driven invasion of cancer cells, *Cancer Cell*, 7(2), pp. 155–165.
19. Buschman, M.D., Bromann, P.A., Cejudo-Martin, P., Wen, F., Pass, I., Courtneidge, S.A. (2009). The novel adaptor protein Tks4 (SH3PXD2B) is required for functional podosome formation, *Mol Biol Cell*, 20(5), pp. 1302–1311.
20. Linder, S., Aepfelbacher, M. (2003). Podosomes: Adhesion hot-spots of invasive cells, *Trends Cell Biol*, 13(7), pp. 376–385.
21. Buccione, R., Orth, J.D., McNiven, M.A. (2004). Foot and mouth: Podosomes, invadopodia and circular dorsal ruffles, *Nature Rev*, 5(8), pp. 647–657.
22. Block, M.R., Badowski, C., Millon-Fremillon, A., Bouvard, D., Bouin A.P., Faurobert, E., Gerber-Scokaert, D., Planus, E., Albiges-Rizo, C. (2008). Podosome-type adhesions and focal adhesions, so alike yet so different, *Eur J Cell Biol*, 87, pp. 491–506.
23. Ghrebi, S., Hamilton, D.W., Douglas, Waterfield, J., Brunette, D.M. (2013). The effect of surface topography on cell shape and early ERK1/2 signaling in macrophages; linkage with FAK and Src, *J Biomed Mater Res A*, 101, pp. 2118–2128.
24. Collin, O., Na, S., Chowdhury, F., Hong, M., Shin, M.E., Wang, F., Wang, N. (2008). Self-organized podosomes are dynamic mechanosensors, *Curr Biol*, 18, pp. 1288–1294.
25. Berton, G., Lowell, C. (1999). Integrin signalling in neutrophils and macrophages, *Cell Signal*, 11, pp. 621–635.
26. Zaveri, T.D., Lewis, J.S., Dolgova, N.V., Clare-Salzler M.J., Keselowsky, B.G. (2014). Integrin-directed modulation of macrophage responses to biomaterials, *Biomaterials*, 35, pp. 3504–3515.
27. Aepfelbacher, M., Essler, M., Huber, E., Czech, A., Weber, P.C. (1996). Rho is a negative regulator of human monocyte spreading, *J Immunol*, 157, pp. 5070–5075.
28. Allen, W.E., Jones, G.E., Pollard, J.W., Ridley, A.J. (1997). Rho, Racand Cdc42 regulate actin organization and cell adhesion in macrophages, *J Cell Sci*, 110(Pt 6), pp. 707–720.
29. Hall, A. (1998). Rho GTPases and the actin cytoskeleton, *Science*, 279, pp. 509–514.
30. Hoppe, A.D., Swanson, J.A. (2004). Cdc42, Racl, and Rac2 display distinct patterns of activation during phagocytosis, *Mol Biol Cell*, 15, pp. 3509–3519.
31. Rich, A., Harris A.K. (1981). Anomalous preferences of cultured macrophages for hydrophobic and roughened substrata, *J Cell Sci*, 50, p. 1–7.
32. Salthouse, T.N. (1984). Some aspects of macrophage behavior at the implant interface, *J Biomed Mater Res*, 18, pp. 395–401.

33. Barth, K.A., Waterfield J.D., Brunette, D.M. (2013). The effect of surface roughness on RAW 264.7 macrophage phenotype, *Biomed Mater Res Part A*, 101, pp. 2679–2688.
34. Ma, Q.L., Zhao, L.Z., Liu, R.R., Jin, B.Q., Song, W., Wang, Y., Zhang, Y.S., Chen, L.H., Zhang, Y.M. (2014). Improved Implant Osseointegration of a Nanostructured Titanium Surface via Mediation of Macrophage Polarization, *Biomaterials*, 35, pp. 9853–9867.
35. Tan, K.S., Qian, L., Rosado, R., Flood, P.M., Cooper, L.F. (2006). The Role of Titanium surface topography on j744a.1 macrophage ınflammatory cytokines and nitric oxide production, *Biomaterials*, 27, pp. 5170–5177.
36. Leporatti, S., Gerth, A., Köhler, G., Kohlstrunk, B., Hauschildt, S., Donath, E. (2006). Elasticity and adhesion of resting and lipopolysaccharide-stimulated macrophages, *FEBS Lett*, 580, pp. 450–454.
37. Féréol, S., Fodil, R., Labat, B., Galiacy, S., Laurent, V.M., Louis, B., Isabey, D., Planus, E. (2006). Sensitivity of alveolar macrophages to substrate mechanical and adhesive properties, *Cell Motil Cytoskeleton*, 63, pp. 321–340.
38. Patel, N.R., Bole, M., Chen, C., Hardin, C.C., Kho, A.T., Mih, J., Deng, L., Butler, J., Tschumperlin, D., Fredberg, J.J., Krishnan, R., Koziel, H. (2012). Cell elasticity determines macrophage function, *PLoS One*, 7, pp. e41024.
39. Beningo, K.A., Wang Y.-l. (2002). Fc-receptor-mediated phagocytosis is regulated by mechanical properties of the target, *J Cell Sci*, 115(4), pp. 849–856.
40. Nemir, S., Hayenga, H.N., West, J.L. (2010). PEGDA hydrogels with patterned elasticity: Novel tools for the study of cell response to substrate rigidity, *Biotechnol Bioeng*, 105, pp. 636–644.
41. Blakney, A.K., Swartzlander, M.D., Bryant, S.J. (2012). The effects of substrate stiffness on the in vitro activation of macrophages and in vivo host response to poly (ethylene glycol)-based hydrogels, *J Biomed Mater Res A*, 100(6), pp. 1375–1386.
42. Previtera, M.L., Sengupta, A. (2015). Substrate stiffness regulates proinflammatory mediator production through tlr4 activity in macrophages, *PLoS One*, 10(12), pp. e0145813.
43. Adlerz, K.M., Aranda-Espinoza, H., Hayenga, H.N. (2016). Substrate elasticity regulates the behavior of human monocyte-derived macrophages, *Eur Biophys J*, 45(4), pp. 301–309.
44. Martin, D., Bootcov, M., Campell, T., French, P., Breit, S. (1995) Human macrophages contain a stretch-sensitive potassium channel that is activated by adherence and cytokines, *J Membr Biol*, 315, pp. 305–315.
45. Pugin, J., Dunn, I., Jolliet, P., Tassaux, D., Magnenat, J.L., Nicod, L.P., Chevrolet, J.C. (1998). Activation of human macrophages by mechanical ventilation in vitro, *Am J Physiol*, 275, pp. L1040–L1050.
46. Wu, J., Yan, Z., Schwartz, D.E., Yu, J., Malik, A.B., Hu, G. (2013). Activation of NLRP3 inflammasome in alveolar macrophages contributes to mechanical stretch-induced lung inflammation and injury, *J Immunol*, 190, pp. 3590–3599.
47. Kurata, K., Uemura, T., Nemoto, A., Tateishi, T., Murakami, T., Higaki, H., Miura, H., Iwamoto, Y. (2001). Mechanical strain effect on boneresorbing activity and messenger RNA expressions of marker enzymes in isolated osteoclast culture, *J Bone Miner Res*, 16, pp. 722–730.
48. McEvoy, A., Jeyam, M., Ferrier G., Evans, C.E., Andrew, J.G. (2002). Synergistic effect of particles and cyclic pressure on cytokine production in human monocyte/macrophages: Proposed role in periprosthetic osteolysis, *Bone*, 30(1), pp. 171–177.
49. Wehner, S., Buchholz, B.M., Schuchtrup, S., Rocke, A., Schaefer, N., Lysson, M., Hirner, A., Kalff, J.C. (2010). Mechanical strain and TLR4 synergistically induce cell-specific inflammatory gene expression in intestinal smooth muscle cells and peritoneal macrophages, *Am J Physiol Gastrointest Liver Physiol*, 299, pp. G1187–G1197.

50. Jetten N., Verbruggen, S., Gijbels, M.J., Post M.J., De Winther, M.P., Donners, M.M. (2014). Anti-inflammatory M2, but not proinflammatory M1 macrophages promote angiogenesis in vivo, *Angiogenesis*, 17, pp. 109–118.
51. Ballotta, V., Driessen-Mol, A., Bouten, C.V.C., Baaijens, F.P.T. (2014). Strain-dependent modulation of macrophage polarization within scaffolds, *Biomaterials*, 35, pp. 4919–4928.
52. Wilkinson, P.C., Lackie, J.M. (1983). The influence of contact guidance on chemotaxis of human neutrophil leucocytes, *Exp Cell Res*, 145, pp. 255–264.
53. Refai, A.K., Textor, M., Brunette, D.M., Waterfield, J.D. (2004). Effect of titanium surface topography on macrophage activation and secretion of proinflammatory cytokines and chemokines, *J Biomed Mater Res*, 70, pp. 194–205.
54. Bota, P.C., Collie, A.M., Puolakkainen, P., Vernon, R.B., Sage, E.H., Ratner, B.D., Stayton, P.S. (2010). Biomaterial topography alters healing in vivo and monocyte/macrophage activation in vitro. *J Biomed Mater Res Part A*, 95, pp. 649–957.
55. Moura, C.C.G., Zanetta-Barbosa, D., Dechichi, P., Carvalho, V.F., Soares, P.B.F. (2014). Effects of titanium surfaces on the developmental profile of monocytes/macrophages, *Brazilian Dental J*, 25, pp. 96–103.
56. Wojciak-Stothard, B., Madeja, Z., Korohoda, W., Curtis, A., Wilkinson, C. (1995). Activation of macrophage-like cells by multiple grooved substrata. Topographical control of cell behaviour, *Cell Biol Int*, 19, pp. 485–490.
57. Chen, S., Jones, J.A., Xu, Y., Low, H.Y., Anderson, J.M., Leong, K.W. (2010). Characterization of topographical effects on macrophage behavior in a foreign body response model, *Biomaterials*, 31, pp. 3479–3491.
58. Schafer, V., von Briesen H., Andreesen, R., Steffan, A.M., Royer, C., Troster, S., Kreuter, J., Rübsamen-Waigmann H. (1992). Phagocytosis of nanoparticles by human immunodeficiency virus (HIV)-infected macrophages: A possibility for antiviral drug targeting, *Pharm Res*, 9, pp. 541–546.
59. Ahsan, F., Rivas, I.P., Khan, M.A., Torres Suarez, A.I. (2002). Targeting to macrophages: Role of physicochemical properties of particulate carriers–liposomes and microspheres – on the phagocytosis by macrophages, *J Control Release*, 79, pp. 29–40.
60. Gimona, M., Buccione R. (2006). Adhesions that mediate invasion, *Int J Biochem Cell Biol*, 38, pp. 1875–1892.
61. Vignery A. (2008). Macrophage fusion: Molecular mechanisms, *Methods Mol Biol*, 475, pp. 149–161.
62. Bartneck, M., Schulte, V.A., Paul, N.E., Diez, M., Lensen, M.C., Zwadlo-Klarwasser G. (2010). Induction of specific macrophage subtypes by defined micro-patterned structures, *Acta Biomaterialia*, 6, pp. 3864–3872.
63. Lensen, M.C., Schulte, V.A., Salber, J., Diez, M., Menges, F., Möller, M. (2008) Cellular responses to novel, micropatterned biomaterials, *Pure Appl Chem*, 80(11) pp. 2479–2487.
64. Grimm, M.C., Elsbury, S.K., Pavli, P., Doe, W.F. (1996). Interleukin 8: Cells of origin in inflammatory bowel disease, *Gut*, 38(1), pp. 90–98.
65. Rosenkilde, M.M., Schwartz, T.W. (2004). The chemokine system – a major regulator of angiogenesis in health and disease, *Apmis*, 112(7–8), pp. 481–495.
66. Martin, D., Galisteo, R., Gutkind, J.S. (2009). CXCL8/IL8 stimulates vascular endothelialgrowth factor (VEGF) expression and the autocrine activation of VEGFR2 inendothelial cells by activating NFjB through the CBM (Carma3/Bcl10/Malt1) complex, *J Biol Chem*, 284(10), pp. 6038–6042.
67. Secchiero, P., Corallini, F., di Iasio, M.G., Gonelli, A., Barbarotto, E., Zauli, G. (2005). TRAIL counteracts the proadhesive activity of inflammatory cytokines in endothelial cells by down-modulating CCL8 and CXCL10 chemokine expression and release, *Blood*, 105(9), pp. 3413–3419.

68. Frangogiannis, N.G. (2004). Chemokines in the ischemic myocardium: From inflammation to fibrosis, *Inflamm Res*, 53(11), pp. 585–595.
69. Sato, E., Fujimoto, J., Toyoki, H., Sakaguchi, H., Alam, S.M., Jahan, I., Tamaya, T. (2007). Expression of IP-10 related to angiogenesis in uterine cervical cancers, *Br J Cancer*, 2007, 96(11), pp. 1735–1739.
70. Melgarejo, E., Medina, M.A., Sanchez-Jimenez, F., Urdiales, J.L. (2009). Monocyte chemoattractant protein-1: A key mediator in inflammatory processes, *Int J Biochem Cell Biol*, 41(5), pp. 998–1001.
71. Paul, N.E., Skazik, C., Harwardt, M., Bartneck, M., Denecke, B., Klee, D, Salber, J., Zwadlo-Klarwasser, G. (2008). Topographical control of human macrophages by a regularly microstructured polyvinylidene fluoride surface, *Biomaterials*, 29(30), pp. 4056–4064.
72. Khang, D., Liu-Snyder, P., Pareta, R., Lu, J., Webster, T.J. (2009). Reduced responses of macrophages on nanometer surface features of altered alumina crystalline phases, *Acta Biomater*, 5(5), pp. 1425–1432.
73. Luu, L.U., Gott, S.C., Woo, B.W.K., Rao, M.P., Liu W.F. (2015). Micro- and nanopatterned topographical cues for regulating macrophage cell shape and phenotype, *ACS Appl Mater Interfaces*, 7, pp. 28665–28672.
74. McWhorter, F.Y., Davi, C.T., Liu, W.F. (2015). Physical and mechanical regulation of macrophage phenotype and function, *Cell Mol Life Sci*, 72, pp. 1303–1316.
75. Vereyken, E.J., Heijnen, P.D., Baron, W., de Vries, E.H., Dijkstra, C.D., Teunissen, C.E. (2011). Classically and alternatively activated bone marrow derived macrophages differ in cytoskeletal functions and migration towards specific CNS cell types, *J Neuroinflammation*, 8, pp. 58.
76. Hulbert, S.F., Morrison, S.J., Klawitter, J.J. (1972). Tissue reaction to three ceramics of porous and non-porous structures, *J Biomed Mater Res*, 6, pp. 347–374.
77. Ward, W.K., Slobodzian, E.P., Tiekotter, K.L., Wood, M.D. (2002). The effect of microgeometry, implant thickness and polyurethane chemistry on the foreign body response to subcutaneous implants, *Biomaterials*, 23, pp. 4185–4192.
78. Sussman, E.M., Halpin, M.C., Muster, J., Moon, R.T., Ratner, B.D. (2013). Porous implants modulate healing and induce shifts in local macrophage polarization in the foreign body reaction, *Ann Biomed Eng*, 42(7), pp. 1508–1516.
79. Almeida, C.R., Serra, T., Oliveira, M.I., Planell, J.A., Barbosa, M.A., Navarro, M. (2014). Impact of 3-D printed PLA- and chitosan-based scaffolds on human monocyte/macrophage responses: Unraveling the effect of 3-D structures on inflammation, *Acta Biomater*, 10(2), pp. 613–622.
80. Steinman, R.M. (1991). The dendritic cell system and its role in immunogenicity, *Annu Rev Immunol*, 9, pp. 271–296.
81. Banchereau, J., Steinman, R.M. (1998). Dendritic cells and the control of immunity, *Nature*, 392(6673), pp. 245–252.
82. Burns, S., Hardy, S.J., Buddle, J., Yong, K.L., Jones, G.E., Thrasher, A.J. (2004). Maturation of DC is associated with changes in motile characteristics and adherence, *Cell Motil Cytoskeleton*, 57(2), pp. 118–132.
83. van Helden, S.F., Krooshoop, D.J., Broers, K.C., Raymakers, R.A., Figdor, C.G., van Leeuwen, F.N. (2006). A critical role for prostaglandin E2 in podosome dissolution and induction of high-speed migration during dendritic cell maturation, *J Immunol*, 177(3), pp. 1567–1574.
84. van Helden, S.F., Oud, M.M., Joosten, B., Peterse, N., Figdor, C.G., van Leeuwen, F.N. (2008). PGE2-mediated podosome loss in dendritic cells is dependent on actomyosin contraction downstream of the RhoA–Rho-kinase axis, *J Cell Sci*, 121(7), pp. 1096–1106.

85. van Helden, S.F., van den Dries, K., Oud, M.M., Raymakers, R.A., Netea, M.G., van Leeuwen, F.N., Figdor, C.G. (2010). TLR4-mediated podosome loss discriminates gram-negative from gram-positive bacteria in their capacity to induce dendritic cell migration and maturation, *J Immunol*, 184(3), pp. 1280–1291.
86. van den Dries, K., van Helden, S.F.G., te Riet, J., Diez-Ahedo, R., Manzo, C., Oud, M., van Leeuwen, F.N., Brock, R., Garcia-Parajo, M. F., Cambi, A., Figdor C.G. (2012). Geometry sensing by dendritic cells dictates spatial organization and PGE 2-induced dissolution of podosomes, *Cell Mol Life Sci*, 69, pp. 1889–1901.
87. Lee, S., Choi, J., Shin, S., Im, Y.M., Song, J., Kang, S.S., Nam, T.H., Webster, T.J., Kim, S.H., Khang, D. (2011). Analysis on migration and activation of live macrophages on transparent flat and nanostructured titanium, *Acta Biomater*, 7, pp. 2337–2344.
88. Van Goethem, E., Poincloux, R., Gauffre, F., Maridonneau-Parini, I., Le Cabec, V. (2010). Matrix architecture dictates three-dimensional migration modes of human macrophages: Differential involvement of proteases and podosome-like structures, *J Immunol*, 184, pp. 1049–1061.
89. Miller, M.J., Wei, S.H., Parker, I., Cahalan, M.D. (2002). Two-photon imaging of lymphocyte motility and antigen response in intact lymph node, *Science*, 296, pp. 1869–1873.
90. Kwon, K.W., Park, H., Doh, J. (2013). Migration of T-cells on surfaces containing complex nanotopography, *PLoS ONE*, 8(9), pp. e73960.
91. Kwon, K.W., Park, H., Song, K.W., Choi, J.C., Ahn, H., Park, M.J., Suh, K.-Y., Doh J. (2012). Nanotopography-guided migration of T-cells, *J Immunol*, 189, pp. 2266–2273.
92. Cao, H., McHugh, K., Chew, S.Y., Anderson, J.M. (2009). The topographical effect of electrospun nanofibrous scaffolds on the ın vivo and ın vitro foreign body reaction, *J Biomed Mater Res Part A*, 93, pp. 1151–1159.
93. Saino, E., Focarete, M.L., Gualandi, C., Emanuele, E., Cornaglia, A.I., Imbriani, M., Visai, L. (2011). Effect of electrospun fiber diameter and alignment on macrophage activation and secretion of proinflammatory cytokines and chemokines, *Biomacromolecules*, 12, pp. 1900–1911.
94. Garg, K., Pullen, N.A., Oskeritzian, C.A., Ryan, J.J., Bowlin, G.L. (2013). Macrophages functional polarization (m1/m2) in response to varying fiber and pore dimensions of electrospun scaffolds, *Biomaterials*, 34, pp. 4439–4451.
95. Sanders, J.E., Stiles, C.E., Hayes, C.L. (2000). Tissue response to single-polymer fibers of varying diameters: Evaluation of fibrous encapsulation and macrophage density, *J Biomed Mater Res*, 52, pp. 231–237.
96. Brodbeck, W.J., Patel, J., Voskerician, G., Christenson, E., Shive, M.S., Nakayama, Y., Matsuda, T., Ziats, N.P., Anderson, J.M. (2002). Biomaterial adherent macrophage apoptosis is increased by hydrophilic and anionic substrates in vivo, *Proc Natl Acad Sci USA*, 16, pp. 10287–10292.
97. Castner, D.G., Ratner, B.D. (2002). Biomedical surface science: Foundations to frontiers, *Surf Sci*, 500 (1–3), pp. 28–60.
98. Schutte, R.J., Parisi-Amon, A., Reichert, W.M. (2009). Cytokine profiling using monocytes/macrophages cultured on common biomaterials with a range of surface chemistries, *J Biomed Mater Res Part A*, 88(1), pp. 128–139.
99. Dadsetan, M., Jones, J.A., Hiltner, A., Anderson, J.M. (2004). Surface chemistry mediates adhesive structure, cytoskeletal organization, and fusion of macrophages, *J Biomed Mater Res Part A*, 2004, 71, pp. 439–448.
100. Jones, J.A., Chang, D.T., Meyerson, H., Colton, E., Kwon, I.K., Matsuda, T., Anderson, J.M. (2007). Proteomic analysis and quantification of cytokines and chemokines from biomaterial surface-adherent macrophages and foreign body giant cells, *J Biomed Mater Res Part A*, 83, pp. 585–596.

101. McBane, J.E., Matheson, L.A., Sharifpoor, S., Santerre J.P., Labow, R.S. (2009). Effect of polyurethane chemistry and protein coating on monocyte differentiation towards a wound healing phenotype macrophage, *Biomaterials*, 30, pp. 5497–5504.
102. Alfarsi, M.A., Hamlet, S.M., Ivanovski, S. (2013). Titanium surface hydrophilicity modulates the human macrophage inflammatory cytokine response, *J Biomed Mater Res Part A*, 102(1), pp. 1–8.
103. Deeg, J., Axmann, M., Matic, J., Liapis, A., Depoil, D., Afrose, J., Curado, S., Dustin, M.L., Spatz J.P. (2013). T-cell activation is determined by the number of presented antigens, *Nano Lett*, 13, pp. 5619e26.
104. Chacko, B.K., Chandler, R., Mundhekar, A.N., Pruitt, H.M., Ramachandran, A., Barnes S., Patel, R.P. (2005). Revealing anti-inflammatory mechanisms of soy-isoflavones by flow: Modulation of leukocyte-endothelial cell interactions, *Am J Physiol*, 289, pp. H908–H915.
105. Tsai, I.Y., Kuo, C.C., Tomczyk, N., Stachelek, S.J., Composto, R.J., Eckmann, D.M. (2011). Human macrophage adhesion on polysaccharide patterned surfaces, *Soft Matter*, 7, pp. 3599–3606.
106. Isik, S., Schuhmann, W. (2006). Detection of nitric oxide release from single cells by using constant-distance-mode scanning electrochemical microscopy, *Angew Chem Int Ed*, 45, 7451–7454.
107. Borgmann, S., Radtke, I., Erichsen, T., Priv.-Doz, A.B., Heumann, R., Schuhmann, W. (2006). Electrochemical high-content screening of nitric oxide release from endothelial cells, *Chembiochem*, 7, pp. 662–668.
108. Inoue, K., Ino, K., Shiku, H., Kasai, S., Yasukawa, T., Mizutani, F., Matsue, T. (2010). Electrochemical monitoring of hydrogen peroxide released from leucocytes on horse-radish peroxidase redox polymer coated electrode chip, *Biosen Bioelectron*, 25, pp.1723–1728.
109. Yan, J., Pedrosa, V.A., Enomoto, J., Simonian, A.L., Revzin A. (2011). Electrochemical biosensors for on-chip detection of oxidative stress from immune cells, *Biomicrofluidics*, 5, pp. 032008.
110. Braden, K., Biran, L.R., Underwood, C.J., Tresco, P.A. (2008). Characterization of microglial attachment and cytokine release on biomaterials of differing surface chemistry, *Biomaterials*, 29, pp. 3289–3297.
111. Kato, K., Umezawa, K., Funeriu, D.P., Miyake, M., Miyake, J., Nagamune T. (2003). Immobilized culture of nonadherent cells on an oleyl poly(ethylene glycol) ether-modified surface, *Biotechniques*, 35, pp. 1014–1021.
112. Sakurai, K., Teramura, Y., Iwata, H. (2011). Cells immobilized on patterns printed in DNA by an inkjet printer, *Biomaterials*, 32, pp. 3596–3602.
113. Yamazoe H., Ichikawa, T., Hagihara, Y., Iwasaki Y. (2016). Generation of a patterned co-culture system composed of adherent cells and immobilized nonadherent cells, *Acta Biomaterialia*, 31, pp. 231–240.
114. Stybayeva, G., Zhu, H., Ramanculov, E., Dandekar, S., George, M., Revzin, A. (2009) Micropatterned co-cultures of T-lymphocytes and epithelial cells as a model of mucosal immune system, *Biochem Biophys Res Commun*, 380, pp. 575–580.
115. Mossman, K., Groves, J. (2007). Micropatterned supported membranes as tools for quantitative studies of the immunological synapse, *Chem Soc Rev*, 36, pp. 46–54.
116. Monks, C.R.F., Freiberg, B.A., Kupfer, H., Kupfer, A. (1998). Three-dimensional segregation of supramolecular activation clusters in T cells, *Nature*, 395, pp. 82–86.
117. Grakoui, A., Bromley, S.K., Sumen, C., Davis, M.M., Shaw, A.S., Allen, P.M., Dustin, M.L. (1999). The immunological synapse: A molecular machine controlling T-cell activation, *Science*, 285, pp. 221–227.

118. Hardy, G., Nayak, R., Zauscher, S. (2013). Model cell membranes: Techniques to form complex biomimetic supported lipid bilayers via vesicle fusion, *Curr Opin Colloid Interface Sci*, 18(5), pp. 448–458.
119. Orth, R.N., Wu, M., Holowka, D.A., Craighead, H.G., Baird, B.A. (2003). Mast cell activation on patterned lipid bilayers of subcellular dimensions, *Langmuir*, 19, pp. 1599–1605.
120. Groves, J.T., Ulman, N., Boxer, S.G. (1997). Micropatterning of fluid lipid bilayers on solid supports, *Science*, 275, pp. 651–653.
121. Groves, J.T., Boxer, S.G. (2002). Micropattern formation in supported lipid membranes, *Acc Chem Res*, 35, pp. 149–157.
122. Grakoui, A., Bromley, S.K., Sumen, C., Davis, M.M., Shaw, A.S., Allen, P.M., Dustin, M.L. (1999). The immunological synapse: A molecular machine controlling T-cell activation, *Science*, 285, pp. 221–227.
123. Faroudi, M., Utzny, C., Salio, M., Cerundolo, V., Guiraud, M., Muller, S., Valitutti, S. (2003). Lytic versus stimulatory synapse in cytotoxic T lymphocyte/target cell interaction: Manifestation of a dual activation threshold, *Proc Natl Acad Sci USA*, 100, pp. 14145–1450.
124. Purbhoo, M.A., Irvine, D.J., Huppa, J.B., Davis, M.M. (2004). T-cell killing does not require the formation of a stable mature immunological synapse, *Nat Immunol*, 5, pp. 524–530.
125. Li, Q.J., Dinner, A.R., Qi, S., Irvine, D.J., Huppa, J.B., Davis, M.M., Chakraborty, A.K. (2004). CD4 enhances T-cell sensitivity to antigen by coordinating Lck accumulation at the immunological synapse, *Nat Immunol*, 5, pp. 791–799.
126. Averbeck, M., Braun, T., Pfeifer, G., Sleeman, J., Dudda, J., Martin, S.F., Kremer, B., Aktories, K., Simon, J.C., Termeer, C. (2004). Early cytoskeletal rearrangement during dendritic cell maturation enhances synapse formation and Ca(2+) signaling in CD8(+) T-cells, *Eur J Immunol*, 34, pp. 2708–2719.
127. Brossard, C., Feuillet, V., Schmitt, A., Randriamampita, C., Romao, M., Raposo, G., Trautmann, A. (2005). Multifocal structure of the T cell–dendritic cell synapse, *Eur J Immunol*, 35, pp. 1741–1753.
128. Balamuth, F., Leitenberg, D., Unternaehrer, J., Mellman, I., Bottomly, K. (2001). Distinct patterns of membrane microdomain partitioning in Th1 and Th2 cells, *Immunity*, 15, pp. 729–738.
129. Hallman, E., Burack, W.R., Shaw, A.S., Dustin, M.L., Allen, P.M. (2002). Immature CD4(+)CD8(+) thymocytes form a multifocal immunological synapse with sustained tyrosine phosphorylation, *Immunity*, 16, pp. 839–848.
130. O'Keefe, J.P., Blaine, K., Alegre, M.L., Gajewski, T.F. (2004). Formation of a central supramolecular activation cluster is not required for activation of naiveCD8(+) T cells, *Proc Natl Acad Sci USA*, 101, pp. 9351–9356.
131. Jin, T., Pennefather, P., Lee, P.I. (1996). Lipobeads: A hydrogel anchored lipid vesicle system, *FEBS Lett*, 397, pp. 70–74.
132. Hu, C.-M.J., Zhang, L., Aryal, S., Cheung, C., Fang, R.H., Zhang, L. (2011). Erythrocyte membrane-camouflaged polymeric nanoparticles as a biomimetic delivery platform, *Proc Natl Acad Sci USA*, 108, pp. 10980–10985.
133. Ashley, C.E., Carnes, E.C., Phillips, G.K., Padilla, D., Durfee, P.N., Brown, P.A., Hanna, T.N., Brinker, C.J. (2011). The targeted delivery of multicomponent cargos to cancer cells by nanoporous particle-supported lipid bilayers, *Nat Mater*, 10, pp. 389–397.
134. Goldstein, S.A., Mescher, M.F. (1986). Cell-sized, supported artificial membranes (pseudocytes): Response of precursor cytotoxic T lymphocytes to class I MHC proteins, *J Immunol*, 137, pp. 3383–3392.

135. Mescher, M.F. (1992). Surface contact requirements for activation of cytotoxic T lymphocytes, *J Immunol*, 149, pp. 2402–2405.
136. Qi, S.Y., Groves J.T., Chakraborty, A.K. (2001). Synaptic pattern formation during cellular recognition, *Proc Natl Acad Sci USA*, 98, pp. 6548–6553.
137. Mossman K.D., Campi, G., Groves J.T., Dustin, M.L. (2005). Altered TCR signaling from geometrically repatterned immunological synapses, *Science*, 310, pp. 1191–1193.
138. Hsu, C.-J., Hsieh, W.-T., Waldman, A., Clarke, F., Huseby, E.S., Burkhardt, J.K., Baumgar, T. (2012). Ligand mobility modulates immunological synapse formation and T cell activation, *Plos One*, 7(2), pp. e32398.
139. Zheng, P., Bertolet, G., Chen, Y., Huang, S., Liu, D. (2015). Super-resolution imaging of the natural killer cell ımmunological synapse on a glass-supported planar lipid bilayer, *J Vis Exp*, 96, pp. e52502.
140. Shen, K., Thomas, K.V., Dustin M.L., Kam L.C. (2008). Micropatterning of costimulatory ligands enhances CD4+ T cell function, *Proc Natl Acad Sci USA*, 105, pp. 7791–7796.
141. Shen, K. Milone, M.C., Dustin, M.L., Kam, L.C. (2009). Nanoengineering of immune cell function, *Mater Res Soc Symp Proc*, 1209, pp. YY03–01.
142. Dustin, M.L., Chakraborty, A.K., Shaw, A.S. (2010). Understanding the structure and function of the immunological synapse, *Cold Spring Harb Perspect Biol*, 2, a002311.
143. Choudhuri, K., Llodrá J., Roth, E.W., Tsai, J., Gordo, S., Wucherpfennig, K.W., Lance K., Stokes, D.L., Dustin M.L. (2014). Polarized release of T-cell-receptor-enriched microvesicles at the immunological synapse, *Nature*, 507, pp. 118–123.
144. Kaizuka, Y., Douglass, A.D., Varma, R., Dustin, M.L., Vale, R.D. (2007). Mechanisms for segregating T cell receptor and adhesion molecules during immunological synapse formation in Jurkat T cells, *Proc Natl Acad Sci USA*, 104, pp. 20296–20301.
145. Irvine, D.J., Doh, J. (2007). Synthetic surfaces as artificial antigen presenting cells in the study of T cell receptor triggering and immunological synapse formation, *Seminars in Immunology*, 19, pp. 245–254.
146. Douglass, A.D., Vale, R.D. (2005). Single-molecule microscopy reveals plasma membrane microdomains created by protein–protein networks that exclude or trap signaling molecules in T cells, *Cell*, 121, pp. 937–950.
147. Groves, J.T., Dustin, M.L. (2003). Supported planar bilayers in studies on immune cell adhesion and communication, *J Immunol Methods*, 278, pp. 19–32.
148. Doh, J., Irvine, D.J. (2006). Immunological synapse arrays: Patterned protein surfaces that modulate immunological synapse structure formation in T cells, *Proc Natl Acad Sci USA*, 103, pp. 5700–5705.
149. Adutler-Lieber, S., Zaretsky, I., Platzman, I., Deeg, J., Friedman, N., Spatz J.N., Geiger, B. (2014). Engineering of synthetic cellular microenvironments: Implications for immunity, *J Autoimmun*, 54, pp. 100e111.
150. Rostam, H.M., Singh, A., Vrana, N.E., Alexander, M.R., Ghaemmaghami, A.M. (2015). Impact of surface chemistry and topography on the function of antigen presenting cells, *J Biomater Sci*, 3, pp. 424–441.
151. Sridharan, R., Cameron, A.R., Kelly, D.J., Kearney, C.J., O'Brien, F.J. (2015). Biomaterial based modulation of macrophage polarization: A review andsuggested design principles, *Materials Today*, 18(6), pp. 313–325.
152. Ishii, M., Wen, H., Corsa, C.A., Liu, T., Coelho, A.L., Allen, R.M., Carson, W.F., Cavassani, K.A., Li, X., Lukacs, N.W., Hogaboam, C.M., Dou, Y., Kunkel, S.L. (2009). Epigenetic regulation of the alternatively activated macrophage phenotype, *Blood*, 114, pp. 3244–3254.

4 The Overview of Titanium and Its Crystalline Phases
The Impact in Biomedical Applications

Miklós Weszl, Liza Pelyhe, Eszter Bognár and Imre Kientzl

CONTENTS

4.1 INTRODUCTION

Implants are an indispensable part of modern medical practice and each year millions of implants are put in patients to replace the function of failing tissues and organs. Titanium is known as a biocompatible material and has long been used for the replacement of bone tissue, while it has recently also been used in some new applications [1], such as in the field of otorhinolaryngology for auricular and tracheal implants [2]. In the last few years the application of titanium implants has also dramatically increased in terms of diversity and quantity. This means that titanium implants are available for more heterogeneous patient populations of broader demographics and clinical conditions than before, improving the quality of life of many human beings. On the other hand, this magnitude of expansion in the volume of indwelling titanium implants has revealed some hidden risks that are associated with the use of titanium in the human body. Immuno-inflammatory tissue reaction and bacterial infection-associated complications of titanium implants have recently become a great concern.

It is still a common occurrence for titanium implants to fail due to bad osseointegration, peri-implantatis, osteolysis etc. This can be due to the effect of particle release from the implant; there is significant literature on the induction of pro-inflammatory cytokine release by immune cells in the presence of titanium wear particles such as IL-6, IL12 or TNF-α. A higher level of IL-6 was detected in synovial fluid of patients with aseptic knee implant loosening compared to control groups [3]. Depending on the target area, the rate of failure can be in the range of 2–10%. Currently, there are only a few generic indicators (such as smoking and diabetes, factors that are known to affect healing overall) that are in use in order to indicate an elevated risk of implant failure; however, several studies are underway to elucidate patient-specific indicators for such adverse effects. For example, aseptic loosening, the failure of particularly orthopaedic implants without contribution of a local infection, can be generally related to the improper fixation of the implant, which results in excessive stress/strain conditions on the surrounding bone tissue. Aseptic loosening accounts for nearly three-quarters of all implant failures for total hip thyroplasty. However, excessive immune reaction related poor integration and osteolysis also contribute to aseptic loosening. Recently, Schoeman et al. demonstrated that there is an inverse relationship between aseptic loosening of knee implants with the levels of IFN-γ in 116 patients [4]. Although the exact role of IFN-γ in bone formation is not well established, there are studies showing an important potentially positive contribution of IFN-γ as shown by significant reduction in bone formation in IFN-γ knock-out mice [5]. Moreover, it was shown that a specific allele (C allele) of MMP1 SNP (single-nucleotide polymorphism) has shown strong correlation with aseptic failure in 91 patients of aseptic loosening following total hip replacement [6]. Thus, beyond lifestyle, co-morbidity- and immune profile-related effects there may also be genetic factors determining implant failure.

Osteolysis has been shown to be directly related with inflammatory reactions, in which the contribution of macrophages is considerable. Bone resorption under homeostasis conditions is carried out by resident macrophage population in the bone osteoclasts. However, in the case of bone damage (as in the case of implant presence) inflammatory macrophages also contribute to the bone resorptive activities. Macrophages are widely found in histological analysis of peri-implant osteolysis cases in close interaction with wear particles from the implants, where TLR receptors are active in the macrophage/wear particle interactions [7]. Moreover, as stated above the release of pro-inflammatory cytokines is one of the main factors in the reaction to titanium implants and it has been shown that the wear particle/macrophage interactions result in the release of IL-1 and IL-6, together with chemokines such as MIP-1 and MCP-1 [8]. The reactions are closely related to the properties of the wear particles, such as their composition, concentration and size. Thus, it is important to consider the relation between the release of wear particles and the surface properties of titanium implants.

In an ageing society, the effects of implant failure have more reverberating effects, as these problems can mean additional health problems for ailing patients. For the time being, the root causes of these complications are not exactly known (as seen above, they are multifactorial); however, some recent scientific findings suggest that the chemical and physical properties of the surface of a titanium implant may significantly affect its biological characteristics. Thus, it is important to understand the underlying properties of the titanium surface for better appreciation of the interactions between implants and host tissues.

Titanium is a metal (atomic number 22) discovered in late eighteenth century. As a strong and relatively corrosion-resistant metal, it has found many applications in industry. Titanium oxide naturally grows on the surface of metallic titanium when it comes into contact with ambient air. The titanium might be present in various oxidation states in this titanium oxide surface, but sixfold coordinated Ti atoms are the most frequent and constitute the most stable form of titanium dioxide (TiO_2). Hence, the titanium oxide layer that covers the surface of titanium implants is often simply referred to as the TiO_2 surface. As a matter of fact, the TiO_2 surface is responsible for the biocompatibility of a titanium implant and, in addition, its quality may significantly affect the mechanical properties of the implant, such as its corrosion and fatigue resistance.

During the last few decades, applied research has been focused mainly on the mechanical aspects of titanium implants, while limited attention has been dedicated to the exploration of the underlying physical and chemical properties of biocompatibility. The objective of this introductory chapter is to draw attention to the scientific achievements in the domain of TiO_2 research, as well as to the untapped opportunities in conjunction with implant applications. A deeper understanding and more precise control over these properties together with a deeper understanding of cellular reaction as a function of surface physical and chemical changes can significantly decrease the complications related to titanium implant/immune system interface [9].

4.2 OVERVIEW ON THE CRYSTALLINE PHASES OF TITANIUM DIOXIDE

In nature, titanium is mostly found in two ores: ilmenite ($FeTiO_3$) and rutile (TiO_2) [10], which are both used in industry for the production of pure TiO_2. Ilmenite contains between 40 and 65% TiO_2, whereas rutile contains about 95% titanium dioxide (TiO_2) [11]. TiO_2 exists in various natural and high-pressure polymorphs, for instance, anatase (tetragonal), rutile (tetragonal), brookite (orthotrombic), akaogiite (monoclinic), columbite (orthotrombic), fluorite-type polymorph (cubic), pyrite-type polymorph (cubic), baddeleyite-type polymorph (monoclinic) and cotunnite (orthotrombic), which is one of the hardest known polycrystalline materials [12,13]. However, at the current level of technology, rutile and anatase only play a role in biomedical applications.

The smallest crystal in the anatase and rutile is called a unit cell, a basic building block that consists of a titanium atom surrounded by six oxygen atoms in a more or less distorted octahedral configuration, which forms tetragonal crystal structures [14]. In the unit cell of rutile, the atoms occupy less space than in the more elongated anatase unit (Figure 4.1). This steric difference of the unit cells may make rutile thermodynamically more stable than anatase under natural conditions, driving phase transformation [15]. From a medical perspective it may be important to note that the phase transformation occurs only at relatively high (transition) temperature, which varies in the range of 400–1200°C [16]. This means that the phase transformation

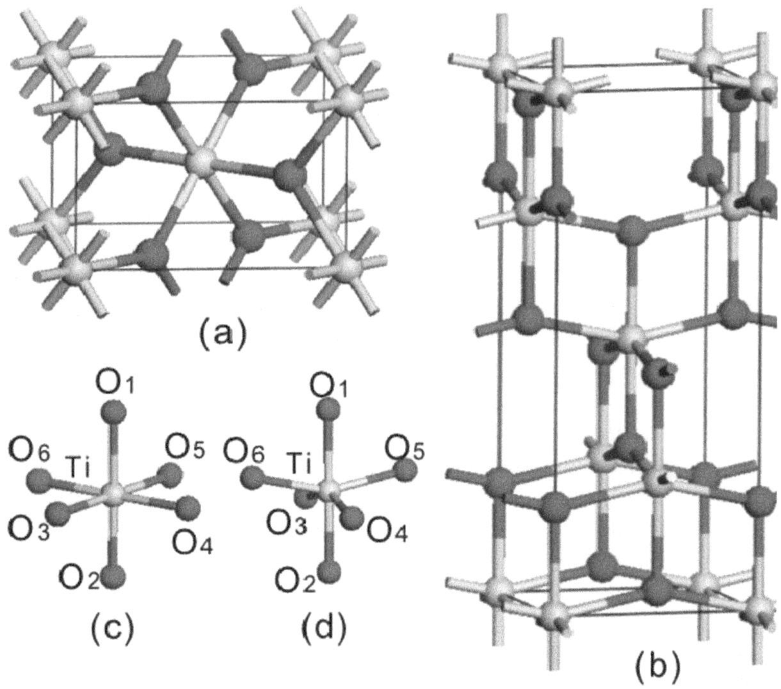

FIGURE 4.1 Schematic representation of the tetragonal crystal cells of: (a) rutile; (b) anatase; and schematic representation of the atomic structures of a TiO_6 octahedron in: (c) rutile; (d) anatase. Reprinted with permission from [14].

will not normally happen under physiologic conditions. Previous studies have shown that the method of preparation, dopant concentration atmosphere and particle size can influence the rate of anatase to rutile phase transformation. Experiments shows that if specific ions are doped into the TiO_2 lattice the anatase-rutile transformation occurs much more easily. Nevertheless, in the presence of transition metallic ions with highly unpaired electron spin as impurities or alloys, like Co^{II} and Ni^{II} the anatase – rutile phase transformation takes place even at room temperature [17]. This may be a peculiar risk factor that would alter the biological characteristics of a TiO_2 surface on an indwelling implant in the lifetime of the device, as it has previously been shown that the osteogenic response to anatase or rutile phase-rich surfaces is different [18].

Recent scientific achievements in the field of the photocatalysis have markedly increased our understanding of the electronic structure of TiO_2, as well as its electrochemical and chemical properties. However, the conversion of those results into viable medical technologies occurs with some lateness. The phase transformation of anatase to rutile entails changes in the electron structure that are responsible for the different chemical properties of those two crystalline forms, which may also affect the biological behaviour of the various TiO_2 surfaces. Concerning photocatalytic applications, the mixed-phase samples of anatase and rutile outperform the individual polymorphs [19]; nonetheless, the biological relevance of the different crystalline phases in conjunction with implant surfaces requires more studies. As the surface phase changes generally involve different surface treatments, the observed effect is mostly multi-factorial, where the micro-retentive properties of the titanium implant surface (such as roughness, presence of micro/nanopatterned structures such as etches or nanotubes obtained via anodisation) should also be taken into account [20]. One important line of research for the biomedical significance of the anatase:rutile ratio is the determination of the effect of the surface crystalline phases on the conformation of the adsorped proteins as the nature of the protein adsorption is an important determinant of the subsequent inflammatory reactions. For example, it has been shown that phosphorus doped rutile titanium oxide surfaces had increased haemocompatibility due to the decreased activation of clotting cascade and diminished platelet adhesion [21].

Some attention has been paid to the TiO_2 polymorphs in publications that deal with the biocompatibility of implant surfaces with a view to exploring possible interrelations with the response of the cells [22]. Nevertheless, there are no reported data in the literature from systematic studies that aim to unfold the causal relationships or correlations between cell responses and the crystalline phases. Such studies would be essential to deepen our understanding of the biological effects of the different TiO_2 polymorphs in a biomedical context. However, the investigation of the sole effect of crystalline phases on cell response might be extremely difficult, especially in case of multiphase samples where the anatase and rutile are present concurrently. During the synthesis of TiO_2 multiple factors may change simultaneously, including but not limited to surface area, surface topography, crystal aspect ratio, grain size, exposure of facets, bulk and surface defects. Although, the effects of all these factors on the cell response are more or less known in the art, the resultant biological effect of all these factors is still vague; therefore, they should be carefully taken into consideration during the appraisal of the results of biocompatibility studies, otherwise the conclusion may be biased.

For example, He et al. used DC reactive magnetron sputtering under different pressure conditions to obtain anatase and rutile-rich or amorphous titanium dioxide layers. As the method utilised enables strong control over the crystalline phase, they compared the effect of different crystalline phases on the behaviour of osteoblasts and observed crystalline phase-specific effects on cell attachment, spreading and alkaline phosphatase activity (where the anatase phase is more permissive to adhesion and spreading) [23] (Figure 4.2). Moreover, it has been shown that the anatase phase is more potent in induction of hydroxyapatite growth in the presence of simulated body fluid (SBF) compared to the amorphous phase [24]. However, the stability of these layers is equally important in biomedical applications as anatase titanium dioxide nanoparticles have been shown to induces ROS secretion (such as superoxide anion) and cytotoxicity at high concentrations [25]; thus, it is crucial to ensure their strength of adhesion on implant surfaces. Recently, we have demonstrated that by utilising a double-anodisation protocol it is possible to obtain highly stable nanopitted surfaces (compared to nanotubes obtained with conventional anodisation) on dental implants [26].

As the presence of TiO_2 nanoparticles released from implant surfaces was also shown to induce pro-inflammatory responses in addition to cell membrane damage and cytotoxicity, it is important to have stable surface layers for reduced immune reactions to modified titanium implant surfaces. At organism level, it has been shown with silkworms that the presence of TiO_2 has a positive effect on the survival

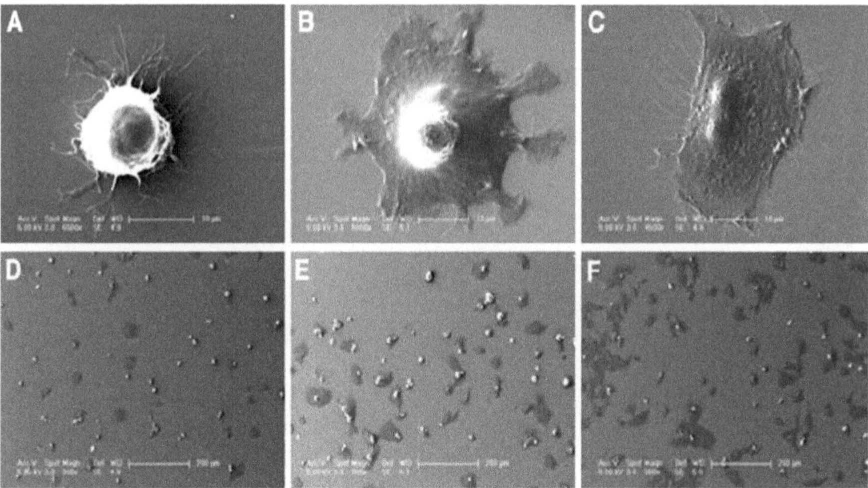

FIGURE 4.2 The effect of the surface crystalline phase on cell attachment on titanium surfaces. By changing the pressure conditions of the deposition, different crystalline phases (anatase, rutile and amorphous) can be obtained using DC reactive magnetron sputtering. Scanning electron microscopy (SEM) micrographs demonstrates that cells are more spread in general on anatase surfaces compared to rutile and amorphous surfaces after eight hours of incubation. (A–C) Representative images of the present cellular morphologies (hemispherical, spread cell with multilple lamellipodia or fully spread cells); (D–F) micrographs of adhered cells on amorphous, rutile-rich and anatase-rich surfaces, respectively. Reprinted with permission from [23].

rate after infection with *Bacillus bombyseptieus*; however, it also induced disruptive effects on apoptosis and had a significant effect on gene expression patterns (more than 15 pathways related to host defence, innate immunity, apoptosis etc.) [27]; thus, the prevention of excessive release of TiO_2 nanoparticles is highly important.

During the synthesis of TiO_2 the formation of the crystalline phase significantly depends on the applied conditions and process parameters (Table 4.1). Concerning medical device applications, recent surface treatment technologies have primarily been optimised for the manipulation of the topography (nano- and micro-roughness) of titanium implants. On the other hand, these technologies may also be effective to the control the formation of the crystalline phase of TiO_2 – however, with certain limitations.

It must be noted that it would be misleading to interpret the biological performance of a TiO_2 surface, or conversely, the response of the cells on the surface, solely in terms of phase composition, since other factors, including but not limited to surface area and topography, may have strong influence on it. Nevertheless, the surface is an important component of a solid-state material because it has the ability to initiate heterogeneous chemical reactions. This property of the surface becomes especially important when the size of the surface is reduced to the nanoscale [28]. The engineering of surface nanostructures – more specifically, deliberately exposing specific crystal facets with high energy and reactivity – has become a promising

TABLE 4.1
Common Synthesis Methods of TiO_2 and Resultant Polymorphs

Synthesis Method	Conditions	Polymorphs				Ref.
		Amorphous	Anatase	Rutile	Anat+Rutile	
Acid-assisted sol-gel method	Synthesis was carried out at 25–80°C		✓			[13]
Anodisation	Carried out at ~27°C in 0.15M NH4F at pH4 supplemented with EDTA applying 20V	✓				[29]
Anodisation	Carried out in 0.5M H2SO4 applying 70–120V from 120–300 sec at room temperature		✓			[30]
Anodisation	Carried out in 0.5M H2SO4 applying 120V for 300 s at room temperature				✓	[31]
Laser ablation	Using second harmonic (532 nm) of a pulsed Nd-YAG laser under 50 mtorr O_2 pressure at 300°C (substrate temperature)			✓		[32]

research direction in recent years in energy conversion and environmental application of TiO_2 [33]. Concerning rutile crystals, the {001} facet has the highest surface energy [12]. As for anatase, the {110} facet is the most stable and the {010}, {101} and {001} facets have the highest surface energies, respectively [33].

Interestingly, Zhao et al. recently predicated, based on density functional theory, that anatase nano-crystals with predominantly exposed {101} facets facilitate the adherence of bacteria in microbial fuel cells because such facets promote the selective adsorption of the carboxyl and hydroxyl groups of bacterial pili at room temperature, which assures their immobilisation [34]. This finding suggests that the mechanical and physicochemical properties, e.g., surface roughness and wettability, are not completely sufficient to predict or explain the biological characteristics of a TiO_2 surface but the electron structure and reactivity of the exposed crystal facets may also have significant effect on cell response. Table 4.2 below shows some methods of controlled growth of TiO_2 nano-crystals that expose high-energy facets. For the time being, anatase has attracted more research interest than rutile and brookite owing to its higher activity in photocatalytic and energy conversion reactions. It can be hypothesised that surface reactivity will also have potential effects on the behaviour of cells and also immune response for TiO_2 surfaces; but this has not yet been widely studied.

TABLE 4.2
Methods of Growing TiO_2 Nano-Crystals with Their High-Energy Facets Exposed

	Conditions	Yield
	Anatase Facets	
{001}	In TiF4 aqueous solution and HF in a Teflon-lined autoclave at 180°C for 2–20 h [35]	Percentage of exposed {001} up to 90%; thickness of nanocrystals is around 8 nm
{100}	Synthetised in the mixed solution of ionic liquid water (BMIM-BF_4) [36]	Percentage of {100} in the total surface varies from 40% to 95%
{010}	Tri-titanate $H_2Ti_3O_7$ nanosheet solution was subjected to hydrothermal treatment in HCl solution for 24 h [37]	Not known
[111]	Synthesised from tri-titanate $H_2Ti_3O_7$ nanosheets by hydrothermal reaction [37]	Not known
	Rutile Facets	
{331}	Titanium-glycolate complex solution was supplemented with picolinic acid and autoclaved at 473K for 24 h [38]	Not known
{111}	Synthetised by solvothermal method at 220°C for 12 h in the solution of HCl and NaF [39]	Depending on Ti-F molar ratio varies between 25 and 98.5%

4.3 EFFECT OF SURFACE DEFECTS ON THE REACTIVITY OF TIO_2 CRYSTALLINE FACETS

Surface defects introduce changes in the electronic structure of TiO_2 that play a role in a variety of surface phenomena. Hence the ability to control the amount and the quality of imperfections, such as point defects and step edges, has attracted a great deal of scientific interest. Concerning step edges, depending on the applied surface treatment and process parameters, the number and size of terraces may vary (for instance, annealing at high temperature, the size of terraces increases with the applied temperature) [40]. Models have been constructed based on autocompensation theory to explain step edges [41], which is illustrated in Figure 4.3.

According to the theory, the most stable surfaces are predicted to be those that are autocompensated, which means that excess charge from cation-derived dangling bonds compensates anion-derived dangling bonds. Thus, the net result is that the cation- and anion-derived dangling bonds are completely empty (full) on stable surfaces [42]. Concerning the formation of a step edge by removing part of the upper terrace the same number of Ti-O and O-Ti bonds need to be broken, as illustrated in Figure 4.4.

Concerning Figure 4.4, the formation of the step edge yields fourfold coordinated Ti atoms (terminating the Ti rows of the upper terrace) and fivefold coordinated Ti atoms (terminating the bridging O rows). The O atoms along the $[1\bar{1}1]$ step edge are alternately threefold (as in the bulk) and twofold coordinated. There are possibilities to change the step orientation that may result in a different coordination number of atoms. This brief insight into step geometries and coordination numbers of atoms at step edges may have significant practical relevance because a decrease in the coordination number of surface atoms often correlates with an enhancement in chemical reactivity. Micro-, but more importantly, nano-size particles naturally exhibit a much

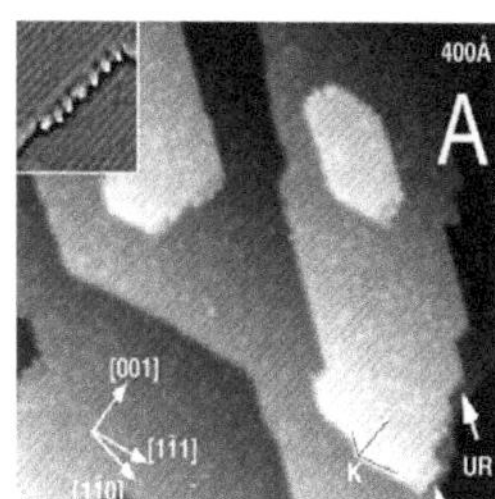

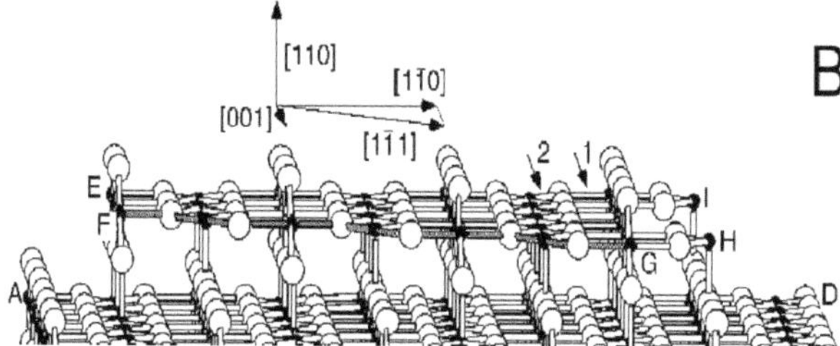

FIGURE 4.3 (A) Scanning tunneling microscope (STM) micrograph of the step structure on a clean stoichiometric TiO_2 {110}-(1x1) surface; (B) the ball-and-stick model representation (black balls: Ti; white balls: O). The imaged surface is produced via sputtering and subsequent annealing at 1100K (in ultra-high vacuum). This resulted in a step structure that is dominated by step edges running parallel to $[1\bar{1}1]$ and [001] directions. Markings: kink site (K); smooth (UR); and rugged (R). The smooth and rugged step edges along [001] in the STM image are attributed to step edges AB and HI in the ball-and-stick model. Reprinted with permission from [12].

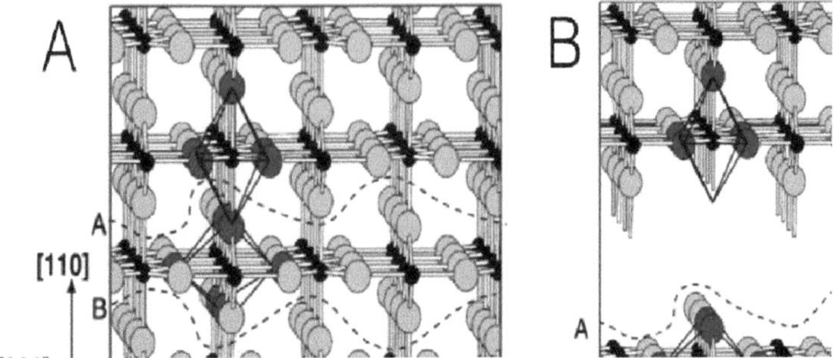

FIGURE 4.4 The ball-and-stick model of an intact (A) and cut (B) rutile crystal structure. The intact structure is an octohedra (with slight distortion). In the cut structure the number of broken Ti-O and O-Ti bonds were the same (autocompensation). Reprinted with permission from [12].

higher step concentration than flat single crystals, hence this topic may be pivotal to understand and consciously control the reactivity of TiO_2. Smaller particles expose a larger fraction of coordinatively unsaturated surface atoms owing to edges, corners and surface defects compared to larger particles [33].

Point defects are of high importance for surface properties, especially oxygen vacancies that may emerge on the surface of TiO_2 in the course of various surface treatments, such as annealing, electron bombardment and UV irradiation [42,43]. At the site of oxygen vacancy $Ti^{4+} \rightarrow Ti^{3+}$ conversion occurs that supports dissociative water adsorption, which increases the wettability of the TiO_2 surface [44]. The coordinatively unsaturated surface Ti^{n+} cations at TiO_2 exhibit Lewis acid sites with the tendency to form chemical bond with soluble basic molecules, while O^{n-} anions exhibit Lewis basic sites with the tendency to absorb soluble acidic molecules. Relying on the density functional calculations of Selloni and co-workers on anatase TiO_2 surfaces, Österlund discerned that: (i) surfaces with a large density of coordinatively unsaturated surfaces sites promote dissociation and bidentate bonding of soluble acidic molecules (i.e., formic acid) due to interactions with basic surface O atoms present on these surfaces; (ii) surface planes exhibiting strained configuration of surface atoms, i.e., large Ti-O-Ti bond angles within the surface plane, make the surface O atom become more or less basic, and hence more or less reactive. It has also been concluded that the in-plane Ti-O-Ti bond angles vary considerably at the {101}, {111}, {100}, {112} and {001} surfaces, with the {101} surface exhibiting the lowest Ti-O-Ti bond angle within the surface plane (along the [101] direction), while the others have a strained angle. All these can potentially have an effect first on the interaction of the titanium surfaces with biological molecules and consequently the potential responses of the cells to the adsorbed proteins in conformations dictated by the surface crystalline phases.

4.4 BIOLOGICAL ASPECTS OF TIO_2 CRYSTALLINE PHASES

The effect of the nanostructuration of titanium surfaces on immune cells has been widely studied. For example, the attachment and spreading of murine macrophages (RAW264.7) have been shown to be strongly correlated with the diameter of the nanotubular TiO_2 [45]. Moreover, on nanotubes with bigger diameters (up to 120 nm) an increased release of bone morphogenetic protein 2 (BMP-2) was also observed. Another study carried out on J744A.1 macrophages demonstrated that 80-nm nanotubes significantly decreased the expression of several pro-inflammatory markers such as TNF-α, MIP-1-α and MCP-1, both at protein and gene-expression level [46].

A more recent study demonstrated the differential response by macrophages to TiO_2 nanotubes produced by application of different voltages. At 20 V, macrophages had more M2-like phenotype with higher arginase and IL-10 expression, whereas, at 10 V, the expression levels of IL-1β, TNF-α and iNOS (induced nitric oxide synthase) were higher [47]. They also demonstrated that this had downstream ramifications as pre-osteoblast osteogenic capacity and vascular endothelial cell capillary sprouting capacities were both enhanced when conditioned media from macrophage cultures came into contact with optimised nanotubular titanium. An *in vivo* study demonstrated the advantage of nanostructured surfaces in the context of titanium implants as implants with nanofeatures induced less inflammatory response (with a significant decrease in TNF-α expression together with the decreased expression of CatK (an osteoclast marker; see Chapter 8 for more information on osteoclasts) in a rat tibia model [48]. Histological analyses showed that there were significantly fewer CD-163+ macrophages (M1 macrophages) around implants with nanofeatures. Another potential benefit of nanostructured surfaces (particularly anodised surfaces) is inherent antimicrobial activity. This would also have secondary beneficial effects as it has been shown that biofilm formation significantly reduces the corrosion resistance of titanium surfaces (Figure 4.5) [49] (More information on biofilm formation will be given in the next chapter).

The literature of comparative studies concerning cell response on the different crystalline phases of TiO_2 is limited at the moment but the published results justify the clinical relevance of this research field.

For example, Yu et al. studied the corrosion behaviour of untreated titanium samples compared to amorphous or anatase-rich nanotubes produced by anodisation and showed that the corrosion resistance of anodised samples was significantly higher in Hank's solution [50]. It has been demonstrated that primary lung epithelial cells respond very differently to anatase and rutile TiO_2 nanoparticles. Interestingly, pure

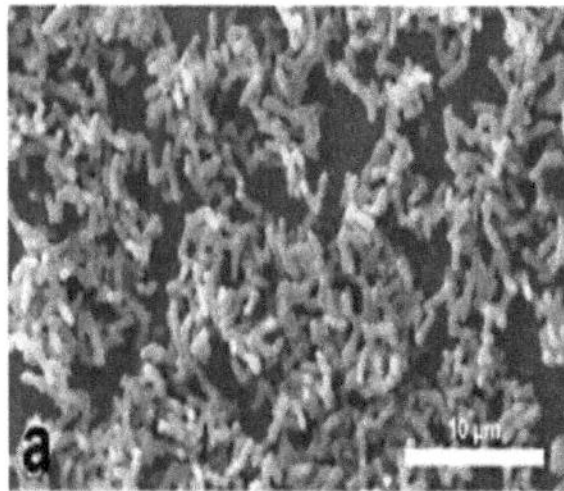

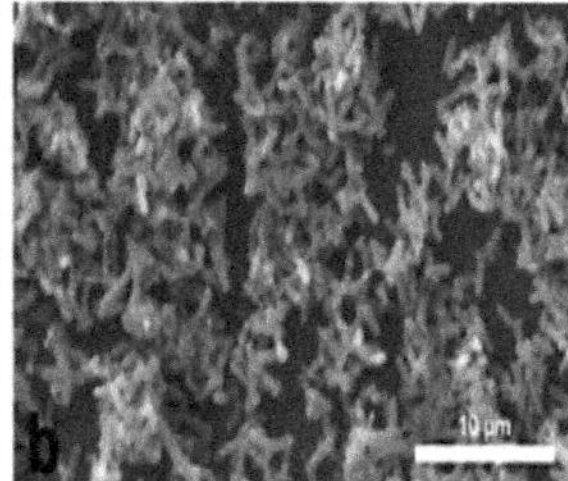

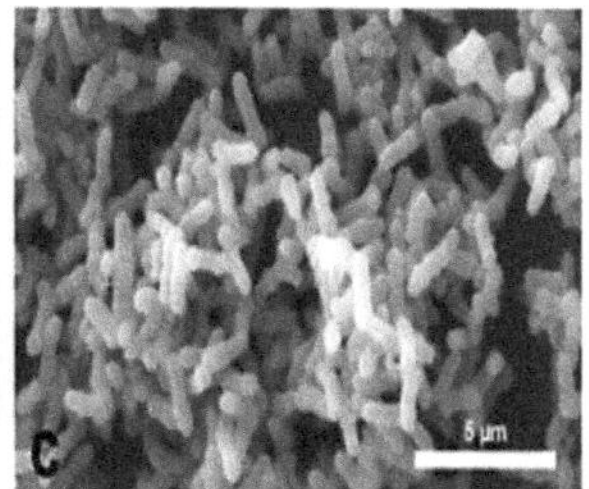

FIGURE 4.5 The growth of *Actinomyces naeslundii* (an oral bacteria) on pure titanium surfaces over the course of seven days: (a) after one day; (b) after three days; and (c) after seven days. The bacteria can form a thick biofilm, which in turn negatively affects the implant's stability. Reprinted with permission from [49].

anatase and rutile particles provoked differential IL-8 response in (A549) epithelial carcinoma cells and no response in (BEAS-2B) immortalised epithelial cells, despite similar formation of ROS. The pure TiO_2 modifications also provoked release of the inflammatory mediators IL-6, G-CSF and VEGF in normal human bronchial epithelial (NHBE) cells but not in the other two cell lines. This supported the conclusion that the responsiveness of lung epithelial cells is strongly dependent on both the physicochemical properties of TiO_2 nanoparticles and the type of responder cells [51]. In an intestinal epithelial cell model (Caco-2), nanoparticles with mixed anatase/rutile phase were more cytotoxic compared to pure anatase phase nanoparticles [52]. Hopefully, these initial results (together with the recent evidence on the effect of crystalline phases on antimicrobial activities of titanium particles and surfaces [53]) will boost the research activity in this field and will uncover the structure-reactivity relation of the various crystalline phases of TiO_2 concerning biocompatibility and unwanted complications, such as immuno-inflammatory tissue reaction or bacterial infection.

4.5 CONCLUSIONS

The current approaches for the enhancement of the TiO_2 surface of implants still rely mainly on conventional metallurgical methods, despite no considerable improvement having been achieved since Branemark explored the biocompatibility of TiO_2. Although a rich amount of experimental data have been generated in conjunction with the structure-activity relation of TiO_2 in the fields of energy conversion and photocatalytic reactivity, these results have not yet been adapted to a large enough extent by biomaterial sciences. However, better understanding of the biological effect of various crystalline phases of TiO_2 and crystal facets may give new momentum to biomaterial research to come out of the deadlock and produce titanium implants with better clinical performance.

As described above, subtle changes in surface nanoscale properties have important effects on the behaviour of immune cells. Thus, another potential advantage of the precise control of surface nanocrystalline states is potential reductions in unwanted immune responses to titanium implants. At the moment, there is no established way of testing the potential immune response of the patients – although there is a generalised test for metal hypersensitivity (MELISA, memory lymphocyte immuno-stimulation assay). However, recently the specificity and sensitivity of the MELISA test was also questioned [54]. For example, a 2007 clinical study showed that out of 56 patients with symptoms related to titanium implants, only 21 (37.5%) tested positive with the MELISA test [55]. Thus, with a limited ability of detection of potential adverse reactions, it is important to develop relatively less inflammatory titanium surfaces via control over surface crystalline phases.

REFERENCES

1. Dean CM, Ahmarani C, Bettez M, Heuer RJ. The adjustable laryngeal implant. *Journal of Voice*. 2001;15(1):141–50.
2. Debry C, Vrana NE, Dupret-Bories A. Implantation of an artificial larynx after total laryngectomy. *New England Journal of Medicine*. 2017;376(1):97–8.

3. Konttinen YT, Xu J, Waris E, Li T-F, Gomez-Barrena E, Nordsletten L et al. Interleukin-6 in aseptic loosening of total hip replacement prostheses. *Clinical and Experimental Rheumatology*. 2002;20(4):485–90.
4. Schoeman MA, Pijls BG, Oostlander AE, Keurentjes JC, Valstar ER, Nelissen RG et al. Innate immune response and implant loosening: Interferon gamma is inversely associated with early migration of total knee prostheses. *Journal of Orthopaedic Research*. 2016;34(1):121–6.
5. Duque G, Huang DC, Dion N, Macoritto M, Rivas D, Li W et al. Interferon-γ plays a role in bone formation in vivo and rescues osteoporosis in ovariectomized mice. *Journal of Bone and Mineral Research*. 2011;26(7):1472–83.
6. Malik MHA, Jury F, Bayat A, Ollier WER, Kay PR. Genetic susceptibility to total hip arthroplasty failure: A preliminary study on the influence of matrix metalloproteinase 1, interleukin 6 polymorphisms and vitamin D receptor. *Annals of the Rheumatic Diseases*. 2007;66(8):1116.
7. Gu Q, Yang H, Shi Q. Macrophages and bone inflammation. *Journal of Orthopaedic Translation*. 2017.
8. Bitar D, Parvizi J. Biological response to prosthetic debris. *World Journal of Orthopedics*. 2015;6(2):172.
9. Barthes J, Ciftci S, Ponzio F, Knopf-Marques H, Pelyhe L, Gudima A et al. The potential impact of surface crystalline states of titanium for biomedical applications. *Critical Reviews in Biotechnology*. 2017:1–15.
10. Meinhold G. Rutile and its applications in earth sciences. *Earth-Science Reviews*. 2010;102(1):1–28.
11. Zhang W, Zhu Z, Cheng CY. A literature review of titanium metallurgical processes. *Hydrometallurgy*. 2011;108(3):177–88.
12. Diebold U. The surface science of titanium dioxide. *Surface Science Reports*. 2003;48(5):53–229.
13. Leyva-Porras C, Toxqui-Teran A, Vega-Becerra O, Miki-Yoshida M, Rojas-Villalobos M, García-Guaderrama M et al. Low-temperature synthesis and characterization of anatase TiO_2 nanoparticles by an acid assisted sol–gel method. *Journal of Alloys and Compounds*. 2015;647:627–36.
14. Yin W-J, Chen S, Yang J-H, Gong X-G, Yan Y, Wei S-H. Effective band gap narrowing of anatase TiO_2 by strain along a soft crystal direction. *Applied Physics Letters*. 2010;96(22):221901.
15. Vu NH, Le HV, Cao TM, Pham VV, Le HM, Nguyen-Manh D. Anatase–rutile phase transformation of titanium dioxide bulk material: A DFT+ U approach. *Journal of Physics: Condensed Matter*. 2012;24(40):405501.
16. Hanaor DA, Sorrell CC. Review of the anatase to rutile phase transformation. *Journal of Materials Science*. 2011;46(4):855–74.
17. Gole JL, Prokes SM, Glembocki OJ. Efficient room-temperature conversion of anatase to rutile TiO_2 induced by high-spin ion doping. *The Journal of Physical Chemistry C*. 2008;112(6):1782–8.
18. Mendonça G, Mendonça DB, Simões LG, Araújo AL, Leite ER, Duarte WR et al. The effects of implant surface nanoscale features on osteoblast-specific gene expression. *Biomaterials*. 2009;30(25):4053–62.
19. Kaplan R, Erjavec B, Pintar A. Enhanced photocatalytic activity of single-phase, nanocomposite and physically mixed TiO_2 polymorphs. *Applied Catalysis A: General*. 2015;489:51–60.
20. Stanford CM. Surface modification of biomedical and dental implants and the processes of inflammation, wound healing and bone formation. *International Journal of Molecular Sciences*. 2010;11(1):354–69.

21. Maitz MF, Pham M-T, Wieser E, Tsyganov I. Blood compatibility of titanium oxides with various crystal structure and element doping. *Journal of Biomaterials Applications*. 2003;17(4):303–19.
22. Li M, Huang G, Qiao Y, Wang J, Liu Z, Liu X et al. Biocompatible and freestanding anatase TiO_2 nanomembrane with enhanced photocatalytic performance. *Nanotechnology*. 2013;24(30):305706.
23. He J, Zhou W, Zhou X, Zhong X, Zhang X, Wan P et al. The anatase phase of nanotopography titania plays an important role on osteoblast cell morphology and proliferation. *Journal of Materials Science: Materials in Medicine*. 2008;19(11):3465–72.
24. Grigal IP, Markeev AM, Gudkova SA, Chernikova AG, Mityaev AS, Alekhin AP. Correlation between bioactivity and structural properties of titanium dioxide coatings grown by atomic layer deposition. *Applied Surface Science*. 2012;258(8): 3415–19.
25. Wang J, Ma J, Dong L, Hou Y, Jia X, Niu X et al. Effect of anatase TiO_2 nanoparticles on the growth of RSC-364 rat synovial cell. *Journal of Nanoscience and Nanotechnology*. 2013;13(6):3874–9.
26. Weszl M, Tóth KL, Kientzl I, Nagy P, Pammer D, Pelyhe L et al. Investigation of the mechanical and chemical characteristics of nanotubular and nano-pitted anodic films on grade 2 titanium dental implant materials. *Materials Science and Engineering: C*. 2017;78:69–78.
27. Xu K, Li Y, Hu J, Li F, Tian J, Xue B et al. Effect of titanium dioxide nanoparticles on silkworm's innate immunity and resistance to bacillus bombyseptieus. *Science of Advanced Materials*. 2016;8(8):1512–22.
28. Chen W, Kuang Q, Wang Q, Xie Z. Engineering a high energy surface of anatase TiO_2 crystals towards enhanced performance for energy conversion and environmental applications. *RSC Advances*. 2015;5(26):20396–409.
29. Lim Y-C, Zainal Z, Tan W-T, Hussein MZ. Anodization parameters influencing the growth of titania nanotubes and their photoelectrochemical response. *International Journal of Photoenergy*. 2012.
30. Diamanti M, Pedeferri M. Effect of anodic oxidation parameters on the titanium oxides formation. *Corrosion Science*. 2007;49(2):939–48.
31. Luo Z, Poyraz AS, Kuo C-H, Miao R, Meng Y, Chen S-Y et al. Crystalline mixed phase (anatase/rutile) mesoporous titanium dioxides for visible light photocatalytic activity. *Chem Mater*. 2015;27(1):6–17.
32. Escobar-Alarcón L, Haro-Poniatowski E, Camacho-López M, Fernández-Guasti M, Jimenez-Jarquin J, Sánchez-Pineda A. Growth of rutile TiO2 thin films by laser ablation. *Surface Engineering*. 1999;15(5):411–14.
33. Österlund L, ed. Structure-reactivity relationships of anatase and rutile TiO2 nanocrystals measured by in situ vibrational spectroscopy. *Solid State Phenomena*; 2010: Trans Tech Publ.
34. Zhao Y-L, Wang C-H, Zhai Y, Zhang R-Q, Van Hove MA. Selective adsorption of l-serine functional groups on the anatase TiO_2 (101) surface in benthic microbial fuel cells. *Physical Chemistry Chemical Physics*. 2014;16(38):20806–17.
35. Yang HG, Sun CH, Qiao SZ, Zou J, Liu G, Smith SC et al. Anatase TiO_2 single crystals with a large percentage of reactive facets. *Nature*. 2008;453(7195):638–41.
36. Zhao X, Jin W, Cai J, Ye J, Li Z, Ma Y et al. Shape-and size-controlled synthesis of uniform anatase Tio_2 nanocuboids enclosed by active {100} and {001} facets. *Advanced Functional Materials*. 2011;21(18):3554–63.
37. Chen C, Ikeuchi Y, Xu L, Sewvandi GA, Kusunose T, Tanaka Y et al. Synthesis of [111]-and {010}-faceted anatase TiO_2 nanocrystals from tri-titanate nanosheets and their photocatalytic and DSSC performances. *Nanoscale*. 2015;7(17):7980–91.

38. Truong QD, Hoa HT, Le TS. Rutile TiO_2 nanocrystals with exposed {331} facets for enhanced photocatalytic CO_2 reduction activity. *Journal of Colloid and Interface Science*. 2017.
39. Lai Z, Peng F, Wang H, Yu H, Zhang S, Zhao H. A new insight into regulating high energy facets of rutile TiO_2. *Journal of Materials Chemistry A*. 2013;1(13):4182–5.
40. Fischer S, Munz AW, Schierbaum K-D, Göpel W. The geometric structure of intrinsic defects at TiO2 (110) surfaces: An STM study. *Surface Science*. 1995;337(1–2):17–30.
41. Diebold U, Lehman J, Mahmoud T, Kuhn M, Leonardelli G, Hebenstreit W et al. Intrinsic defects on a TiO_2 (110)(1× 1) surface and their reaction with oxygen: A scanning tunneling microscopy study. *Surface Science*. 1998;411(1):137–53.
42. Shultz AN, Jang W, Hetherington W, Baer DR, Wang L-Q, Engelhard MH. Comparative second harmonic generation and X-ray photoelectron spectroscopy studies of the UV creation and O_2 healing of Ti3+ defects on (110) rutile TiO_2 surfaces. *Surface Science*. 1995;339(1–2):114–24.
43. Park K-H, Koak J-Y, Kim S-K, Heo S-J. Wettability and cellular response of UV light irradiated anodized titanium surface. *The Journal of Advanced Prosthodontics*. 2011;3(2):63–8.
44. Hugenschmidt MB, Gamble L, Campbell CT. The interaction of H_2O with a TiO_2 (110) surface. *Surface Science*. 1994;302(3):329–40.
45. Sun S, Yu W, Zhang Y, Jiang X, Zhang F. Effects of TiO_2 nanotube layers on RAW 264.7 macrophage behaviour and bone morphogenetic protein-2 expression. *Cell Proliferation*. 2013;46(6):685–94.
46. Lü W, Wang N, Gao P, Li C, Zhao H, Zhang Z. Effects of anodic titanium dioxide nanotubes of different diameters on macrophage secretion and expression of cytokines and chemokines. *Cell Proliferation*. 2015;48(1):95–104.
47. Wang J, Qian S, Liu X, Xu L, Miao X, Xu Z et al. M2 macrophages contribute to osteogenesis and angiogenesis on nanotubular TiO_2 surfaces. *Journal of Materials Chemistry B*. 2017;5(18):3364–76.
48. Karazisis D, Ballo AM, Petronis S, Agheli H, Emanuelsson L, Thomsen P et al. The role of well-defined nanotopography of titanium implants on osseointegration: Cellular and molecular events in vivo. *International Journal of Nanomedicine*. 2016;11:1367.
49. Zhang S-M, Qiu J, Tian F, Guo X-K, Zhang F-Q, Huang Q-F. Corrosion behavior of pure titanium in the presence of Actinomyces naeslundii. *Journal of Materials Science: Materials in Medicine*. 2013;24(5):1229–37.
50. Yu W-q, Qiu J, Xu L, Zhang F-q. Corrosion behaviors of TiO_2 nanotube layers on titanium in Hank's solution. *Biomedical Materials*. 2009;4(6):065012.
51. Ekstrand-Hammarström B, Akfur CM, Andersson PO, Lejon C, Österlund L, Bucht A. Human primary bronchial epithelial cells respond differently to titanium dioxide nanoparticles than the lung epithelial cell lines A549 and BEAS-2B. *Nanotoxicology*. 2012;6(6):623–34.
52. Gerloff K, Fenoglio I, Carella E, Kolling J, Albrecht C, Boots AW et al. Distinctive toxicity of TiO_2 rutile/anatase mixed phase nanoparticles on Caco-2 cells. *Chemical Research in Toxicology*. 2012;25(3):646–55.
53. Liu N, Chang Y, Feng Y, Cheng Y, Sun X, Jian H et al. {101}–{001} Surface heterojunction-enhanced antibacterial activity of titanium dioxide nanocrystals under sunlight irradiation. *ACS Applied Materials & Interfaces*. 2017;9(7):5907–15.
54. Vadalà M, Laurino C, Palmieri B. The memory lymphocyte immunostimulation assay in immune system disorders: Is useful or useless? *Journal of Laboratory Physicians*. 2017;9(4):223.
55. Muller K, Valentine-Thon E. Hypersensitivity to titanium: Clinical and laboratory evidence. *Neuroendocrinology Letters*. 2006;27(1):31–5.

5 Bacterial Attachment and Biofilm Formation on Biomaterials
The Case of Dental and Orthopaedic Implants

Lia Rimondini and Michael Gasik

CONTENTS

5.1 INTRODUCTION

The key challenges in developing medical devices are device efficacy, suitability and patient safety. The main issue related to orthopaedic implants is strongly connected to bone quality, design of the implant and the interface between implant and bone tissue. Demand for orthopaedic implants has grown astronomically over the last several decades as an ageing but lively generation searches for ways to remain active. Better understanding about the technology of implantation among patients will contribute to this demand for the next 20 to 30 years. As with any surgery, implantation might have complications, of which those associated with acute and delayed prosthetic joint infections (PJI) remain a high concern.

Periprosthetic joint infections (PJIs) are a devastating complication after arthroplasty and are associated with substantial patient morbidity [1]. PJIs can drastically compromises patients' quality of life, causing pain, immobility and generally necessitating additional operations, leading to significant potential tissue loss. Additional time in hospital and operations also increase the risk of further nosocomial infections with potentially highly resistant pathogens, which can result in further complications and can eventually be fatal (a rate of 25% was given for revision surgeries due to such secondary infections [2,3]). The prevalence of lifestyle-related diseases such as diabetes, obesity etc. is on the rise and contributes to the increase in complication rates. They are expected to increase by 673% for total hip and 174% for total knee arthroplasties in the USA alone by 2030, with the annual revision costs to US hospitals increased ranging from $320 million to $566 million during 2001–2009, projected to exceed $1,620 million by 2020 [4]. Many "aseptic loosening" cases in the past were actually improperly identified or reported, in more than 70% of cases being caused by bacteria [5,6].

The most alarming issue in PJI is fast-growing resistance of bacterial strains against all known antibiotics and antibacterial drugs. Recent discovery [7] of the fast-spreading polymyxin-resistant mcr-1 gene in bacteria present in live feedstock and environment leaves little space of success for any antibiotics to treat possible PJI [8].

Total joint arthroplasties have a substantial rate for infections [9–13], and concurrent infections at spinal surgery may manifest months or years later, with 5–10% of patients developing deep infections after 11–45 months. The longer the amount of time before surgery, the harder it is to cure an infection without removing the implant. The rising number of implantations means more patients will potentially suffer from these infections unless that rate is significantly reduced. This also put a huge burden of cost on the healthcare system and patients, as the direct costs of treatments due to PJI in the USA are estimated to be $25,000–90,000 (depending on severity of the case), and, on average, £75,000 in the UK per infection case, causing losses of more than $800 million (USA) and more than £170 million (UK) every year [14–16].

Infections are becoming more common due to the increasing prevalence of multi-drug-resistant bacteria in hospital settings. The reported death rates due to MRSA (methicillin-resistant *S. aureus*) infections are of 20,000–40,000 mortalities annually in the USA and ~25,000 in the EU [17]. Most micro-organism-caused infections are present in the host flora (including those on skin) and cannot be fully avoided [18]. Common biofilm-related medical device infections (including dental cases [19,20]) are due to the Gram-negative *Pseudomonas aeruginosa*, *Pseudomonas fluorescens* or *Escherichia coli*, or to the Gram-positive *Staphylococcus epidermidis*, *Staphylococcus aureus* or *enterococci*. Staphylococci are associated with metallic and polymer orthopaedic implants and an antibiotic treatment application is common practice [9–13,21,22]. Treatment of *S. aureus*-infected implants with antibiotics in general necessitates their removal [21]. Due to the favourable surface provided by the implant, the *S. aureus* minimal infecting dose is significantly increased [9].

Hospitals are a source of special pathogens that are under continuous change that has a considerable effect on their pathogenicity [23]. This is an underlying reason for the threat of multi-drug resistance (MDR) by hospital bacteria, which increases the risks of peri implant infections. At the moment of this publication, the collectively known MDR strains under the acronym of "ESKAPE" were identified species *Enterococcus faecium*, *S. aureus*, *Klebsiella pneumoniae*, *Acinetobacter baumannii*, *P. aeruginosa*, and *Enterobacter spp.* The common human skin bacterium *S. epidermidis*, once considered harmless, has become one of the most important pathogens causing chronic infection in immunocompromised, immunosuppressed and long-term hospitalised hosts, as well as one of the leading causes of infections of implanted medical devices [24].

In addition to broad variation between bacterial species, each individual species contains many strains that differ from each other in a small but definable way [25]. For example, *S. aureus* infections may be present in two patients; however, one of these infections could be susceptible to commonly used antibiotics, whilst the other is resistant – for example, MRSA. This therefore makes it difficult to characterise bacterial-biomaterial interactions without studying an array of clinically relevant species and strains [26].

Fungal species are also a potential infection source. In vascular catheter infections, the fungus *Candida albicans* has been isolated on a regular basis [27]. Fungal infections (mycoses) are significantly increasing due to the use of broad-spectrum antibodies and immunosuppressive therapies, as well as the presence of foreign bodies (implants) [28]. Sepsis due to fungal infection increased by over 200% in the USA alone between 1979 and 2000 [29].

Fungal sepsis is chiefly secondary to candidemia (especially *C. glabrata* and *C. albicans*), accounting for 70–80% of yeasts isolated from patients [30]. Candida species grow as unicellular yeasts, but they can convert to multicellular, filamentous forms of growth, pseudohyphae and pseudomycelium, with *C. albicans* and *C. dubliniensis* able to form true hyphae. Candida were reported to be the fourth-most common organism recovered from bloodstream infections in the USA, associated with a crude mortality rate of about 40%. Several Candida virulence factors contribute to their ability to cause infection, including surface molecules that permit adherence of the organism to other structures (human cells, extracellular matrix, prosthetic devices). Within the hospital setting, areas with the highest rates of candidemia include intensive care units (ICUs), surgical units, trauma units and neonatal ICUs. In fact, the application of anti-biotics increases colonisation of the GI tract by Candida from ~30% in normal immunocompetent adults to nearly 100% colonisation rates in patients receiving antibiotics [31].

Mycoses in orthopaedic applications due to candidiasis are increasing problems in spine (vertebral and intravertebral disk), wrist, femur, humerus and osteochondral junctions. Patients with underlying joint disease (e.g., rheumatoid arthritis, prosthetic joints) are at increased risk. Candida arthritis can occur in any joint and is usually monoarticular (knee), but has been reported to affect multiple joints in up to 25%

of cases. Infection resembles bacterial septic arthritis, but chronic infection often develops with secondary bone involvement because of the delay in diagnosis and suboptimal treatment [31].

5.2 FORMATION OF BIOFILM AND PROGRESS OF MEDICAL DEVICE-ASSOCIATED INFECTION

5.2.1 What Is a Biofilm?

Biofilms are phenotypically diverse populations of bacteria and/or fungi, embedded in the mainly autogeneous extracellular slime matrix [32,33]. Other components in the biofilm include multivalent cations, inorganic particles and colloidal and dissolved compounds. For bacteria, the advantages of biofilm formation are protection from antibiotics, or other "unpleasant" factors, and variations in dynamic environments. Intercellular communications ("quorum sensing") within a biofilm rapidly stimulate the regulation of gene expression enabling temporal adaptation such as phenotypic variation and the ability to survive in "harsh" conditions. Bacteria quorum sensing engages chemical molecules, acting as messages that their infectious agents are able to recognise.

Quorum sensing can not only occur within a bacterial species but also between diverse species, and can regulate different processes, serving as a communication network. Not surprisingly, about 99% of the world's population of bacteria has been found in the form of a biofilm at various stages of growth and the films are as diverse as the bacteria are numerous [34]. The physiology and molecular nature of biofilm formation varies greatly between organisms. Biofilms play a vital role in both the persistence of infection and the failure of treatment regimens (the two key clinical features of BRI). They can be considered to be stable microenvironments in which bacteria are protected from host-defence mechanisms and most therapeutic agents [35].

Upon implantation, a biomaterial is coated by the surrounding body fluids (saliva, blood, tissue fluid etc.), which results in a pre-conditioning film. This film, containing proteins such as fibronectin and fibrinogen, enables the attachment of bacteria [36]. The surface properties of the biomaterial are an important determinant of this process [22]. Other physicochemical factors that can affect the bacterial adhesion include oxygen tension, pH, surface energy, wettability, topography etc.

An and Friedman [22] described adhesion as a situation where bacteria adhere firmly to a surface by complete physicochemical interactions between them, including an initial phase of reversible physical contact and a time-dependent phase of irreversible chemical and cellular adherence (i.e., where energy is involved in the formation of an adhesive junction between the bacteria and surfaces). Adherence is a general description of bacterial adhesion (the initial process of attachment of bacteria directly to a surface) and is a less scientific term for bacterial adhesion. Attachment can be defined as the initial stage of bacterial adhesion, referring more to physical contact than to complicated chemical and cellular interactions, and is usually reversible. Bacterial adhesion is a complex process related to several parameters such as the presence of proteins, bacterial species, material surface properties etc. [22,37]. The intrinsic chemical nature and superficial topography of implant materials can indeed influence (to a certain extent) an early microbial adhesion and the chances of eventual colonisation of the prosthesis [38,39].

Following the initial attachment phase (once the biomaterial surface is ready), the microorganisms adopt a highly characteristic metabolic state, when they begin to produce enzymes and encapsulate the thick extracellular polymeric matrix from glycoside residues, which they synthesise intracellularly. This protects the bacteria against the host immune system and provides an adhesion site for further bacterial attachment [40,41]. Inside this matrix, bacteria divide and eventually form a three-dimensional community [42]. This mucoid substance consists mainly of high-molecular-mass polysaccharide, which appears to determine both the structure and cohesive strength of biofilms by promoting bacterial cell-to-cell associations and the development of thick layers of bacteria [43].

A more detailed description of the biofilm formation phases also takes into account biofilm topology and time evolution scale (Figure 5.1). For example [44], five biofilm phases have been described: the initial binding (adhesion) is stage I (attachment may still be reversible, as some cells can detach). Stage II starts when the adhesion becomes irreversible (some minutes after stage I). After the initial adhesion to the epithelial surface, the bacteria start to multiply while emitting chemical signals that inter-communicate between the bacterial cells – a process known as "quorum sensing". Once the signal intensity exceeds a certain threshold, the genetic mechanisms underlying exopolysaccharide (EPS) production are activated, leading to the entrapment of nutrients and other planktonic bacteria [45]. During stage II, aggregates are formed and bacterial motility is decreased, forming progressively layered stacks of 10–50 μm (the biofilm stage III). When the biofilm reaches its ultimate thickness (generally > 100–150 μm), it goes into stage IV, indicating its maximal mechanical stability. During stage V, bacterial dispersion becomes notable as some bacteria return to the planktonic phenotype and leave the biofilm. This begins several days after stage IV [46].

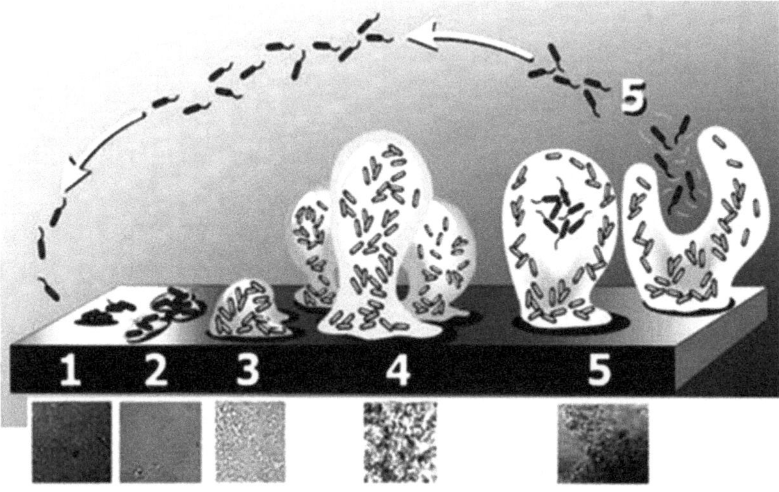

FIGURE 5.1 Schematic model of the phases involved in formation based on information in [37,47,48].

5.2.2 Why and How Does Biofilm Cause Infection?

The first step in the development of biomaterial-associated infection is considered the trigger to formation of a multilayered community of bacteria embedded in a self-produced matrix of extracellular polymeric substance, i.e., a biofilm [12,40,49]. The concept of the biofilm phenotype explains the persistence of bacterial infection and the need to remove the implant to eradicate infection (Figure 5.2). The extremely stable and virulent biofilm is formed after attachment and colonisation of bacteria embedded in extracellular products (EPS slime), making bacteria thousands of times more resistant to antibiotics [21,37,50,51].

The course of infections involves three major preparatory phases, as shown above: (1) microbial adhesion; (2) microbial proliferation; and (3) final formation of a bacterial biofilm. However, the simple existence of biofilm does not yet mean the course of infection, when the biofilm is still in its more or less latent state. After some time, bacteria in biofilm start to generate toxic metabolic products and release planktonic bacteria by rolling, spreading or other mechanisms, triggering immune and inflammatory responses.

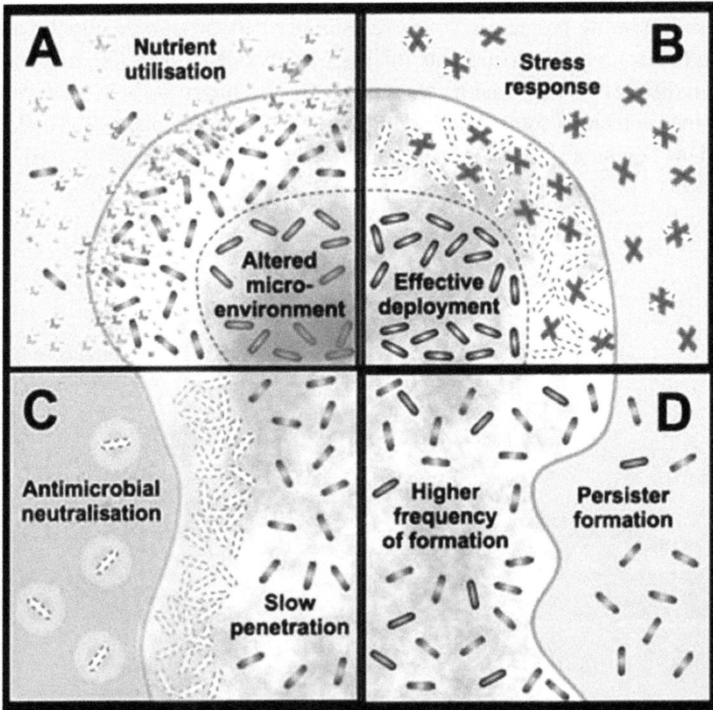

FIGURE 5.2 Reactive responses schematic of bacteria in different areas of biofilm based on the information in [47].

The pathogenesis of peri-implant infections differs from that of other post-surgical infections for a series of phenomena that are strictly related to the presence of foreign bodies – biomaterials [13]. The interstitial milieu surrounding prosthetic implants is known to represent a region of local immune depression and an immuno-incompetent fibro-inflammatory zone [52], highly susceptible to microbial colonisation and favourable to the instauration of infections [22,53,54]. The critical dose of contaminating microorganisms required to produce infection is much lower when a foreign material (implant surface) is present at the site [13,55–58]. For instance, it was reported that only ~100 bacteria CFU are sufficient to contaminate completely a sterile orthopaedic implant vs. ~10000 CFU without this foreign-body presence [59]. Permanent implants do also produce additional disturbances like debris due to micromotions, corrosion and mechanical wear. This can damage the tissues surrounding the implant, creating conditions where the immune defences are mostly depleted. The local immuno-depression present in the peri-prosthetic tissue generally facilitates the establishment of an infection for all implant materials (these issues are addressed in more detail in the below materials-specific sections).

It was also suggested that biofilm's ability to cause chronic infections by periodically releasing planktonic species (which are recognised by the host immune system) is the optimal way for pathogens to survive [60].

It is now understood that chronic inflammatory diseases result from infection with a large microbiota of chronic biofilm and L-form bacteria (Th1 pathogens). Some bacterial L-forms, lacking cell walls, are able to reside inside macrophages, which makes them "invisible" to immune response, thus circumventing their detection by identification of the proteins on their cell walls [61]. Many of the Th1 pathogens are capable of creating substances that bind and inactivate the vitamin D receptor – a fundamental receptor of the body that controls the activity of the innate immune system [62]. The formation of biofilms may contribute to immune dysfunction; as patients acquire a more virulent form of Th1 pathogens and other persistent bacterial forms, it becomes easy for biofilms to form on any tissue surface of the human body.

5.3 BIOFILMS ON IMPLANT SURFACES

5.3.1 General Features of Biofilms on Implants

The links between host-related and local environmental factors and biofilm infections are generally known, but the link between them and prosthetic biomaterials is not very clear. The clinical data is limited on the influence of different biomaterials on prosthetic BRI. The international consensus group [63] concluded that, based on the available medical literature, the incidence of such infections does not vary, regardless of whether cemented arthroplasty components (without antibiotics) or uncemented arthroplasty components are used.

The structure of biofilm varies greatly depending on the bacterial nature, biomaterial, surface properties and the conditions. Some typical features of the biofilm formed on the implant sur-face are schematically shown in Figure 5.3. Besides the biofilm core itself, the topology might have voids and channels for fluid flow and may exhibit tails or streamers, from which separate bacteria or their clusters leave for

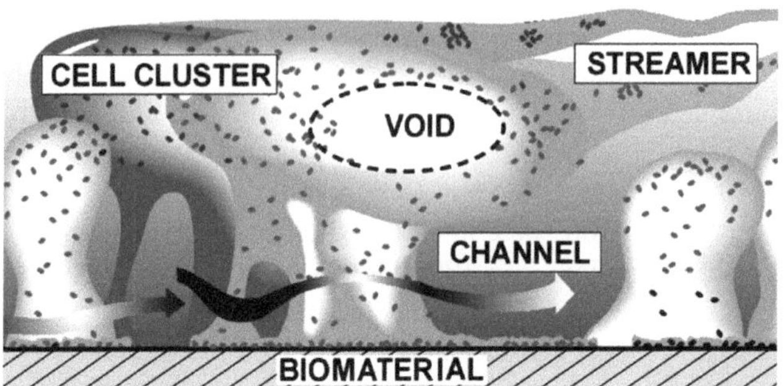

FIGURE 5.3 Main components of the biofilm structure on the surface of a biomaterial. (Drawn with data modified from Van Eldere, J., Gasthuisberg, U.Z., Pathogenesis and clinical importance of biofilms. Presentation (29 June 2006), REGA Institute and Katholieke Universiteit Leuven (Belgium), 2006.)

expansion into other areas. This periodic release of planktonic bacteria from some biofilms may be the cause of many relapsing infections.

Most available implants have rough surfaces, as roughness improves the stability and integration of the implant in the hard tissue. However, biofilms grow more easily on rough surfaces [64]. The roughness threshold for biofilm formation in the oral cavity has been shown [65] to be Ra ~0.2 μm: below this threshold, for Ra values within the microscale, there is no significant improvement in inhibiting bacterial adhesion [66]. In contrast, at the nanoscale, rough and geometrically determined surfaces can have antifouling properties [67]. However, other variables such as the nature and the quantity of adsorbed proteins [68], surface energy and short-range interactions are also important [10].

The behaviour of biofilm on flat surfaces is also different from those biofilms residing inside very rough surfaces on in porous bodies [9,69] (coatings or similar). Implants with highly rough and porous surface structures are in general prone to greater bacterial adhesion in comparison to devices presenting smooth surfaces. The most logical explanation to these findings is due to the much larger surface area accessible for adhesion [37]. However, the monitoring of biofilm formation in porous structures is difficult with the currently available techniques [70]. Besides the "optimal" implant anti-bacterial function (not considering specific drug-carrying surfaces), the requirements for osteoblast fixation, mechanical and biomechanical constraints set additional challenges for implant development.

In addition to orthopaedic joint prosthetics (internal implants), percutaneous implant devices also suffer from a lack of successful skin integration around the biomaterial exit site due to bacteria invasion [71]. As bacteria colonise the implant surface and adjacent damaged tissue, biomaterial exit sites become the gateway to infection [10,72–74], indicating higher occurrence of osteomyelitis after insertion of an external fixator.

For all types of implants and surfaces, it is important to note that biofilm formation does not happen independently of reactions between the implant surface (foreign body), host tissue cells and the whole system, including immune response. One of the concepts employed in such analysis [75] is "race for surface": microbes are racing against the tissue cells to occupy the clean, sterilised surface of the biomaterial. If bacteria win this race, as usually happens since bacteria start the race earlier, contaminating the surface during surgery and *in vivo* placement, biofilm is formed and tissue cells have little chance to establish a proper interface [76]. When the surface generates an inflammatory reaction, immune system activation might hinder biofilm formation to some extent.

In addition, it should be considered that the essential notion found in the literature of favouring the hydrophilic over the hydrophobic forces is likely oversimplifying, considering the complexity of biological communications in the region of an implant. Moreover, the physical-chemical parameters are often not adequately measured – hydrophilicity may be measured with different techniques (sessile drop contact angle method using different liquids, using one liquid or two liquids in static or dynamic conditions or using Wilhelmy's plate dynamic method) and the results are not easily comparable. Finally, many physicochemical properties have a reciprocal influence. For instance, roughness strongly affects the superficial charges and hydrophilicity properties: the same materials may display different wetting properties in relation to the roughness as described by Wenzel's or Cassie-Baxter's wetting models. All these aspects make it difficult to find a sound explanation of what is experimentally or clinically observed.

It is clear that further researches are needed in co-cultures of cells and bacteria on realistic implant surfaces to understand the synergy and the mechanism of surface colonisation in proper conditions. There are numerous reasons why biofilms are extremely difficult to culture; due to diffusion of liquid through a biofilm, the fluid and mechanical forces acting on a biofilm must be known to be cultured correctly [77]. Taking into account the three-dimensional structure of biofilm and tissues, we prefer to talk about "the race for space" instead of just surface alone, as it is evident the dynamics and proliferation of the biofilm and tissues are clearly not limited to surface characteristics alone. Also, very little has thus far been studied about anisotropy of structures and properties of biofilms, which can have great value in different cases, such as in the contamination of stents and catheters.

5.3.2 Biomechanics of Biofilms and Their Interaction with Implants and Environment

Analysis of the mechanical properties of biofilms, such as biofilm deformation under shear or multidirectional stress [78], is an important aspect in their treatment [79]. Some examples of such forces are for oral cavity tongue movements and tooth brushing, blood flow for vascular implants and the interstitial fluid and biomaterial movements in orthopaedic implants [78].

When detachment forces acting on a biofilm exceed the forces acting between different organisms in a biofilm, the latter is overloaded, leading to its failure. When detachment forces exceed the forces by which the initially adhering organisms connect with a substrate, the entire biofilm dislodges from the substrate [80]. Increased fluid-related or mechanical shear [81], the presence of locking cations [82] (such as Ca^{2+}), increased EPS production [83], EPS composition [84] and changes in quorum sensing [85] are all known to affect the strength and stiffness of bacterial biofilms. These and other studies suggest that biofilms behave as viscoelastic materials [80,81], and even though values of the elastic and viscous properties vary by many orders of magnitude, viscoelasticity is common for biofilms [86]. The relaxation time constant for a collection of biofilms (*S. aureus*, *S. mutans* etc.) was found to be about 18 min. As the bacterial doubling times are in similar ranges [87], the relaxation of biofilms is tightly related with their survival under transient stresses. However, there are as yet no extensive consistent studies of viscoelasticity of biofilms, which might be very different for biofilm inside porous or on a rough surface implants, where traditional rheology test methods are not suitable.

In terms of the general behaviour of viscoelastic materials, they might be approximated to some extent with a modified biphasic theory used for biomechanical description of highly hydrated tissues such as cartilage [88]. Their solid and fluid constituents might be presented as nearly idealised solid and fluid, linked with share of stresses between the phases, whilst keeping the compliance in deformation and shear rate. Experiments confirm biofilms themselves being highly compressible [89], and since water is almost incompressible at physiological conditions, water is squeezed out of the channels. This process may also constitute the reason as to why biofilm elasticity and viscosity is dependent of the mode of stress application [78]. Here, one would observe the size effect caused by the diameter of the indenter or a compression plate, as boundary conditions for such test would be less predictable; that is why use of indentation the method (e.g., as used in the analysis of cartilage biomechanics) is not recommended for biofilms.

More consistent, physiologically relevant test protocols were developed for application of simple unconfined dynamic compression (as closer to many implant applications) with ~1 Hz frequency and strain-controlled deformation, immersed in the corresponding media [90]. Upon programmed strain increase and measurement of the force required and resulting phase shift it is possible to extract biomechanical parameters of biofilms and tissues with much higher precision. Addition of other variables like drug input or change in media can also assist in understanding how specific biofilms react to environmental changes. One has to be cautious in defining testing conditions for biofilms, as improper selection of combination of specimen thickness, frequency and amplitude of deformation may give substantial artifacts [91]. However, when such studies are made with realistic contaminated biomaterials surfaces, this may also give valuable information for the implementation of associated therapeutic measures [78]. In *C. albicans* fungal biofilms hyphal content was found to be a determining parameter for the strength of biofilms [92]; a high hyphal content shows more resistance of the biofilm to compression. This makes removal of such biofilms more difficult using vortexing and sonification. In that study neither polysaccharides nor proteins were found to contribute significantly to biofilm strength. Additionally, there was no correlation between biofilm thickness and hydrophobicity in that study.

Beyond biofilm formation on implant surfaces, bacterial activities can also directly affect implants by degrading the biomaterials or by inducing corrosion [93]. The reduction of pH in the titanium implant microenvironment in the presence of biofilms can significantly decrease titanium's corrosion resistance [94]. The presence of lactic acid-producing bacteria such as *S. mutans* can increase the corrosion risk of titanium-based implants.

The effect of biofilms in sliding was studied previously [95] for titanium implants covered with biofilms containing *S. mutans* and *C. albicans*. It was shown that the biofilm presence can act as a lubricant, with important ramifications as the decrease in the friction between the implant and the surrounding tissue, due to the presence of the biofilm, can have important effects on implant loosening.

The degradation and wear debris from the damaged implant have been clearly correlated with surrounding microenvironment physiological alterations: this often causes the innate and adaptive immunity reaction that bring to a massive macrophage and lymphocyte T-activation [96]. This inflammatory phase usually compromises the implanted tissue and facilitates bacteria adhesion and colonisation of the device and, sometimes, of the related and surrounding tissues. This seems to be of the most concern in metal-on-polymer (MoP) joint implants, such as metallic alloys vs. cross-linked polyethylene. A significant time-dependent surface degradation was reported for MoP where particles of different size and character are released from the implants surfaces.

Wear particles, pro-adhesive molecules recruitment and stimulation of the immune system are some examples of the impaired devices-surrounding tissue networks due to the metal and polymeric particles release. This situation often favours bacteria implant colonisation, leading to severe infections and the need for device replacement. Stimulation of cellular immune responses results in superoxide radical and cytokine-mediated tissue damage which increases susceptibility to implant infection or aseptic loosening, with initiation of a cytokine cascade. A self-perpetuating, immunoincompetent fibro-inflammatory zone develops around implants, which features tissue cell damage, increases susceptibility to infection and results in failure of the implant [52].

The combined impact of biofilms on corrosion, erosion and wear of biomaterials remains unclear, although there are clinical indications in orthopaedic practice that there is a potential link between the type of bearing surface and the subsequent PJI [97]. This is accompanied by increased potential risk because of the ability of metal debris particles to modulate the immune system and bacterial growth [98]. Although as yet based only on limited data, Parvizi reported [99] that the incidence of infection was significantly higher with metal-on-polyethylene surfaces (1.1%) compared to patients with ceramic-on-polyethylene (0.87%) or ceramic-on-ceramic surfaces (0.54%).

MoM implant degradation has been shown in correlation to other severe side effects: increase of cytokine release (IL-6 and TNF-α) from immune effector cell, up-regulation of TNF-α gene in osteocytes, viability decrease of fibroblasts, dissemination in different body sites (such as liver and spleen) via lymphatic system and induction of immune system [100]. This large spectrum of side effects is due to the toxicity not only of the delivered particles, but also of the emanated ions (derived from chromium oxide). In fact, ions have a genotoxic effect thanks to their ability to penetrate the cell membrane and to rapidly enter cells metabolic activities. If the particle concentration is very high, serious DNA damage is possible, leading to a severe carcinogenic risk.

5.3.3 Biofilms on Different Biomaterials

5.3.3.1 Metallic Biomaterials

Several metallic alloys are being widely employed in orthopaedic and dental cases, of which the majority are titanium alloys, stainless steels, cobalt-chromium-based alloys and noble metal alloys, with a lesser share of shape memory alloys and different composites [101]. Of these, titanium-based materials have been widely used as dental and orthopaedic implant materials because of their mechanical strength, corrosion resistance and biocompatibility [102–104]. However, biofilm formation still poses as a potential failure mechanism [105–107]. Even though the effect of certain parameters such as hydrophilicity is known to be a potential way of decreasing biofilm formation, the actual situation is complex, with multiple parameters related to bacteria and the biomaterial concerned contributing to biofilm formation [108–113]. As an example, streptococci species are not sensitive to hydrophilic surface modifications of titanium [114].

Orthopaedic titanium implant surfaces exhibit different roughness types [10,115], surface treatment and other features, usually designed to promote osseointegration and mechanical contact between the implant and host tissues [116,117]. All titanium (in general all metallic) implants might be roughly divided into ones with a highly porous surface (normally coating such as vacuum plasma-sprayed (VPS) titanium) and without it (polished, sandblasted, etched or otherwise treated). Furthermore, the implants can be additionally coated with an external layer (hydroxyapatite, bioactive glass etc.) and it general knowledge that such modification would critically affect surface roughness, porosity, wettability and consequently cell and bacterial adhesion [118]. Rough titanium surfaces enhance the formation of focal contacts by cells for stronger adhesion, and they guide cytoskeletal assembly and membrane receptor organisation [119–121].

For example, in a study [10], the adhesion of *S. aureus*, *S. epidermidis* and *P. aeruginosa* was examined on conventional titanium surfaces, "nanorough" surfaces (produced by electron beam evaporation) and nanotubular and nanotextured surfaces (by two different anodisation processes). The two latter cases had an amorphous TiO_2 layer generated during anodisation, on the contrary to conventional and nanorough surfaces, where the TiO_2 layer was crystalline. In that case, the nanorough Ti surfaces produced by electron beam evaporation decreased the adherence of the bacteria the most, taking into account similarity of the surface chemistries.

Whereas anatase, an amorphous or nanocrystalline thin film TiO_2 layer, is employed on a titanium surface [122], it may have its own antibacterial effect, the magnitude of which might depend even on how long this surface was exposed, for example, to sunlight or whether an antibiotic is also present [123]. Different concentrations of nano-scale TiO_2 were tested in a study [124] to find out the best concentration that can have the most effective antibacterial property against the MRSA culture. In the case of nalidixic acid, TiO_2 nanoparticles showed a synergic effect on the antibacterial activity of this antibiotic against a test MRSA strain. Thus, TiO_2 nanoparticles were empowered the antimicrobial action of ß-lactams, cephalosporins, aminoglycosides, glycopeptides, macrolids, lincosamides and tetracycline in combination effect against MRSA.

The effect of multiple parameters such as surface treatments, porosity and topography of titanium implants on bacteria and cell attachment [125] demonstrated that highly porous materials pose a higher risk of biofilm formation (with a threshold of 47% porosity) regardless of surface modifications. These experimental data indicate the possibility of decreasing the biofilm formation by 80–90% for flat substrates versus untreated, vacuum plasma-sprayed porous titanium and by 65–95% for other porous titanium coatings. It has also been shown that optimised surfaces also enhance cell proliferation and differentiation.

The use of different surface modifications for the purpose of simultaneous ossteo-integration and anti-biofilm resistance improvement was analysed *in vivo* for bioactive glass (BAG)-coated and hydrothermally treated (with anatase TiO_2 film) titanium [118]. It was observed that coating type behaves differently on "flat" and "porous" surfaces. For non-porous specimens little differences have been observed, but thin BAG coating behaves somewhat better, especially at longer implantation times. For porous specimens, the opposite seems to hold, as a BAG-treated specimen has worse behaviour than others, whereas hydrothermally treated titanium shows rather stable data for all implantation times for all parameters. This behaviour of specimens correlates well with the previous *in vitro* tests [125], which have proven to also ensure better condition for simultaneous bacteria repelling and promotion of osteogenic cells reactions.

Cobalt-chromium-molybdenum (CoCrMo) alloys are another type of metallic biomaterials used in several applications as implantable devices (including MoM and MoP combinations). As for other metals, they are also subject to corrosion and wear, and can be colonised with bacterial biofilms. The presence of pores due to degradation dramatically decreases the bacteria-anti-adhesive ability of metal alloy. A porous CrCoMo surface required a concentration of *S. aureus* 40 times smaller to become contaminated in comparison to the same polished material when implanted in a rabbit [126]. Moreover, CrCoMo results in a more bacteria-friendly surface than titanium, requiring an *S. aureus* suspension 15 times less concentrated to contaminate porous de-vices in comparison with the polished ones. Metal ions and particles are often the reason of delayed-type IV T-cell mediated immune response. In fact, the presence of metal ions can induce the release of IL-1, IL-6 TNF-α and IFN-ɣ from macrophages with a subsequent activation of T-lymphocytes. Intermediate-size particles can be recognised by macrophages as foreign bodies; as a consequence, they activate the antigen-presenting cell pathway, leading to a massive immune response and consequent implant failure [127]. The presence of metal particles has been also associated with prolonged infections.

It could be also advised that more details of the biomaterials have to be reported together – for example, listing of surface wettability only does not help to decide about the biofilm resistance ability if the means of its achievement would not be provided. Similar consistency is desirable for other physical parameters such as porosity, topography or roughness, as there is always a risk of insufficient information when the implant processing data were confined into few values.

5.3.3.2 Polymer Biomaterials

The types of polymer applied in orthopaedic and dental implants are usually limited to polyethylene (PE) with different density and molecular weight, polymethylmetacrylate

(PMMA) for bone cement and fluorinated polymers such as the PTFE and polyetheretherketone (PEEK) families [128–131]. In cartilage repair, biodegradable polylactic acid isomer (PLA, PLLA, PLDA)-based materials and composites are also used [132,133].

The surface topography is also important for polymeric implants for bacterial adhesion [26,134]. Due to the presence of plasticisers, differences in crystallinity etc., the variance in surface properties of polymers is higher temporally compared to metallic implants [135,136], such as diffusion of non-polymerised polymers into the surrounding tissue and having cytotoxic effects [137]. Moreover, release of polymeric debris, such as cross-linked polyurethane, causes macrophage activation and pro-inflammatory cytokine release, which can lead to adverse immune reactions and can even result in bone resorption [138].

As the majority of different polymers is extensively used in other medical products like blood and urinal catheters, studies were made to determine to what extent indigenous bacteria, lactobacilli, could colonise prosthetic devices *in vivo* and *in vitro* and could attach to specific polymer surfaces *in vitro.* Intrauterine devices (IUDs) are such a class of medical devices, which are continuously exposed to periodic and extreme conditions, shifting from more to less acidic or anaerobic, and linked with the cervical and vaginal flora, whose composition and contamination level are hardly predictable [139]. "Normal" vaginal flora typically shows a predominance of *Lactobacillus spp*, believed to promote a healthy milieu by providing numerical dominance and by producing lactic acid to maintain an acid environment, inhospitable to many bacteria [140,141]. Lactobacilli also produce hydrogen peroxide (H_2O_2), antibiotic toxic hydroxyl radicals, bacteriocins and probiotics [142,143]. In one study, polyethylene IUDs in place for two years were removed from six women who were asymptomatic and free of signs of cervical or uterine infection [144]. Lactobacilli were found well attached to the IUDs, demonstrating that bacterial biofilms consisting of indigenous bacteria can occur on prosthetic devices without inducing a symptomatic infection. *In vitro* studies for polyethylene specimens found well-documented lactobacilli strains *L. acidophilus* T-13, *L. casein* GR-1, GR-2 and RC-17 and *L. fermentum* A-60. These organisms were found to adhere to IUDs and polymer urinary catheters within 24 hours.

An interesting observation in that study was that adhesion of *L. acidophilus* T-13 to specific polymer surfaces was optimal at fluorinated ethylene propylene incubated for 9 h at 37°C in phosphate-buffered saline (pH 7.1). Besides, lactobacilli adhered well to polyethyleneterephthalate (PET), polystyrene (PS), sulfonated polystyrene and to silicone-latex catheter materials. The adherence *in vitro* to these polymers was linearly linked with increased hydrophobicity.

The effects of polymer component machining and molding on bacterial attachment, adhesion and biofilm formation were also studied on polyetheretherketone (PEEK), which is one of the most used polymers in different applications, including orthopaedics [26]. Rougher-machined PEEK surfaces provide a better milieu for bacterial attachment compared to moulded PEEK. Having surface features of the same order of magnitude as the adhering bacteria generally promotes adhesion; thus, individual surface structures with dimensions between 0.5–1.0 μm should generally be avoided to reduce bacterial adhesion [145–147].

One of the methods to influence bacterial attachment to polymer surfaces is to make their wettability more extreme. For example, the grafting of polyethylene glycol to polyurethane surfaces to increase wettability has been shown to dramatically decrease *E. coli* and *S. epidermidis* adhesion [148]. Surface thiocyanation has also been used to decrease wettability, leading to a 90% reduction in bacterial adhesion attributed to the altered surface chemistry without cytotoxicity [149]. However, the relationship between surface wettability and bacterial adhesion is not always clear due to the broad variation of bacterial adhesions and the complexity of physicochemical interactions in different media. Cunliffe et al. [150] found that bacterial adhesion was more species- than surface hydrophobicity-dependent. Nevertheless, due to a huge variety of polymer forms, surfaces, molecular and mechanical properties and degradability, it is difficult to predict in general whether or not some specific biomaterial would be less or more prone to bio-film formation.

Antibiotic-loaded cements (PMMA and similar) are commonly used for the prevention and treatment of orthopaedic infections [151]. However, recent data have emphasised that bacteria can persist and colonise antibiotic-impregnated bone cement [152]. For different antibiotic cement types (gentamicin, vancomycin), *S. epidermidis*, *S. aureus* and MRSA were the most frequent organisms identified in this study. It was found that *S. epidermidis* had persisted only on gentamicin-loaded beads, while MRSA could grow on gentamicin-vancomycin-impregnated cement as well. According to the Norwegian Arthroplasty Register, the further insertion of antibiotics into porous cements was not effective in preventing surgical site infection [153]. The persistence of bacterial growth on bone cement is a hazardous problem in orthopaedic surgery, as it can lead to the emergence of bacterial resistance to antibiotics and might result in clinical recurrence of infection [154].

5.3.3.3 Ceramic Biomaterials

The bioceramics types used in modern implants could be classified as bioinert and bioresorbable. The first group consists mainly of alumina, zirconia and composites based on them, whereas in the second class there are calcium phosphates [155] (hydroxyapatite, tricalcium phosphate, apatite, fluoroapatite), bioactive glass [156] (BAG), composites like apatite-wollastonite (AW) and BAG-ceramics [157]. These ceramics are of the most widespread use in clinical practice. Bioceramics is also widely applied in the form of coatings, manufactured by a variety of methods (plasma spray, sol-gel, chemical deposition, in situ synthesis, anodisation etc.). The most common are hydroxyapatite as an external coating [158] and TiO_2 (anatase) as generated on titanium alloy surfaces. The performance and effect of the latter on bacterial adhesion and biofilm formation was discussed above when considering titanium alloy substrates. However, the behaviour of TiO_2, which is produced separately (not grown from titanium), somewhat differs from the previous materials.

The photocatalytic inactivation of microorganisms seeded on formed TiO_2 surfaces on aluminium was studied [159] using ultra-violet LED illumination (388 nm). Such surfaces were found to be highly effective at eradicating *P. aeruginosa*, *S. aureus* and *C. albicans* cells, showing no obvious dependence on cell density. As for titanium-based TiO_2, a possible mechanism for inactivation based upon oxidation and reduction of cell membranes/walls is by photo-generated OH radicals. Those species with relatively thicker and complex cell wall structures (*C. albicans* and *S. aureus*) were destroyed more slowly than *P. aeruginosa*, which has a thinner cell wall. On the other hand, there are data indicating that the short-wave light itself is capable of destroying MRSA [160]. At the modern level of knowledge, anatase (TiO_2) antibacterial activity might be considered a proven mechanism that relies on generation of free and sufficiently long-lived radicals generating higher oxidative stress to bacterial species.

However, bioceramics can also be colonised by bacteria [64], even though there is a certain level of observed reduction in biofilm formation. A study with yttria-stabilised zirconia has shown that *S. mutans* attachment to zirconia was less than with titanium [161], with similar observations *in vivo* [162].

Generally speaking, no porous and high-mechanical-performance ceramics materials seem to have intrinsic antibacterial properties. For instance, no differences in biofilm formations were observed between glazed and polished yttrium-stabilised tetragonal zirconia polycrystal ceramic for dental prosthetic reconstructions. The slightly lower amount of bacteria recovered on polished surfaces was probably due to the superior surface smoothness, confirming what was previously debated about surface roughness importance in first bacteria adhesion [163].

Another key factor to be considered is the strong wear resistance of a ceramic surface in comparison with metallic and polymeric ones. Implant surface degradation is known to lead to severe alterations in micro- and nano-structures, potentially causing micro-cracks and surface charge variations. If devices are coated, the loss of the coating is also very common when surface degradation occurs. Polyethylene-based devices are frequently affected by structural yielding, causing high risk of failure due to structural cracks, which in addition are easily colonised by bacteria. Ceramic devices are strongly resistant to surface cracks, thus inhibiting the formation of bacteria-friendly regions versus polymers.

These factors have also been studied for the case of resorbable bioceramics such as hydroxyapatite [164]. Strains of *S. mutans* were applied on different hydroxyapatite disks and the adsorption of basic proteins was found to have a slightly enhanced effect on bacterial adhesion, whereas acidic proteins were observed to decrease it. The zeta-potential of hydroxyapatite was found correlated with absorbed molecule and the environment. It was, however, noted that interaction is more complex than could be expected based solely on electrostatic (Coulomb) interactions, as proteins absorbed onto hydroxyapatite were engaged in both short- and long-range interactions. The reduction of bacterial adherence with acidic proteins (poly-L-glutamate, phosvitin, caseins) was attributed to an increase in repulsion between electrical double layers surrounding the bacterium and the ceramic surface.

Some ceramics are also used as antibiotic carriers, which are intended for release of the active agent in the vicinity of the implant-tissue interface [165,166]. For example, silica nanoparticles (SiO_2) can be used as elegant carriers of antibiotics that prolong antibiotics release and decrease the frequency of administration [167]. Pure silica has no antimicrobial role independent of its size but in nano-powder form it can work as an effective drug carrier. Antimicrobial studies of hybrid SiO_2-gentamicin nanoparticles were shown to be especially effective against Gram-positive *B. subtilis*.

5.3.3.4 Other Biomaterial Types

Various elastomers and hydrogels as well as composites are some of the most used biomaterials in modern medical practice [168,169]. Hydrogels are polymeric materials that swell in water and retain a significant fraction of water within the three-dimensional network (cross-linked structures) without dissolving [170,171]. Earlier, they were less relevant to orthopaedic and dental implants, but recently application of elastomeric scaffolds to induce secondary bone healing is described as a paradigm shift in the approach to healing bone defects, which has traditionally involved matching hard bone with a rigid material that has stiffness similar to bone [172]. Despite these materials being "soft", they nevertheless show tendency to be contaminated with bacteria and form biofilms, which probability increases depending on the time the hydrogel is present in the site and not yet biodegraded.

To date, most of the issues related to biofilm-related infections with hydrogels were studies for soft tissue repair applications [173–175]. Such infections are generally bacterial (but can be fungal or viral), either acute (inflammation or abscesses at the site of injection, typically due to *S. aureus* or *S. pyogenes*), or delayed-onset chronic infections, which generally develop two or more weeks later, possibly involving an atypical organism (such as mycobacteria or *Escherichia coli*) [176]. The biofilm-related infections in such biomaterials are usually of delayed type, as virulent biofilms need some time to set up [177,178]. Common skin bacteria include *S. aureus*, coagulase-negative *Staphylcococcus spp*, *Streptococcus spp*, *Propionibacterium acnes* and possibly *Enterobacteriaceae* and *P. aeruginosa* [179,180]. The origin of infection of the hydrogel could be a contaminated implant, "surgical" environment, patient skin or seeding of the hydrogel from a remote infection source.

An example for the analysis of hydrogels to bacterial response *in vitro* was performed by Alijotas-Reig et al. [181] for soft tissue implants, such as hyaluronic acid, hydroxyapatite-based filler, polyalkylimide and polyacrylamide with *E. coli* as a bacterial strain. It was observed that non-degradable biomaterials did not allow bacterial growth over the biomaterial itself. This sounds logical, as more "solid" (nondegradable) biomaterials simply have fewer options to provide diffusive and mobility paths for cells and nutrients. Degradable hyaluronic and hydroxyapatite compounds thus allowed bacterial colonisation over the biomaterial (noting that behaviour for *S. aureus* or *Staphylcococcus spp* might possibly be different). However, as was pointed out, the behaviour of isolated or medium bacteria in suspension differ from that usually observed in biofilms (Figure 5.2). Permanent implants have an increased risk of low-grade infection due to a biofilm around them [182]. Thus, permanent hydrogels are more prone to biofilm formation. Logically, fillers with a higher water proportion should have a higher rate of fluid exchange with the surrounding tissue fluids, giving the gel a biomechanical stimulus, which disturbs the integrity of the biofilm [183].

5.4 COMBATING IMPLANT-ASSOCIATED BIOFILM INFECTIONS

As previously discussed, the eradication of biofilm from contaminated surfaces is still very challenging for clinicians and disappointing results in antibiotics therapies often lead to device replacement. Therefore, intense research in orthopaedics and other fields (such as materials science) are now focused on device surface modification in order to prevent bacteria adhesion [184]. Because biofilm is able to propagate the infection to the surrounding tissues, an ideal device design must forecast the prevention of biofilm formation and thus protect nearby (and sometimes distant) tissues. The general approaches are thus: (i) incorporation of potential bacteria-killing agents such as antibiotics, silver etc.; or (ii) suppression or prevention of biofilm matrix development by dispersing agents, quorum sensing silencing or other combined cues. The most recent and attractive techniques to induce antibacterial properties onto implant surfaces are briefly discussed below.

5.4.1 Utilisation of Bacteria-Killing Methods

For some biomaterials, one option is grafting/doping other metal ions capable of reduction of biofilm formation. Ions like silver, copper, bismuth and zinc are known to have oligodynamic effect (toxic effect on living organisms) on microorganisms. Silver is recognised as a powerful bacteria killer agent as it is able to bind DNA, RNA and phosphoproteins, causing a direct stop through genetic interference [185]. Moreover, silver was shown to be able to interpose bacteria metabolism through the binding of thiol groups [186] and by causing the production of reactive oxygen species [187]. Silver in nanoparticles is able to kill both Gram-negative and Gram-positive organisms [188], as demonstrated in studies involving *E. coli*, *Enterococcus spp* and *S. aureus* [189] and in pre-clinical *in vivo* studies [190].

Zinc has been extensively studied [191], but its efficacy was clear only for planktonic cells and not for complex biofilm communities [192]. Zinc activity is related to its ability to increase bacterial membrane permeability and subsequent cell damage by disrupting the bacterial cell wall. Most of the metallic implant studies are usually centred on modifying the titanium implant surface with these ions [193]. Similarly, zirconium-doped titanium presents antimicrobial activity beside high epithelial cell attraction and mediates healthy cell proliferation to promote the formation of an epithelial cell barrier over the implant surface, similar to titanium-free biomedical zirconium-niobium alloys [194].

In *in vitro* study [195] biomimetic antibacterial silver and gallium surface modification treatments were developed for titanium implants. In particular, the morphological, physico-chemical, biological and antibacterial characterisation features of silver- and gallium-modified titanium surfaces were reported. The antibacterial properties of silver, as shown above, are well-known [196] and have been extensively studied [197], despite some concerns on cell toxicity [198]; but more recently gallium has also been shown to have antibacterial properties, since it replaces Fe^{3+} in bacterial metabolism. Gallium anti-resorptive effects on bone and bone fragments show that it is adsorbed onto the surface of bone, where it is effective in blocking osteoclast resorption, without appearing to be cytotoxic to osteoclasts, or inhibiting cellular metabolism [199].

Antibiotics (despite the growing concerns about resistance) application remains one of the main therapeutic actions for biofilm-related infections, whether administrated locally, systemically or by prophylaxis. As mentioned earlier, traditional protocols might be rather ineffective in treatment that relates to lower efficacy of antibiotics for bacteria residing in biofilms. In dentistry, infection rates as high as

30% were reported despite prophylaxis [200]. Instead of massive, continuous antibiotic procedure, very low, pulsed doses of bacteriostatic antibiotics, additionally varying the order of their administration, were shown to be rather effective against biofilms and other Th1 pathogens [61]. The mechanism used in the Marshall protocol (which uses of a total of five bacteriostatic antibiotics [62]) is that a first wave of antibiotic will eradicate the bulk of the biofilm cells, leaving persister cells (the most resistant) intact and allowing them to grow again when the antibiotic supply is suspended. However, the persister bacteria cannot accumulate sufficient resistance to the drug and they cannot manage to form a new, more virulent biofilm before the second application of the antibiotic [61]. That should then completely eliminate the persister cells, which are still in planktonic state.

Recently, more data have been obtained on the activity of dormant (persister) population within biofilms, known as quiescence cells. For example, the MRSA biofilm mislays its antibiotic resistance when it disaggregates in fresh antibiotic-free liquid medium, while the resistance is re-acquired once clusters are exposed again to the same drugs [201]. So, these data also raise the question of whether affecting quiescence cells could improve the raising of more virulent phenotypes. It has been revealed that the cytoplasmic protease ClpP can be activated in *S. aureus* by antibiotic acyldepsipeptide (ADEP4) to kill persister cells by causing them to digest themselves.

On the local level (implant surface) there are several options for antibiotics administration. Antibiotics fixing to device surfaces is a common strategy to prevent or treat bacteria adhesion for orthopaedic implants. In general, vancomycin and gentamycin are the most commonly used, with proven efficacy [202]. Steel and titanium implants with vancomycin covalently bound to the surface were found to reduce bacterial colonisation in an ovine model. However, the limitation of this strategy is clearly related to the short time of drug loading and the limited neighbouring area of influence. In fact, antibiotics are not delivered and the efficacy is strictly related to the reservoir capability; also, without an operative delivery system, a drug's effects are limited to the tissue(s) in direct contact with the doped device and no or little protection is provided for surrounding tissues that can still be affected by infection. Very limited data are available for long-period assays regarding this kind of treatment, leading to a remarkable lack of information regarding bacteria adhesion prevention and possible immunological reactions.

To overcome these limitations, device surfaces can be optimised to deliver the engaged drugs (e.g., some mouldable materials or coatings can be designed with particular bead-like structures aimed to contain and deliver antibiotics). The usual goal is that these materials can deliver high local concentrations of antibiotics to the surgical site. By combining the mechanical stability and the long-lasting properties with the possibility to controlled drug delivery, it is possible to obtain materials that are able to maintain tissue integrity and sterility for very long periods after surgery.

Despite the noticeable advantages provided by these materials, the control of drug release still represents a challenging step due to the burst release of drugs. In this situation, one risk is that not all surrounding bacteria are killed, leaving a possible contamination source. Rapid drug release can also lead to the fast mutation of surviving bacteria to a drug-resistant strain (persisters), amplifying the possibility of strongly decreasing antibiotic efficacy. However, a very slow and sparing drug release is not effective, being unable to kill planktonic bacteria remaining in the surgical site. Therefore, clinical evidence pointing to the optimal parameters required for infection control are difficult to interpret [203]. This is a rationale for why alternative administration, like the Marshall protocol shown above, is a worthwhile option to override such challenges.

Nowadays, bioresorbable materials, such as calcium sulphate and calcium phosphates, have regained the interest for their readiness to mould them to the surgical site and to carry antibiotics during the production steps [204]. These materials have elution characteristics that can be better controlled by bead size and composition [205], and they do not provide a permanent surface for bacterial adhesion due to abruption and have been shown to be effective against osteomyelitis [206]. These solutions might be employed in the cases where sufficient mechanical properties are not required and thus they could not be used for long-period implants.

5.4.2 Utilising Preventive Methods

It is tempting to design and produce a surface capable of completely repelling bacterial and attracting only proper host tissue cells only by using topographical cues. However, while smooth surfaces decrease bacterial adhesion, they also are known to promote fibrotic capsule formation compared to rougher surfaces [207,208]. One potential way of circumventing this trade-off is through nanoscale topographies [209]. Nanoscale topographical features may be suitable for increasing eukaryotic cell adhesion through specific adhesion structures, yet too small to promote bacterial adhesion. The effect of nanotopographies is feature-dependent [51,210] and can decrease [10] or increase bacterial adhesion [211,212]. It is likely that (nano)topography should not be considered independently of the surface material, structure, chemistry and eventually biofilm-specific features [213].

However, it is very important to remember that the level of anti-adhesive properties has to respect and not overcome the purpose of a particular type of orthopaedic implant surface. For example, a deep anti-adhesive mono- or multi-layer could interfere with new bone formation, leading to early mechanical failure. Ideally, the best coating technology would be able to retain required host cell interactions and at the same time selectively prevent bacterial adhesion. Moreover, device properties might not only reduce bacteria adhesion but also prevent biofilm phenotype conversion [214].

A possible strategy of reducing bacterial adhesion is to bind molecules capable of modifying the hydrophilic properties of devices. Molecules like glycolipids, lipopeptides, polysaccharide–protein complexes, phospholipids, fatty acids and neutral lipids could be combined as single or mixed layers, forming a smooth sheet where bacteria are no longer able to adhere and start the recruitment of other floating planktonic cells [215]. However, it has also been demonstrated that such biosurfactants, like antibiotics, can be strain-specific and have a limited effectiveness towards multiple bacterial strains community [216]. As an example, literature showed that positively charged materials were able to reduce Gram-negative but not Gram-positive bacterial adhesion [217]. More promising results were obtained by binding macromolecules (heparin and heparin and polypeptides) to improve hydration of devices surfaces; with this strategy, biofilm formation was reduced by interfering with bacteria adhesion [218].

Since extracellular polysaccharides (EPS) represent a very important tool for bacteria aggregation and protection from drugs and the immune system, they are an important target to develop anti-biofilm strategies. DNase I is an effective DNA-digesting enzyme capable of breaking down eDNA *in vitro* [219]. As eDNA is a major component of biofilms [220], its digestion disrupts the biofilm [221]. The polysaccharides are the second target of disaggregating agent-based strategies. However, as opposed to eDNA, the degradation of species or genus specific polysaccharides require specific enzymes. As an example, Staphylococci are the most common pathogens related to orthopaedic infections; they can produce poly-N-acetylglucosamine that is successfully digested by dispersin B. The use of the latter was successful in eradicating biofilm from polyurethanes and catheters [222]. Disaggregating agents are therefore promising but still presenting a problem for patients as disaggregated single colonies are not inhibited and are free to float into the bloodstream. Thus, antibiotics therapy must be coupled with the use of disaggregating agents to prevent the propagation of the infection towards other locations.

Next, as biofilm formation and the gaining of virulence are often regulated by quorum sensing, it raises the question of whether quorum sensing could be effectively silenced. One of the most common signalling pathways was identified as the acetylated homoserine lactone-based (Las) system. There, an acetylated homoserine lactone is secreted into the surroundings, where it can be taken up by adjacent bacteria to bind with the LasR transcriptional regulator. Therefore, it should be possible to impose signalling silencing by the use of LasR inhibitors, targeting the Las quorum sensing system. This was proven in *P. aeruginosa* biofilms, accelerated bacterial clearance and reducing pathology in a mouse model of lung infection [223]. Encouraging results have been achieved also in a *Caenorhabditis elegans* model of infection [224]. Despite these promising results, the use of quorum sensing inhibitors has not yet been tested in clinical trials, probably due to the lacking information of how this silencing method could influence other pathways.

This signalling could also be affected to inhibit aggregation between adherent and floating bacteria. The principle is very similar to disaggregating agents, but in this case the activity is not directly targeted but is based on a genetic switch-off. To date, two signals that show the greatest promise are nanomolar nitric oxide (NO) and cis-2-decanoic acid, a fatty acid messenger. Cis-2-decanoic acid has been demonstrated to reduce biofilm formation by several pathogens [225], However, for NO and cis-2-decanoic acid, the optimal delivery system (intended as amount and rate) must be still clarified.

5.5 CONCLUDING REMARKS

Material science can provide proofs and strategies to study and modify biomaterial surface in terms of bacteria adhesion, whether with or without antibacterial drugs. It was earlier believed that hydrophilic, highly hydrated or non-charged surfaces could be the best choice. Such bio-materials surfaces have been indeed shown *in vitro* to prevent the adhesion of many bacterial species by limiting the contact between bacteria cells and device surfaces. Host cell attachment, however, may also be negatively affected by certain surface treatments, topography, adhesion kinetics and significant variations in the environment. It is not possible to make a one-for-all strategy for anti-bacterial implant surfaces and combined measures are required depending on the implant design, purpose and patient conditions. What are certainly required are additional studies to understand various clinically relevant biofilm properties, evolution and interaction with biomaterials and tissues to elaborate an optimal strategy for the prevention of biofilm-related prosthetic infections.

REFERENCES

1. Gbejuade, H.O., Lovering, A.M., Webb, J.C. (2015). The role of microbial biofilms in prosthetic joint infections, *Acta Orthopaed*, 86, pp. 147–158.
2. Kapadia, B.H., Berg, R.A., Daley, J.A., Fritz, J., Bhave, A., Mont, M.A. (2015). Periprosthetic joint infection. *Lancet*, 387, pp. 386–394.
3. Kurtz, S.M., Lau, E., Watson, H., Schmier, J.K., Parvizi, J. (2012). Economic burden of periprosthetic joint infection in the United States. *J Arthroplasty*, 27 (Suppl. 1), pp. 61–65.
4. Baek, S.H. (2014). Identification and preoperative optimization of risk factors to prevent periprosthetic joint infection. *World J Orthop*, 5, pp. 362–367.
5. Perdreau-Remington, F., Stefanik, D., Peters, G., Ludwig, C., Riitt, J., Wenzel, R., Pulverer G. (1996). A four-year prospective study on microbial ecology of explanted prosthetic hips in 52 patients with "aseptic" prosthetic joint loosening. *Eur J Clin Microbiol Infect Dis*, 15, pp. 160–165.
6. Portillo, M.E., Salvadó, M., Alier, A., Sorli, L., Martínez, S., Horcajada, J.P., Puig, L. (2013). Prosthesis failure within 2 years of implantation is highly predictive of infection. *Clin Orthop Relat Res*, 471, pp. 3672–3678.
7. Liu, Y., Wang, Y., Walsh, T.R., Yi, L., Zhang, R., Spencer, J., Doi, Y., Tian, G., Dong, B., Huang, X., Yu, L., Gu, D., Ren, H., Chen, X., Lv L., He, D., Zhou, H., Liang, Z., Liu, J., Shen, J. (2016). Emergence of plasmid-mediated colistin resistance mechanism MCR-1 in animals and human beings in China: A microbiological and molecular biological study. *Lancet*, 16, pp. 161–168.
8. O'Toole, G.A. (2002). Microbiology: A resistance switch. *Nature*, 416, pp. 695–696.
9. Simchi, A., Tamjid, E., Pishbin, F., Boccaccini, A.R. (2011). Recent progress in inorganic and composite coatings with bactericidal capability for orthopaedic applications. *Nanomedicine*, 7, pp. 22–39.
10. Puckett, S.D., Raimondo, T., Webster, T.J. (2010). The relationship between the nanostructure of titanium surfaces and bacterial attachment. *Biomaterials*, 31, pp. 706–713.
11. von Recum, A. (ed.) (1998). *Handbook of Biomaterials Evaluation* (Taylor-Francis, USA), p. 916.
12. Donlan, R.M. (2001). Biofilms and device-associated infections. *Emerg Infect Dis*, 7, pp. 277–281.
13. Campoccia, D., Montanaro, L., Arciola, C.R. (2006). The significance of infection related to orthopedic devices and issues of antibiotic resistance. *Biomaterials*, 27, pp. 2331–2339.
14. Fenwick, E., Claxton, K., Sculpher, M. (2001). Representing uncertainty: The role of cost-effectiveness acceptability curves. *Health Econ*, 10, pp. 779–787.
15. Karlsson, G., Johannesson, M. (1996). The decision rules of cost-effectiveness analysis. *Pharmacoecon*, 9, pp. 113–120.

16. Meani, E., Romanò, C., Crosby, L., Hofmann, G., Calonego, G. (eds) (2007). *Infection and local treatment in orthopedic surgery* (Springer, Berlin Heidelberg), 396 p.
17. http://ec.europa.eu/dgs/health_food-safety/amr/index_en.htm.
18. Rogers, K. (ed.) (2011). *Bacteria and Viruses* (Britannica Educational Publishing, UK), 216 p.
19. De Ryck, T., Grootaert, C., Jaspaert, L., Kerckhof, F.M., Van Gele, M., De Schrijver, J., Van der Abbeele, P., Swift, S., Bracke, M., Van de Wiele, T., Vanhoecke, B. (2014). Development of an oral mucosa model to study host-microbiome interactions during wound healing. *Appl Microbiol Biotechnol*, 98, pp. 6831–6846.
20. Millhouse, E., Jose, A., Sherry, L., Lappin, D.F. Patel, N., Middleton, A.M., Pratten, J., Culshaw, S., Ramage, G. (2014). Development of an in vitro periodontal biofilm model for assessing antimicrobial and host modulatory effects of bioactive molecules. *BMC Oral Health*, 14, pp. 80.
21. Pye, A.D., Lockhart, D.E.A., Dawson, M.P., Murray, C.A., Smith, A.J. (2009). A review of dental implants and infection. *J Hospital Infect*, 72, pp. 104–110.
22. An, Y.H., Friedman, R.J. (1998). Concise review of mechanisms of bacterial adhesion to biomaterial surfaces. *J Biomed Mater Res*, 43, pp. 338–348.
23. Bereket, W., Hemalatha, K., Getenet, B. et al. (2012). Update on bacterial nosocomial infections. *Eur Rev Med Pharmacol Sci*, 16, pp. 1039–1044.
24. Rohde, H., Frankenberger, S., Zähringer, U., Mack, D. (2010). Structure, function and contribution of polysaccharide inter-cellular adhesin (PIA) to Staphylococcus epidermidis biofilm formation and pathogenesis of biomaterial-associated infections. *Eur J Cell Biol*, 89, pp. 103–111.
25. Schito, G.C. (2006). The importance of the development of antibiotic resistance in staphylococcus aureus. *Clin Microbiol Infect*, 12, Suppl. 1, pp. 3–8.
26. Rochford, E.T.J., Jaekel, D.J., Hickok, N.J., Richards, R.G., Moriarty, T.F., Poulsson, A.H.C. (2012). Chapter Bacterial Interactions with polyaryletheretherketone, in *PEEK Biomaterials Hand-book*, Kurtz, S.M. (ed.) (William Andrew / Elsevier, Amsterdam), pp. 93–117.
27. Hampton, A.A., Sherertz, R.J. (1998). Vascular-access infections in hospitalized patients. *Surg Clin North Am*, 68, pp. 57–71.
28. Hospenthal, D.R., Rinaldi, M.G. (eds) (2015). *Diagnosis and Treatment of Fungal Infections*, 2nd ed. (Springer), 300 p.
29. Martin, G.S., Mannino, D.M., Eaton, S., Moss, M. (2003). The epidemiology of sepsis in the United States from 1979 through 2000. *N Engl J Med*, 348, pp. 1546–1554.
30. Calderone, R.A. (2001). *Candida and candidiasis* (ASM Press, Washington, DC).
31. Sobel, J.D. (2015). Candidiasis, in *Diagnosis and Treatment of Fungal Infections*, 2nd ed., Hospenthal, D.R., Rinaldi M.G. (eds), (Springer), pp. 101–117.
32. Garrett, T.R., Bhakoo, M., Zhang, Z. (2008). Bacterial adhesion and biofilms on surfaces. *Prog Nat Sci*, 18, pp. 1049–1056.
33. Costerton, J.W. (1999). Introduction to biofilm. *Int J Antimicrob Agents*, 11, pp. 217–221.
34. Dalton, H.M., March, P.E. (1998). Molecular genetics of bacterial attachment and biofouling. *Curr Opin Biotechnol*, 9, pp. 252–255.
35. Maki, D.G., Stolz, S.M., Wheeler, S., Mermel, L.A. (1997). Prevention of central venous catheter-related bloodstream infection by the use of an antiseptic-impregnated catheter – a randomized, controlled trial. *Ann Intern Med*, 127, pp. 257–266.
36. Green, R.J., Davies, M.C., Roberts, C.J., Tendier, S.J.B. (1999). Competitive protein adsorption as observed by surface plasmon resonance. *Biomaterials*, 20, pp. 385–391.
37. Katsikogianni, M., Missirlis, Y.F. (2004). Concise review of mechanisms of bacterial adhesion to biomaterials and of techniques used in estimating bacteria-material interactions. *Europ Cells Mater*, 8, pp. 37–57.

38. Dougherty, S.H. (1988). Pathobiology of infection in prosthetic devices. *Rev Infect Dis*, 10, pp. 1102–1117.
39. Gristina, A.G., Naylor, P.T., Myrvik, Q.N. (1990). Musculosceletal infection, microbial adhesion, and antibiotic resistance. *Infect Dis Clin N Am*, 4, pp. 392–408.
40. Donlan, R.M. (2002). Biofilms: Microbial life on surfaces. *Emerg Infect Dis*, 8, pp. 881–890.
41. Liu, Y., Li, J. (2008). Role of Pseudomonas aeruginosa biofilm in the initial adhesion, growth and detachment of Escherichia coli in porous media. *Environ Sci Technol*, 42, pp. 443–449.
42. Mack, D., Fischer, W., Krokotsch, A., Leopold, K., Hartmann, R., Egge, H., Laufs, R. (1996). The intercellular adhesin involved in biofilm accumulation of Staphylococcus epidermis is a linear beta-1,6-linked glucosaminoglycan: Purification and structural analysis. *J Bacterial*, 178, pp. 175–183.
43. Christensen, B.E., Charaklis, W.G., Charaklis, K.C. (1990) *Physical and Chemical Properties of Biofilms* (Wiley, USA), pp. 93–130.
44. John, G.T., Donald, C.L. (2007). Biofilms: Architects of disease, in *Textbook of Diagnostic Microbiology*. 3rd ed., Connie, R.M., Donald, C.L., George, M. (eds) (Saunders), pp. 884–895.
45. Costerton, J.W., Stewart, P.S., Greenberg, E.P. (1999). Bacterial biofilms: A common cause of persistent infections. *Science*, 284, pp. 1318–1322.
46. Aparna, M.S., Sarita, Y. (2008) Biofilms: Microbes and disease. Brazil. *J Infect Dis*, 12, pp. 526–530.
47. Van Eldere, J., Gasthuisberg, U.Z. (2006). Pathogenesis and clinical importance of biofilms. Presentation (29 June 2006), REGA Institute and Katholieke Universiteit Leuven (Belgium).
48. Vuong, C., Otto, M. (2000). Staphylococcus epidermidis infections. *Microbes Infect*, 4, pp. 481–489.
49. Raulio, M., Salkinoja-Salonen, M., Wilhelmson, A., Laitila, A. (2009). Ultrastructure of biofilms formed on barley kernels during malting with and without starter culture. *Food Microbiol*, 26, pp. 437–443.
50. Truong, V.K., Lapovok, R., Estrin, Y.S., Rundell, S., Wang, J.Y., Fluke, C.J., Crawford, R.J., Ivanova, E.P. (2010). The influence of nano-scale surface roughness on bacterial adhesion to ultrafine-grained titanium. *Biomaterials*, 31, pp. 3674–3683.
51. Mendonça, G., Mendonça, D.B., Aragão, F.J., Cooper, L.F. (2008). Advancing dental implant surface technology – from micron- to nanotopography. *Biomaterials*, 29, pp. 3822–3835.
52. Gristina, A.G. (1994). Implant failure and the immuno-incompetent fibroinflammatory zone. *Clin Orthop Relat Res*, 298, pp. 106–118.
53. Steckelberg, J.M., Osmon, D.R. (1994). Prosthetic joint infections, in *Infection Associated with Indwelling Medical Devices*, Bisno, A.L., Waldvogel, F.A. (eds) (Washington, DC, American Society for Microbiology), pp. 259–901.
54. Schierholz, J.M., Beuth, J. (2001). Implant infections: A haven for opportunistic bacteria. *J Hospital Infect*, 49, pp. 87–93.
55. Elek, S.D. (1956). Experimental staphylococcal infections in the skin of man. *Ann NY Acad Sci*, 65, pp. 85–90.
56. Cordero, J., Munuera, L., Folgueira, M.D. (1996). Influence of bacterial strains on bone infection. *J Orthop Res*, 14, pp. 663–667.
57. Schierholz, J.M., Beuth, J., Rump, A., Konig, D.P., Pulverer, G. (2001). Novel strategies to prevent catheter-associated infections in oncology patients. *J Chemother*, 1, pp. 239–250.
58. Southwood, R.T., Rice, J.L., McDonald, P.J., Hakendorf, P.H., Rozenbilds, M.A. (1985). Infection in experimental hip arthroplasties. *J Bone Joint Surg Br*, 67, pp. 229–231.

59. Gehrke, T., Breusch, S.J. (2007). Management of TKA infection – One-stage exchange, in *Infection and Local Treatment in Orthopedic Surgery*, Meani, E., Romanó, C., Crosby, L., Hofmann G., Calonego, G. (eds) (Springer), pp. 272–285.
60. Parsek, M.R., Singh, P.K. (2003). Bacterial biofilms: An emerging link to disease pathogenesis. *Ann Rev Microbiol*, 57, pp. 677–701.
61. Lewis, K. (2001). Riddle of biofilm resistance. *Antimicrob Agents Chemoth*, 45, pp. 999–1007.
62. Marshall, T.G., Marshall, F.E. (2004). Sarcoidosis succumbs to antibiotics–implications for autoimmune disease. *Autoimmun Rev*, 3, pp. 295–300.
63. Cats-Baril, W., Gehrke, T., Huff, K., Kendoff, D., Maltenfort, M., Parvizi, J. (2013). International consensus on periprosthet-ic joint infection: Description of the consensus process. *Clin Orthop Relat Res Oct,* (E-Pub).
64. Rimondini, L., Cochis, A., Varoni, E., Azzimonti, B., Carrassi, A. (2015). Biofilm formation on implants and prosthetic dental materials, in *Handbook of Bioceramics and Biocomposites*, Antoniac, I.V. (ed.) (Springer), pp. 991–1027.
65. Rimondini, L., Farè, S., Brambilla, E., Felloni, A., Consonni, C., Brossa, F, Carrassi, A. (1997). The effect of surface roughness on early in vivo plaque colonization on titanium. *J Periodontol*, 68, pp. 556–562.
66. Teughels, W., Van Assche, N., Sliepen, I., Quirynen, M. (2006). Effect of material characteristics and/or surface topography on biofilm development. *Clin Oral Implants Res*, 17 (Suppl 2), pp. 68–81.
67. Crick, C.R., Ismail, S., Pratten, J., Parkin, I.P. (2011). An investigation into bacterial attachment to an elastomeric super-hydrophobic surface prepared via aerosol assisted deposition. *Thin Solid Films,* 519, pp. 3722–3727.
68. Badihi Hauslich, L., Sela, M.N., Steinberg, D., Rosen, G., Kohavi, D. (2013). The adhesion of oral bacteria to modified titanium surfaces: Role of plasma proteins and electrostatic forces. *Clin Oral Implants Res*, 24, pp. 49–56.
69. Raulio, M., Järn, M., Ahola, J., Peltonen, J., Rosenholm, J.B., Tervakangas, S., Kolehmainen, J., Ruokolainen. T., Narko, P., Salkinoja-Salonen, M. (2008). Microbe-repelling coated stainless steel analysed by field emission scanning electron mi-croscopy and physicochemical methods. *J Ind Microbiol Biotechnol*, 35, pp. 751–760.
70. Donlan, R.M. (2005). New approaches for the characterization of prosthetic joint biofilms. *Clin Orthop Relat Res*, 437, pp. 12–19.
71. Donlan, R.M., Costerton J.W. (2002). Biofilms: Survival mechanisms of clinically relevant microorganisms. *Clin Microbiol Rev*, 15, pp. 167–193.
72. Moroni, A., Vannini, F., Mosca, M., Giannini, S. (2002). State of the art review: Techniques to avoid pin loosening and infection in external fixation. *J Orthop Trauma*, 16, pp. 189–195.
73. Rimondini, L., Fini, M., Giardino, R. (2005). The microbial infection of biomaterials: A challenge for clinicians and re-searchers. A short review. *J Appl Biomater Biomech*, 3, pp. 1–10.
74. Liu, Y., Zhao, Q. (2005). Influence of surface energy of modified surfaces on bacterial adhesion. *Biophysic Chem*, 117, pp. 39–45.
75. Gristina, A.G. (1987). Biomaterial-centered infection: Microbial adhesion versus tissue integration. *Science*, 237, pp. 1588–1595.
76. Subbiahdoss, G., Kuijer, E., Grijpma, D., van der Mei, H.C., Busscher, H.J. (2009). Microbial film growth vs. tissue integration: "the race for surface" experimentally studied. *Acta Biomater*, 5, pp. 1399–1404.
77. Hall-Stoodley, L., Costerton, J.W., Stoodley, P. (2004). Bacterial biofilms: From the natural environment to infectious diseases. *Nat Rev Micro*, 2, pp. 95–108.

78. Peterson, B.W., He, Y., Ren, Y., Zerdoum, A., Libera, M.R., Sharma, P.K., van Winkelhoff, A.-J., Neut, D., Stoodley, P., van der Mei, H.C., Busscher, H.J. (2015). Viscoelasticity of biofilms and their recalcitrance to mechanical and chemical challenges. *FEMS Microbiology Rev*, 39, pp. 234–245.
79. Volfson, D., Cookson, S., Hasty, J., Tsimring, T.S. (2008). Biomechanical ordering of dense cell populations. *PNAS*, 105, pp. 15346–15351.
80. Towler, B.W., Rupp, C.J., Cunningham, A.B. et al. (2003). Viscoelastic properties of a mixed culture biofilm from rheometer creep analysis. *Biofouling*, 19, pp. 279–285.
81. Stoodley, P., Cargo, R., Rupp, C.J., Wilson, S., Klapper, I. (2002). Biofilm material properties as related to shear-induced deformation and detachment phenomena. *J Ind Microbiol Biotechnol*, 29, pp. 361–367.
82. Korstgens, V., Flemming, H.C., Wingender, J., Borchard, W. (2001). Influence of calcium ions on the mechanical properties of a model biofilm of mucoid Pseudomonas aeruginosa. *Water Sci Technol*, 43, pp. 49–57.
83. Flemming, H.-C., Wingender, J., Mayer, C., Korstgens, V., Borchard, W. (2000). Cohesiveness in biofilm matrix polymers, in *Community Structure and Cooperation in Biofilms*, Allison, D., Gilbert, P., Lappin-Scott, H.M., Wilson, M. (eds) (Cambridge University Press, UK), pp. 87–105.
84. Wloka, M., Rehage, H., Flemming, H.-C., Wingender, J. (2005). Structure and rheological behaviour of the extracellular polymeric substance network of mucoid Pseudomonas aeruginosa biofilms. *Biofilms*, 2, pp. 275–283.
85. Davies, D.G., Parsek, M.R., Pearson, J.P., Iglewski, B.H., Costerton, J.W., Greenberg, E.P. (1998). The involvement of cell-to-cell signals in the development of a bacterial biofilm. *Science*, 280, pp. 295–298.
86. Shaw, T., Winston, M., Rupp, C.J., Klapper, I., Stoodley, P. (2004). Commonality of elastic relaxation times in biofilms. *Phys Rev Lett*, 93, pp. 98102.
87. Gottenbos. B., Van der Mei, H.C., Busscher, H.J., Grijpma, D.W., Feijen, J. (1999). Initial adhesion and surface growth of Pseudomonas aeruginosa on negatively and positively charged poly(methacrylates). *J Mater Sci Mater Med*, 10, pp. 853–855.
88. Bilotsky, Y., Gasik, M. (2015). Modelling of poro-viscoelastic biological systems. *J Phys Conf Series*, 633, pp. 21234–021238.
89. Peterson, B.W., Busscher, H.J., Sharma, P.K., van der Mei, H.C. (2012). Environmental and centrifugal factors influencing the visco-elastic properties of oral biofilms in vitro. *Biofouling*, 28, pp. 913–920.
90. Gasik, M. (2014). New BEST – Biomaterials Enhanced Simulation Test. *J Tissue Sci Eng*, 5, pp. 66.
91. Ewoldt, R.H., Johnston, M.T., Caretta, L.M. (2015). Exper-imental challenges of shear rheology: How to avoid bad data, in *Complex Fluids in Biological Systems*, Spagnolie, S. (ed.) (Springer).
92. Paramonova, E., Krom, B.P., van der Mei, H.C., Busscher, H.J., Sharma, P.K. (2009). Hyphal content determines the com-pression strength of Candida albicans biofilms. *Microbiology*, 155, pp. 1997–2003.
93. Cadosch, D., Al-Mushaiqri, M.S., Gautschi, O.P., Meagher, J., Simmen, H.P., Filgueira, L. (2010). Biocorrosion and uptake of titanium by human osteoclasts. *J Biomed Mater Research*, 95A, pp. 1004–1010.
94. Souza, J.C.M., Henriques, M., Oliveira, R., Teughels, W., Celis, J.P., Rocha, L.A. (2010). Do oral biofilms influence the wear and corrosion behavior of titanium? *Biofouling*, 26, pp. 471–478.
95. Souza, J.C.M., Henriques, M., Oliveira, R., Teughels, W., Celis, J.P., Rocha, L.A. (2010). Biofilms inducing ultra-low friction on titanium. *J Dent Res*, 26, pp. 471–478.
96. Hallab, N.J. (2009). A review of the biologic effects of spine implant debris: Fact from fiction. *SAS J*, 3, pp. 143–160.

97. Parvizi, J., Gehrke, T., Chen, A.F. (2013). Proceedings of the international consensus on periprosthetic joint infection. *Bone Joint J*, 95, pp. 1450–1452.
98. Hosman, A.H., van der Mei, H.C., Bulstra, S.K., Busscher, H.J., Neut, D. (2010). Effect of metal-on-metal wear on the host immune system and infection in hip arthroplasty. *Acta Orthop*, 81, pp. 526–534.
99. Parvizi, J. (2014). Periprosthetic joint infection: Could bearing surface play a role? *CeraNews*, 1, p. 11.
100. Vasconcelos, D.M., Santos, S.G., Lamghari, M., Barbosa, M.A. (2016). The two faces of metal ions: From implants rejection to tissue repair/regeneration. *Biomaterials*, 84, pp. 262–275.
101. Niinomi, M. (ed.) (2010). *Metals for Biomedical Devices* (Woodhead Publishing, UK), 420 pp.
102. Okazaki, Y., Rao, S., Tateishi, T., Ito, Y. (1998). Cytocompatibility of various metal and development of new titanium alloys for medical implants. *Mater Sci Eng*, A243, pp. 250–256.
103. Long, M., Rack, H.J. (1998). Titanium alloys in total joint replacement – A materials science perspective. *Biomaterials*, 19, pp. 1621–1639.
104. Niinomi, M. (2008). Biologically and mechanically biocompatible titanium alloys. *Mater Trans*, 49, pp. 2170–2178.
105. Wu, Y., Zitelli, J.P., TenHuisen, K.S., Yu, X., Libera, M.R. (2011). Differential response of Staphylococci and osteoblasts to varying titanium surface roughness. *Biomaterials*, 32, pp. 951–960.
106. Puleo, D.A., Nanci, A. (1999). Understanding and controlling the bone-implant interface. *Biomaterials*, 20, pp. 2311–2321.
107. Omori, S., Shibata, Y., Arimoto, T., Igarashi, T., Baba, K., Miyazaki, T. (2009). Microorganism and cell viability on anti-microbially modified titanium. *J Dent Res*, 88, pp. 957–962.
108. Nakazato, G., Tsuchiya, H., Sato, M., Yamauchi, M. (1989). In vivo plaque formation on implant materials. *Int J Oral Maxillofac Implants*, 4, pp. 312–316.
109. Leonhardt, A., Gröndahl, K., Bergström, C., Lekholm, U. (2002). Longterm follow-up of osseointergrated titanium implants using clinical, radiographic and microbiological parameters. *Clin Oral Implants Res*, 13, pp. 123–132.
110. McCollum, J., O'Neal, R.B., Brennan, W.A., Van Dyke, T.E., Horner, J.A. (1992). The effect of titanium implant abutments surface irregularities on a plaque accumulation in vivo. *J Periodontol*, 63, pp. 802–805.
111. Asshe, N., Sliepen, I., Quirynen, M., Listgarten, M.A. (2006). Effect of material characteristics and/or surface topography on biofilm development. *Clin Oral Implants Res*, 17, pp. 8–12.
112. Siegrist, B.E., Brecx, M.C., Gusberti, F.A., Joss, A., Lang, N.P. (1991). In vivo early human dental plaque formation on different supporting substances. A scanning electron microscopic and bacteriological study. *Clin Oral Implants Res*, 2, pp. 38–46.
113. Oga, M., Arizaono, T., Sugioka, Y. (1993). Bacterial adherence to bioinert and bioactive materials studied in vitro. *Acta Orthop Scand*, 64, pp. 68–81.
114. Mabboux, F., Ponsonnet, L., Morrier, J.J., Jaffrezic, N., Barsotti, O. (2004). Surface free energy and bacterial retention to saliva-coated dental implants materials: An in vitro study. *Colloids Surf B: Biointerfaces*, 38, pp. 199–205.
115. Li, B., Zhou, M., Yuan, R., Cai, L. (2008). Fabrication of titanium-based microstructured surfaces and study on their superhydrophobic stability. *J Mater Res*, 23, pp. 2491–2499.
116. Shibata, Y., Tanimoto, Y., Maruyama, N., Nagakura, M. (2015). A review of improved fixation methods for dental implants. Part I: Surface optimization for rapid osseointegration. *J Prostodont Res*, 59, pp. 20–33.

117. Shibata, Y., Tanimoto, Y., Maruyama, N., Nagakura, M. (2015). A review of improved fixation methods for dental implants. Part II: Biomechanical integrity at bone–implant interface. *J Prostodont Res*, 59, pp. 84–95.
118. Gasik, M., Braem, A., Chaudhari, A., Duyck, J., Vleugels, J. (2015). Titanium implants with modified surfaces: Meta-analysis of in vivo osteointegration. *Mater Sci Eng C*, 49, pp. 152–158.
119. Wall, I., Donos, N., Carlqvist, K., Jones, F., Brett, P. (2009). Modified titanium surfaces promote accelerated osteogenic differentiation of mesenchymal stromal cells in vitro. *Bone*, 45, pp. 17–26.
120. Borsari, V., Giavaresi, G., Fini, M., Torricelli, P., Tschon, M., Chiesa, R. et al. (2005). Comparative in vitro study on ultra-high roughness and dense titanium coating. *Biomaterials*, 26, pp. 4948–4955.
121. Stevens, M.M., George, J.H. (2005). Exploring and engineering the cell surface interface. *Science*, 310, pp. 1135–1138.
122. Scarano, A., Piatelli, A., Polimeni, A., DiIorio, D., Carinci, F. (2010). Bacterial adhesion on commercially pure titanium and anatase-coated titanium healing screws: An in vivo human study. *J Periodont*, 81, pp. 1466–1471.
123. Shiraishi, K., Koseki, H., Tsurumoto, T. et al. (2008). Antimicrobial metal implant with a TiO_2-conferred photocatalytic bactericidal effect against Staphylococcus aureus. *Surf Inter Anal*, 41, pp. 17–21.
124. Roy, A.S., Parveen, A., Koppalkar, A.R., Prasad, A. (2010). Effect of nano-titanium dioxide with different antibiotics against methicillin-resistant Staphylococcus aureus. *J Biomater Nanobiotechn*, 1, pp. 37–41.
125. Gasik, M., Van Mellaert, L., Pierron, D., Braem, A., Hofmans, D., de Waelheyns, E., Anné, J., Harmand, M.-F., Vleugels, J. (2012). Reduction of biofilm infection risks and promotion of osteointegration for optimized surfaces of titanium implants. *Adv Healthcare Mater*, 1, pp. 117–127.
126. Cordero, J., Munuera, L., Folgueira, M.D. (1994). Influence of metal implants on infection. An experimental study in rabbits. *J Bone Joint Surg Br*, 76, pp. 717–720.
127. Goodman, S., Konttinen, Y.T., Takagi, M. (2014). Joint replacement surgery and the innate immune system. *J Long Term Eff Med Implants*, 24, pp. 253–257.
128. Wong, J.Y, Bronzino, J.D. (2007). *Biomaterials* (CRC Press, Taylor & Francis), 296 p.
129. Kurtz, S.M. (ed.) (2012). *PEEK Biomaterials Handbook* (Elsevier), 300 p.
130. Agrawal, C.M., Parr, J.E., Lin, S.T. (eds) (2000). *Synthetic Biodegradable Polymers for Implants*, ASTM STP1396, 174 p.
131. Hubbell, J.A. (1995). Biomaterials in tissue engineering. *Nature Biotechnol*, 13, pp. 565–576.
132. Lansman, S., Paakko, P., Ryhanen, J. et al. (2006). Poly-L/D lactide(PLDLA) 96/4 fibrous implants: Histological evaluation in the subcutis of experimental design. *J Craniofac Surg*, 17, pp. 1121–1128.
133. Haaparanta, A.M., Jarvinen, E., Cengiz, I.F. et al. (2014). Preparation and characterization of collagen/PLA, chitosan/PLA, and collagen/chitosan/PLA hybrid scaffolds for cartilage tissue engineering. *J Mater Sci Mater Med*, 25, pp. 1129–1136.
134. Whitehead, K.A., Verran, J. (2006). The effect of surface topography on the retention of microorganisms. *Food Bioproducts Process*, 84, pp. 253–259.
135. Harris, L.G., Meredith, D.O., Eschbach, L., Richards, R.G. (2007). Staphylococcus aureus adhesion to standard micro-rough and electropolished implant materials. *J Mater Sci Mater Med*, 18, pp. 1151–1156.
136. Verheyen, C.C.P.M., Dhert, W.J.A., de Blieck-Hogervorst, J.M.A., van der Reijden, T.J.K., Petit, P.L.C., de Groot, K. (1993). Adherence to a metal, polymer and composite by Staphylococcus aureus and Staphylococcus epidermidis. *Biomaterials*, 14, pp. 383–391.

137. DiGiulio, M., D'Ercole, S., Zara, S., Cataldi, A., Cellini, L. (2011). Streptococcus mitis/ human gingival fibroblasts co-culture: The best natural association in answer to the 2-hydroxoethyl methacrylate release. *Acta Pathol Microbiol Immunol Scand*, 120, pp. 139–146.
138. Hosman, A.H., Bulstra, S.K., Sjollema, J. et al. (2012). The influence of Co-Cr and UHMWPE particles on infection persistence: An in vivo study in mice. *J Orthop Res*, 30, pp. 341–347.
139. Haukkamaa, M., Stranden, P., Jousimies-Somer, H., Siitonen, A. (1986). Bacterial flora of the cervix in women using dif-ferent methods of contraception. *Amer J Obstetr Gynecol*, 154, pp. 520–524.
140. Skarin, A., Sylwan, J. (1986). Vaginal lactobacilli inhibiting growth of Gardnerella vaginalis, Mobiluncus and other bacteri-al species cultured from vaginal content of women with bacterial vaginosis. *Acta Pathol Microbiol Immunol Scand*, 94, pp. 399–403.
141. Lamont, R.F., Sobel, J.D., Akins, R.A., Hassan, S.S., Chaiworapongsa, T., Kusanovic, J.P., Romero, R. (2011). The vaginal microbiome: New information about genital tract flora using molecular based techniques. *BJOG*, 118, pp. 533–549.
142. Hawes, S.E., Hillier, S.L., Benedetti, J., Stevens, C.E., Koutsky, L.A., Wolner-Hanssen, P. et al. (1996). Hydrogen peroxide-producing lactobacilli and acquisition of vaginal infections. *J Infect Dis*, 174, pp. 1058–1063.
143. Aroutcheva, A.A., Simoes, J.A., Faro, S. (2001). Antimicrobial protein produced by vaginal Lactobacillus acidophilus that inhibits Gardnerella vaginalis. *Infect Dis Obstet Gynecol*, 9, pp. 33–39.
144. Reid, G., Hawthorn, L.-A., Mandatori, R., Cook, R.L., Beg, H.S. (1988). Adhesion of lactobacilli to polymer surfaces in vivo and in vitro. *J Microbial Ecology*, 16, pp. 241–251.
145. Whitehead, K.A., Colligon, J., Verran, J. (2005). Retention of microbial cells in substratum surface features of micrometer and submicrometer dimensions. *Colloids Surf B: Biointerfaces*, 41, pp. 129–138.
146. Sagomonyants, K.B., Jarman-Smith, M.L., Devine, J.N., Aronow, M.S., Gronowicz, G.A. (2008). The in vitro response of human osteoblasts to polyetheretherketone (PEEK) substrates compared to commercially pure titanium. *Biomaterials*, 29, pp. 1563–1572.
147. von Recum, A.F., van Kooten, T.G. (1995). The influence of micro-topography on cellular response and the implications for silicone implants. *J Biomater Sci Polym Ed*, 7, pp. 181–198.
148. Ki, D.P., Young, S.K., Dong, K.H., Young, H.K., Eun, H.B.L., Hwal, S. et al. (1998). Bacterial adhesion on PEG modified polyurethane surfaces. *Biomaterials*, 19, pp. 851–859.
149. James, N.R., Jayakrishnan, A. (2003). Surface thiocyanation of plasticized poly(vinyl chloride) and its effect on bacterial adhesion. *Biomaterials*, 24, pp. 2205–2212.
150. Cunliffe, D., Smart, C.A., Alexander, C., Vulfson, E.N. (1999). Bacterial adhesion at synthetic surfaces. *Appl Environ Microbiol*, 65, pp. 4995–5002.
151. Van De Belt, H., Neut, D., Uges, D.R.A. et al. (2000). Surface roughness, porosity and wettability of gentamicin-loaded bone cements and their antibiotic release. *Biomater*, 21, pp. 1981–1987.
152. Anagnostakos, K., Hitzler, P., Pape, D., Kohn, D., Kelm, J. (2008). Persistence of bacterial growth on antibiotic-loaded beads. Is it actually a problem? *Acta Orthop*, 79, pp. 302–307.
153. Dale, H., Skramm. I., Lower, H.L. et al. (2011). Infection after primary hip arthroplasty: A comparison of 3 Norwegian health registers. *Acta Orthop*, 82, pp. 646–654.

154. Neut, D., Hendriks, J.G.E., Van Horn, J.R., Van der Mei, H.C., Busscher, H.J. (2005). Pseudomonas aeruginosa biofilm for-mation and slime excretion on antibiotic-loaded bone cement. *Acta Orthop Scand*, 76, pp. 109–114.
155. Dorozhkin, S.V. (2013). Calcium orthophosphate-based bioceramics. *Materials*, 6, pp. 3840–3942.
156. Zhao, Y.F., Ma, J. (2008). Mesoporous bioactive glasses: Synthesis, characterization and in vitro bioactivity. *J Biomimetics Biomater Tissue Eng*, 1, pp. 37–47.
157. Kokubo, T. (ed.) (2008). *Bioceramics and their clinical applications* (Woodhead Publishing, UK), 760 p.
158. Dorozhkin, S.V. (2012). Calcium orthophosphate coatings, films and layers. *Progress in Biomater*, 1, pp. 1–40.
159. MacFarlane, J.W., Jenkinson, H.F., Scott, T.B. (2011). Sterilization of microorganisms on jet spray formed titanium dioxide surfaces. *Appl Catal B: Environmental*, 106, pp. 181–185.
160. Enwemeka, C.S., Williams, D., Hollosi, S., Yens, D., Enwemeka, S.K. (2008). Visible 405 nm SLD light photo-destroys methicillin-resistant Staphylococcus aureus (MRSA) in vitro. *Lasers in Surg Medic*, 40, pp. 734–737.
161. Rimondini, L., Cerroni, L., Carrasi, A., Torricelli, P. (2002). Bacterial colonization of zirconia ceramic surfaces: An in vitro and in vivo study. *Intern J Oral Maxillofac Implants*, 17, pp. 793–798.
162. Scarano, A., Piattelli, M., Caputi, S., Favero, G.A., Piattelli, A. (2004). Bacterial adhesion on commercially pure titanium and zirconium oxide disks: An in vivo human study. *J Periodontol*, 75, pp. 292–296.
163. Scotti, R., Kantorski, K.Z., Monaco, C., Valandro, L.F., Ciocca, L., Bottino, M.A. (2007). SEM evaluation of in situ early bacterial colonization on a Y-TZP ceramic: A pilot study. *Int J Prosthodont*, 20, pp. 419–422.
164. Reynolds, E.C., Wong, A. (1983). Effect of adsorbed protein on hydroxyapatite zeta potential and Streptococcus mutans adherence. *Infection Immunity*, 39, pp. 1285–1290.
165. Gao, P., Nie, X., Zou, M., Shi, Y., Cheng, G. (2011). Recent advances in materials for extended-release antibiotic delivery system. *J Antibiotics*, 64, pp. 625–634.
166. Zilberman, M., Elsner, J.J. (2008). Antibiotic-eluting medical devices for various applications. *J Control Release*, 130, pp. 202–215.
167. Mossely, D.A., Ge, Y., Gasik, M., Nordström, K., Natri, O., Hannula, S.P. (2016). Silica-gentamicin nanohybrids: Synthesis and antimicrobial action. *Materials*, 9, pp. 170–185.
168. Gabride, P., Harris, J. (2014). Regenerating the future of biomaterials in orthopedics. *Medical Design Briefs*, 10.
169. Shi, J., Xing, M.M., Zhong, W. (2012). Development of hydrogels and biomimetic regulators as tissue engineering scaffolds. *Membranes*, 2, pp. 70–90.
170. Huglin, M.R. (1986) *Hydrogels in Medicine and Pharmacy* (CRC Press, USA).
171. Geckil, H., Xu, F., Zhang, X., Moon, S., Demirci, U. (2010). Engineering hydrogels as extracellular matrix mimics. *Nanomedicine*, 5, pp. 469–484.
172. Zaky, S.H., Lee, K.W., Gao, J., Jensen, A., Close, J., Wang, Y., Almarza, A.J., Sfeir, C. (2014). Poly(glycerol sebacate) elastomer: A novel material for mechanically loaded bone regeneration. *Tissue Eng*, 20A, pp. 45–53.
173. Alhede, M., Er, Ö., Eickhardt, S., Kragh, K., Alhede, M., Christensen, L.D., Poulsen, S.S., Givskov, M., Christensen, L.H., Høiby, N., Tvede, M., Bjarnsholt, T. (2014). Bacterial biofilm formation and treatment in soft tissue fillers. *Pathogens and Disease*, 70, pp. 339–346.
174. Christensen, L., Breiting, V., Bjarnsholt, T. et al. (2013). Bacterial infection as a likely cause of adverse reactions to poly-acrylamide hydrogel fillers in cosmetic surgery. *Clin Infect Dis*, 56, pp. 1438–1444.

175. Funt, D., Pavicic, T. (2013). Dermal fillers in aesthetics: An overview of adverse events and treatment approaches. *Clin Cosmet Invest Dermatol*, 6, pp. 295–316.
176. de Boulle, K., Heydenrych, I. (2015). Patient factors influencing dermal filler complications: Prevention, assessment, and treatment. *Clin Cosmet Invest Dermatol*, 8, pp. 205–214.
177. Christensen, L.H. (2009). Host tissue interaction, fate, and risks of degradable and nondegradable gel fillers. *Dermatol Surg*, 35, pp. 1612–1619.
178. Dayan, S.H., Arkins, J.P., Brindise, R. (2011). Soft tissue fillers and biofilm. *Fac Plast Surg*, 27, pp. 23–28.
179. Pittet, B., Montandon, D., Pittet, D. (2005). Infection in breast implants. *Lancet Infect Dis*, 5, pp. 94–106.
180. Brand, K.G. (1993). Infection of mammary prostheses: A survey and the question of prevention. *Ann Plast Surg*, 30, pp. 289–295.
181. Alijotas-Reig, J., Miró-Mur, F., Planells-Romeu, I., Garcia-Aranda, N., Garcia-Gimenez, V., Vilardell-Tarrés, M. (2010). Are bacterial growth and/or chemotaxis increased by filler injections? Implications for the pathogenesis and treatment of filler-related granulomas. *Dermatol*, 221, pp. 356–364.
182. Christensen, L.H., Breiting, V.B., Vuust, J. et al. (2006). Adverse reactions following injections with permanent facial filler, polyacrylamide hydrogel (Aquamid): Causes and treatment. *Eur J Plast Surg*, 28, pp. 464–471.
183. Christensen, L., Breiting, V., Janssen, M. et al. (2005). Adverse reactions to injectable soft tissue permanent fillers. *Aesthetic Plast Surg*, 29, pp. 34–48.
184. Arciola, C.R., Campoccia, D., Speziale, P., Montanaro, L., Costerton, J.W. (2012). Biofilm formation in Staphylococcus implant infections. A review of molecular mechanisms and implications for biofilm-resistant materials. *Biomaterials*, 33, pp. 5967–5982.
185. Clement, J.L., Jarrett, P.S. (1994). Antibacterial silver. *Metal Based Drugs*, 1, pp. 467–482.
186. Liau, S.Y., Read, D.C., Pugh, W.J., Furr, J.R., Russell, A.D. (1997). Interaction of silver nitrate with readily identifiable groups: Relationship to the antibacterial action of silver ions. *Lett Appl Microbiol*, 25, pp. 279–283.
187. Matsumura, Y., Yoshikata, K., Kunisaki, S., Tsuchido, T. (2003). Mode of bactericidal action of silver zeolite and its comparison with that of silver nitrate. *Appl Environ Microbiol*, 69, pp. 4278–4281.
188. Fayaz, A.M., Girilal, M., Yadav, R., Kalaichelvan, P.T., Venketesan, R. (2010). Biogenic synthesis of silver nanoparticles and their synergistic effect with antibiotics: A study against Gram-positive and Gram-negative bacteria. *Nanomedicine*, 6, pp. 103–109.
189. Roe, D., Karandikar, B., Bonn-Savage, N., Gibbins, B., Roullet, J.B. (2008). Antimicrobial surface functionalization of plastic catheters by silver nanoparticles. *J Antimicrob Chemother*, 61, pp. 869–876.
190. Secinti, K.D., Ozalp, H., Attar, A., Sargon, M.F. (2011). Nanoparticle silver ion coatings inhibit biofilm formation on titanium implants. *J Clin Neurosci*, 18, pp. 391–395.
191. Huang, Z., Zheng, X., Yan, D. et al. (2008). Toxicological effect of ZnO nanoparticles based on bacteria. *Langmuir*, 24, pp. 4140–4144.
192. Seil, J.T., Webster, T.J. (2011). Reduced Staphylococcus aureus proliferation and biofilm formation on zinc oxide nanoparticle PVC composite surfaces. *Acta Biomater*, 7, pp. 2579–2584.
193. Yoruç, A.B.H., Şener, B.C. (2012). Biomaterials, in *A Roadmap of Biomedical Engineers and Milestones*, Kara, S. (ed.) (Intechopen), pp. 67–114.
194. Gasik, M., Nomura, N., Kondo, R., Hanawa, T. (2013). Thermal analysis, transformations and properties of Pt- and Pd-Alloyed Zr-Nb Alloys. Proc. 18th Plansee Seminar (Plansee, Austria), pp. 91–98.

195. Cochis, A., Azzimonti, B., Della Valle, C., De Giglio, E., Bloise, N., Visai, L., Cometa, S., Rimondini, L., Chiesa, R. (2016). The effect of silver and gallium doped titanium against the multidrug-resistant Acinetobacter baumannii. *Biomaterials*, 80, pp. 80–95.
196. Alt, V., Bechert, T., Steinrucke, P., Wagener, M., Seidel, P., Dingeldein, E., Domann, E., Schnettler, R. (2004). An in vitro assessment of the antibacterial properties and cytotoxicity of nanoparticulate silver bone cement. *Biomaterials*, 25, pp. 4383–4391.
197. Mirzajani, F., Ghassempour, A., Aliahmadi, A., Esmaeili, M.A. (2011). Antibacterial effect of silver nanoparticles on Staphylococcus aureus. *Res Microbiol*, 162, pp. 542–549.
198. Bao, H., Yu, X., Xu, C. et al. (2015). New toxicity mechanism of silver nanoparticles: Promoting apoptosis and inhibiting proliferation. *PLoS One*, 10, pp. 1–10.
199. Cochis, A., Azzimonti, B., Della Valle, C., Chiesa, R., Arciola, C.R., Rimondini, L. (2015). Biofilm formation on titanium implants counteracted by grafting gallium and silver ions. *J Biomed Mater Res*, 103A, pp. 1176–1187.
200. Esposito, M., Grusovin, M.G., Loli, V., Coulthard, P., Worthington, H.V. (2010). Does antibiotic prophylaxis at implant placement decrease early implant failures? A Cochrane systematic review. *Eur J Oral Implantol*, 2, pp. 101–110.
201. Conlon, B.P., Nakayasu, E.S., Fleck, L.E. et al. (2013). Activated ClpP kills persisters and eradicates a chronic biofilm infection. *Nature*, 503, pp. 365–370.
202. Dunbar, M.J. (2009). Antibiotic bone cements: Their use in routine primary total joint arthroplasty is justified. *Orthopedics*, 32, 9.
203. Patti, B.N., Lindeque, B.G. (2011). Antibiotic-loaded acrylic bone cement in the revision of septic arthroplasty: Where's the evidence? *Orthopedics*, 34, pp. 210.
204. Mousset, B., Benoit, M.A., Delloye, C., Bouillet, R., Gillard, J. (1995). Biodegradable implants for potential use in bone infection. An in vitro study of antibiotic-loaded calcium sulphate. *Int Orthoped*, 19, pp.157–161.
205. Roberts, R., McConoughey, S.J., Calhoun, J.H. (2013). Size and composition of synthetic calcium sulphate beads influ-ence dissolution and elution rates in vitro. *J Biomed Mater Res B Appl Biomater*, 102, pp. 667–673.
206. Kluin, O.S., Van Der Mei, H.C., Busscher, H.J., Neut, D. (2013) Biodegradable vs non-biodegradable antibiotic delivery devices in the treatment of osteomyelitis. *Expert Opin Drug Deliv*, 10, pp. 341–351.
207. Gittens, R.A., McLachlan, T., Olivares-Navarrete, R., Cai, Y., Berner, S., Tannenbaum, R. et al. (2011). The effects of combined micron/submicron-scale surface roughness and nanoscale features on cell proliferation and differentiation. *Biomaterials*, 32, pp. 3395–3403.
208. Garcia, A.J., Keselowsky, B.G. (2002). Biomimetic surfaces for control of cell adhesion to facilitate bone formation. *Crit Rev Eukaryot Gene Expr*, 12, pp. 151–162.
209. Anselme, K., Davidson, P., Popa, A.M., Giazzon, M., Liley, M., Ploux, L. (2010). The interaction of cells and bacteria with surfaces structured at the nanometre scale. *Acta Biomater*, 6, pp. 3824–3846.
210. Levon, J., Myllymaa, K., Kouri, V.-P., Rautemaa, R., Kinnari, T., Myllymaa, S., Konttinen, Y.T., Lappalainen, R. (2010). Patterned macroarray plates in comparison of bacterial adhesion inhibition of tantalum, titanium and chromium com-pared with diamond-like carbon. *J Biomed Mater Res A*, 92, pp. 1606–1613.
211. Ivanova, E.P., Truong, V.K., Wang, J.Y., Berndt, C.C., Jones, R.T. et al. (2010). Impact of nanoscale roughness of titanium thin film surfaces on bacterial retention. *Langmuir*, 26, pp. 1973–1982.
212. Park, M.R., Banks, M.K., Applegate, B., Webster, T.J. (2008). Influence of nanophase titania topography on bacterial attachment and metabolism. *Int J Nanomed*, 3, pp. 497–504.

213. Ferraris, S., Venturello, A., Miola, M. et al. (2014). Antibacterial and bioactive nanostructured titanium surfaces for bone integration. *Appl Surf Sci*, 311, pp. 279–291.
214. Costerton, J.W., Montanaro, L., Arciola, C.R. (2005). Biofilm in implant infections: Its production and regulation. *Int J Artif Organs*, 28, pp. 1062–1068.
215. Bryers, J.D. (2008). Medical biofilms. *Biotechnol Bioengin*, 100, pp. 1–18.
216. Hetrick, E.M., Schoenfisch, M.H. (2206). Reducing implant-related infections: Active release strategies. *Chem Soc Rev*, 35, pp. 780–789.
217. Gottenbos, B., Grijpma, D.W., Van Der Mei, H.C., Feijen, J., Busscher, H.J. (2001). Antimicrobial effects of positively charged surfaces on adhering Gram-positive and Gram-negative bacteria. *J Antimicrob Chemother*, 48, pp. 7–13.
218. Arciola, C.R., Radin, L., Alvergna, P., Cenni, E., Pizzoferrato, A. (1993). Heparin surface treatment of poly(methyl-methacrylate) alters adhesion of a Staphylococcus aureus strain: Utility of bacterial fatty acid analysis. *Biomaterials*, 14, pp. 1161–1164.
219. Peterson, B.W., Van Der Mei, H.C., Sjollema, J., Busscher, H.J., Sharma, P.K. (2013). A distinguishable role of eDNA in the viscoelastic relaxation of biofilms. *MBio*, 4, pp. e00497–e0049713.
220. Hall-Stoodley, L., Nistico, L., Sambanthamoorthy, K. et al. (2008) Characterization of biofilm matrix, degradation by DNase treatment and evidence of capsule downregulation in Streptococcus pneumoniae clinical isolates. *BMC Microbiol*, 8, p. 173.
221. Tetz, V.V., Tetz, G.V. (2010). Effect of extracellular DNA destruction by DNase I on characteristics of forming biofilms. *DNA Cell Biol*, 29, pp. 399–405.
222. Donelli, G., Francolini, I., Romoli, D. et al. (2007). Synergistic activity of dispersin B and cefamandole nafate in inhibition of staphylococcal biofilm growth on polyurethanes. *Antimicrob Agents Chemother*, 51, pp. 2733–2740.
223. Wu, H., Song, Z., Hentzer, M. et al. (2004). Synthetic furanones inhibit quorum-sensing and enhance bacterial clearance in Pseudomonas aeruginosa lung infection in mice. *J Antimicrob Chemother*, 53, pp. 1054–1061.
224. Papaioannou, E., Wahjudi, M., Nadal-Jimenez, P., Koch, G., Setroikromo, R., Quax, W.J. (2009). Quorum-quenching acylase reduces the virulence of Pseudomonas aeruginosa in a Caenorhabditis elegans infection model. *Antimicrob Agents Chemother*, 53, pp. 4891–4897.
225. Jennings, J.A., Courtney, H.S., Haggard, W.O. (2012). Cis-2-decenoic acid inhibits S. aureus growth and biofilm in vitro: A pilot study. *Clin Orthoped Relat Res*, 470, pp. 2663–2670.

6 Biomaterial Surface Properties

Implications in Immune Response

Tuğba Endoğan Tanır, Güneş Esendağlı and Eda Ayşe Aksoy

CONTENTS

6.1 GENERAL CONCEPTS IN IMMUNE RESPONSES

Upon recognition of foreign molecules (non-self-antigens), the immune system takes action to "eradicate", "isolate" or "clear" from the body, especially if they are dangerous to the host. The decision is made according to the stress signals (such as produced upon recognition of tissue damage, metabolic intermediates, microbial products and hypoxia) generated during a non-physiological intervention that disrupts tissue homeostasis. The immunogenicity of a molecule together with stress signals drives the behaviour of the immune cells and results in a specific type and magnitude of inflammatory response.

The most intensive response is given when the antigen is of pathogenic microorganisms. In general, if the foreign mass is large and/or does not induce high levels of inflammatory stress (e.g., extracellular parasites) its contact to the tissues is restricted through a reaction involving both immune and stromal cells. In this case, a boundary is drawn to limit exposure to the foreign materials; nevertheless, the immune cells continue to attack and to interact with the material continuously. On the other hand, if the foreign mass is small enough to be easily removed from the body (e.g., dust and pollens), inflammatory responses are accompanied by mechanical movements and excretion. In these cases, both innate and adaptive immune responses are active against the foreign body encountered.

Although the primary function of the immune system is protection of the organism, it should also be emphasised that the immune system not only evolved to protect the organism against invading microorganisms (i.e., bacteria, viruses, fungi, and parasites) but also plays important roles in tissue regeneration and wound healing. Immune cells practise continuous surveillance and they seek distressed areas where locally produced mediators induce their recruitment and activation. In addition, there are immune cell types that are concentrated in the tissues frequently exposed to particles, microorganisms and other environmental stress factors, such as the respiratory epithelium. These resident immune cells are highly adept at recognising foreign antigens and are responsible for giving an initial response and alarming the body's defence mechanisms. In order not to assault and also to protect the healthy (i.e., non-stressed, non-transformed, non-infected or non-damaged) cells of the host organism, the immune cells are either cannot recognise self-antigens, as in the case of the cells of innate immunity, or are "non-responders to self", as in the case of the cells of adaptive immunity. Therefore, in the absence of tissue damage and other factors that would stress the organism, substances that resemble self-antigens or that avoid recognition by the immune system may prevail in the body. On the other hand, once an antigen is recognised as foreign (non-self), especially both by innate and adaptive arms, the persistence or re-exposure of a cell or a material carrying that antigen is more actively targeted and attacked. Recognition of an antigen by the cells of adaptive immunity (e.g., T- and B-lymphocytes) is more complex and happens in a longer timescale, but they possess capacity to remember and give more prompt and stronger responses upon reencounter. Innate immunity (e.g., monocytes, macrophages, natural killer cells (NKs), dendritic cells (DCs) and granulocytes) has the advantage of directly recognising antigens and taking action in case of stress, but the repertoire of innate immunity is limited for recognition of foreign molecules.

T-lymphocytes need to be primed by antigens of peptidic nature. Antigen-presenting cells (APCs) are specialised for ensuring and facilitating the encounter of T-cells with the antigens, which in turn modulate the nature of T-cell responses. DCs, B-lymphocytes and macrophages are the principal APCs that collect, process and introduce the peptide antigens to T-lymphocytes. Upon recognition of the antigens, cytotoxic T-lymphocytes (CTL) or helper T-lymphocytes (Th) become responsive to that particular protein whether it is carried on a cell or structure (such as a particle, or a fibre in the case of biomaterials). Of the APCs, DCs are particularly important due to their ability to capture antigens and to actively transport them to the lymphoid tissues (lymph nodes) populated by T-cells. When an appropriate amount of an antigen is presented by APCs in the company of additional (co-stimulatory) signals, T-cells become activated and begin to proliferate (i.e., clonally expand). This cross-talk between T-cells and APCs mediated by the antigens results in the acquisition of a specific functional phenotype by the T-cells, which can be destructive (Th1, Th17, CTL subtypes) or regulatory/compensatory (Th2 or Treg subtypes) due to the phenotypic plasticity of immune cells. Th lymphocytes assist and modulate both adaptive and innate immune responses; depending on their subtype, they can augment or alleviate the magnitude of reactions. For example, Th1 cells increase the secretion of degradation enzymes, and the production of reactive intermediates and phagocytosis in macrophages and neutrophils. Th1 also supports cytotoxic T-lymphocytes to kill the cells that present target proteins.

Once the antigens arrive in the lymph nodes, the B-cells are simultaneously activated with T-cells. B-cells, adaptive immunity cells with antibody production, antigen memory and antigen-presenting roles, can recognise soluble, concentrated antigens in the lymph nodes directly (i.e., without a need for an antigen-presenting cell unlike T-cells). In fact, B-cells internalise the antigen for presentation to T-cells. B-cells recognise antigens by membrane-bound Igs (surface antibodies). After being activated, B-cells also produce antibodies in soluble form for antigen elimination. B-lymphocytes are another critical subset that need help from T-cells to react more specifically and efficiently. Once a Th1-type immune response is initiated, activated B-cells start to produce more IgGs than IgMs, which are more effective and specified in immunity. Some of the B-cells differentiate into plasma cells (which have significant longevity) with a high capacity to produce antibodies. Binding of the secreted antibodies with the antigens with high specificity and affinity results in the triggering of cytotoxic activities towards the invading organisms containing the given antigen. The antibody coating of the target cells or materials can be easily recognised by phagocytes such as NKs and they are subsequently eliminated by a process defined as "antibody-dependent cellular cytotoxicity (ADCC)". Moreover, antibodies can also trigger other defence mechanisms such as induced apoptosis and complement-mediated cell lysis. In addition to T- and B-lymphocytes, there are other minor subsets of adaptive immune cells with different capacities to discriminate between foreign and self-antigens.

As lymphoid members of the innate immune system, natural killer (NK) cells can give rapid responses without prior sensitisation. This is regulated by the balance between inhibitory and activated signals. NK cells efficiently destroy stressed cells (i.e., with intracellular infection or cells that has undergone transformation) and avoid harming healthy (non-stressed) cells. An activated NK cell can attach to the target cells' membrane and lead to the target cell's death by secretion of enzymes (such as perforins and granzymes) from their granules and by inducing apoptosis. Additionally, cytokine secretions of the activated NK cells are destructive in immune reactions.

In response to local stress signals that alarm the immune system, monocytes leave the blood circulation and migrate through the connective tissue towards the source of the signals. Upon arrival within the tissues, they differentiate and mature into macrophages. Alternatively, there are tissue-resident macrophages that contribute locally and promptly to the immune reactions. Differentiated macrophages are phagocytes that clear cell debris and macromolecular antigens in wound sites. They produce a big arsenal of biologically active products starting from simple molecules such as ROSs to chemokines, enzymes (proteases), complement components, growth factors and cytokines. According to the microenvironment where the macrophages are found, they can basically differentiate into two functional subsets, either with destructive and pro-inflammatory characters (M1) or with repairing and anti-inflammatory characters (M2). M1 macrophages can result in collateral tissue damage through the production of ROSs, nitric oxide (NO) and various proteolytic enzymes. Furthermore, if the stress factor is originated from a dangerous microorganism (e.g., *Mycobacterium tuberculosis*), M1 macrophages become implicated in the formation of granulomas where they are observed as giant multi-nucleated cells and they contribute to the formation of boundaries around the infected zones. On the other hand, the M2 subtype of macrophages are identified in the healing tissues or in the areas where a stress factor is isolated or being cleared out. They can contribute to the remodelling of the extracellular matrix, angiogenesis, clearance of tissue debris and immune suppression.

Polymorphonuclear neutrophils (PMN) are the most abundant type of leukocytes in the blood. Even though they have a short life-span, they are a vital part of the immune system. PMNs are the most motile leukocytes with their high capacity to easily travel through the stroma and they are usually the first to reach to the site of injury, especially in the acute phase of inflammation. Neutrophils respond to any type of stress including infections, cancer, trauma, heat changes, sterile inflammation, changes in the oxygen levels and pH and other disorders and disruptions of homeostasis. Similar to other phagocytic cells (i.e., macrophages), neutrophils are indispensable in fighting against extracellular bacteria through phagocytosis, releasing reactive molecules and enzymes to remove the invading microorganisms. In the context of biomaterials, neutrophils are also one of the first cell types that interact with biomaterial surfaces upon implantation.

Other than the cellular elements, soluble factors, i.e., plasma proteins, are also an important component of the innate immune system. These factors possess an affinity to bind foreign structures either to directly kill, neutralise (render them non-functional) or convert them into better targets for phagocytic cells. A family of small proteins, the complement system, is one of the most efficient soluble factors which are not only cytotoxic and opsonising but also have capacities to recruit additional leukocytes to the site of inflammation. When an antigen becomes opsonised by circulating factors such as complement, pentraxin, collectin and ficolin proteins, an antigen becomes marked for immune response or simply for clearance from the tissue (e.g., dead cells). Antibodies that are produced against a specific antigen can also opsonise, trigger complement reactions and neutralise the target.

Inflammatory signals produced in the injured tissue have a substantial role to initiate and regulate the healing process. During the inflammatory phase, pathogenic organisms and debris are cleared, the wound bed is sealed by clot formation and tissue repair mechanisms are simultaneously triggered. Immune cells that are recruited into the site of inflammation regulate the proliferation and maturation of stromal and parenchymal cells that re-establish and maintain homeostasis. Nevertheless, tissue healing can be hindered by the presence of infections, foreign bodies and ischemia. In the case of biomaterial-based applications, the presence of the biomaterial-based structures becomes an important component on the type, intensity and length of immune responses.

6.2 BIOMATERIALS AND BIOINTERFACES

Biomaterials are mostly originated from natural or synthetic materials and their design is influenced in order to meet the needs of clinical applications with the development of new manufacturing and processing technologies. In a recent Consensus Conference of the ESB (European Society for Biomaterials), a biomaterial was defined as "a material intended to interface with biological systems to evaluate, treat, augment or replace any tissue, organ or function of the body" [1]. Biomaterials can be ranged from bioinert materials to regenerative materials that can interact *in vivo* to influence the biological processes towards tissue regeneration. In the current biomaterial definition, the term "interface" emphasises the biointerface between a biomaterial and cell, tissue or any living material. Schematic representation of biointerface is shown in Figure 6.1. The interactions between cells, tissues and biomaterial at the tissue-implant interface are almost always related with surface phenomena. These biointerface reactions directly or indirectly determine the fate of biomaterial and affect healing process.

6.2.1 Biomaterial Surface Properties

Generally, surface properties of biomaterials differ from their bulk properties due to unbalanced surface forces and surface energy. Either environmental contaminants or biological contaminants can adsorb on biomaterial surfaces. Also, upon biomaterial implantation there can be enhanced molecular mobility and orientation of surface domains. Active molecules, compounds or impurities can desorb from bulk phase of biomaterial. Chemical changes like those that can be caused by sterilisation techniques can result in oxidation or cross-linking of surface-active groups. All of these challenging situations may occur at biointerface, and they all affect and change the surface properties of biomaterials. Thus, for any *in vitro* or *in vivo* application of biomaterials, the definition and characterisation of the surface properties are crucial. Chemical composition, surface charge, surface reactions, surface energy, surface thermodynamics and surface morphology etc. are highly relevant surface properties with respect to the immune response to biomaterials as they affect protein, cell, blood, bacteria and tissue biomaterial interactions [2].

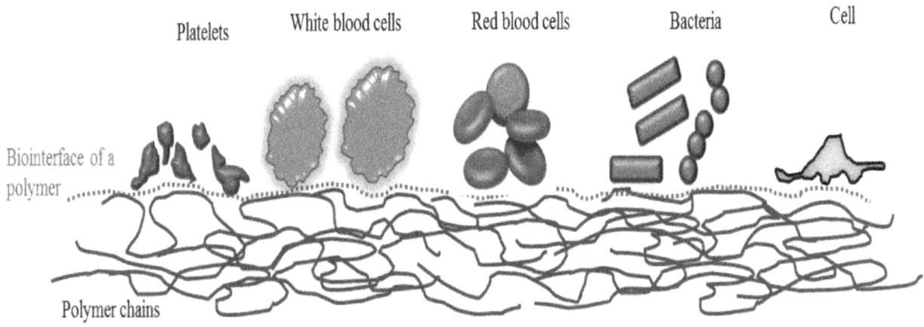

FIGURE 6.1 Illustration of a polymer biointerface: contact with platelets, white blood cells, red blood cells, bacteria and cells, respectively.

Surface chemistry, surface free energy and surface hydrophilicity are dominant properties and they play a critical role in the establishment of an adsorbed biomolecule layer within a few seconds of implantation. The atomic composition of the surface can be defined by surface chemistry and may differ for each biomaterial due to the type of chemical bonding and spatial arrangement of surface atoms. Surface atomic composition directly affects tissue-material interactions. More specifically, surface chemistry determines the type of electrostatic or chemical interactions between proteins and surface molecules [3]. The chemical composition of biomaterial surfaces can be characterised by spectroscopic surface analysis tools such as electron spectroscopy for chemical analysis etc. Surface hydrophilicity or the degree of wettability are other important surface properties and can be quantified by contact angle values of wetting liquid or water droplets on biomaterial surface [2,4]. The surface chemistry of functional groups determines the wettability and water contact angle values of biomaterials. In the case of polymer-based biomaterials, we can predict the surface functional groups according to the type of polymer. Polymers are high-molecular-weight macromolecules composed of covalently bonded specific repeating units. In this manner, generally polymer-based biomaterials may contain several of well-known hydrophilic functional groups such as -OH, $-NH_2$, -COOH, $-OSO_3H$ or non-polar hydrophobic functional groups ($-CH_2$, $-CH_{3}$.(Si-O)-CH_3-, $-CF_2$ etc.). The presence of hydrophilic functional groups leads to high-energy surfaces and results in unusual surface characteristics. Due to unbalanced intermolecular interactions and forces across the surface, more energetic properties are observed on the surface layer rather than the bulk phase. Surface free energy, the energy required to change the surface chemistry of a material per unit area, can be determined by goniometer measurements with proper multiple test liquids. Surface free energy has polar, dispersive, acidic and basic components, and they are also very important for biomaterial-tissue interactions. The surface hydrophilicity of biomaterial firstly affects the protein adsorption upon implantation. When a hydrophobic biomaterial is implanted *in vivo*, within the few seconds water molecules detach from the solid surface biointerface and re-arrangement of proteins take place. These conformational changes generally result in continuous adsorption of protein layers on the biomaterial surface. A tight and irreversible protein binding mostly occurs on biointerface. In the case of a hydrophilic biomaterial surface, desorption of the water from the biointerface is thermodynamically non-favourable. In this case, proteins stay within a solvation shell, and protein adsorption mainly takes place on the surface through this hydration layer. Due to the hydration layer, protein adsorption on hydrophilic surfaces is generally weak and reversible. Moreover, biomaterials that have very high hydrophilic surface properties may expel protein molecules and inhibit protein adsorption. It is clear that optimisation of surface hydrophilicity by controlling surface chemistry is necessary in order to obtain more precise control of protein adsorption [2,5,6].

6.3 IMMUNE RESPONSES TO BIOMATERIALS

Biocompatibility can be described as the capability of a given biomaterial to cause acceptable host response when implanted in the body for a specific application.

Acceptable host response comprises absence of blood clotting, no bacterial growth and appropriate healing. Body recognition, tolerance and biocompatibility are very significant issues starting upon implantation of a biomaterial and lasting during the whole *in vivo* lifetime. A major concern is adverse reactions to the biomaterial, which can frequently result in complication or rejection. Therefore, after implantation immune response should be assessed in order to demonstrate that biomaterial functions as designed and induces no significant damage to the surrounding tissue.

When biomaterials are implanted into the body, within two to three weeks several host responses occur which sequentially can be given as: (i) injury; (ii) initial blood-material interactions; (iii) provisional matrix deposition; (iv) acute inflammation; (v) chronic inflammation; (vi) granulation tissue formation (foreign body reaction); and (vii) fibrosis/fibrous capsule development, respectively [7]. Generally, when an implant comes into contact with blood, protein adsorption takes place based on the surface properties of the biomaterial and followed by macrophage adhesion, release of chemokines and acute inflammation. Then chronic inflammation may occur due to ineffective resolution of acute inflammation causing foreign body giant cell formation and eventually fibrous encapsulation of the biomaterial. It is important to understand these immune reactions that arise at the biomaterial and tissue interface in order to improve implant integration and to guarantee acceptance of the implant by the body.

Implantation of a biomaterial causes injury to adjacent tissues, which initiates a cascade of events leading to wound healing. The response of the body to injury depends on several factors such as its degree, level of damage to the basement membrane, level of provisional matrix formation, hypoxia conditions, level of necrotic cells and the degree of immune response [8]. After implantation, initially complement proteins are activated and due to the cell damage or existence of pathogens, cellular pattern recognition receptors are stimulated. Then, the production of inflammatory cytokines and chemokines (such as MCP-1, IL-8) triggers recruitment of PMNs, monocytes and eventually fibroblasts respectively to the site of injury. Neutrophils at the wound zones are responsible for eliminating pathogens and cellular debris formed during the injury [9]. They disappear one or two days after the injury, to be replaced by monocytes. As mentioned previously, after extravasation from circulation monocytes in the injury microenvironment differentiate into macrophages, which stay in the wounded area for a period lasting up to months. The M2 subtype of macrophages, which are responsible for tissue remodelling and repair, are polarised by the cytokines released by mast cells (a myeloid cell type that resides in the tissues, especially the skin, and gives a prompt response to tissue damage) and later by type 2 helper T-cells (Th2) [7].

The surgical stress and tissue injury upon implantation of a foreign material can induce a strong inflammatory response, which can eventually lead to a foreign body reaction. In the later stages, macrophages fuse to form multinucleated, foreign body giant cells with high phagocytic activity and the implant is surrounded by a granulation tissue. Unless the inflammation is resolved, macrophages and foreign body giant cells further induce attraction and stimulation of other immune cells and also stromal cells such as fibroblasts. This is followed by recessive ECM deposition and encapsulation of the implanted biomaterial [10]. The series of events described, the steps of immune response to a biomaterial, are represented in Figure 6.2.

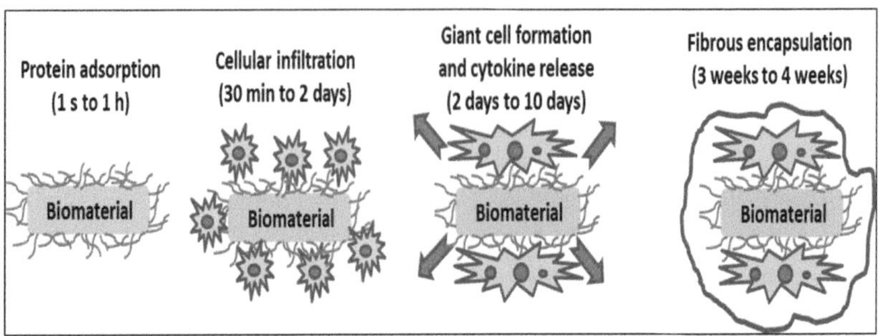

FIGURE 6.2 Representation of immune response to biomaterial.

At the chronic inflammation stage, withdrawal of some macrophages and PMNs take place in the injury site, together with the infiltration of plasma cells (B-cells) and lymphocytes. In order to repair the wound, local extracellular matrix (ECM) is remodelled and new ECM components are secreted by fibroblasts proliferating at the injury site. The extent and length of the chronic response, which induces further cytokine secretion and results in granulation tissue formation, affects the remodelling of ECM and eventually plays a decisive role in tissue regeneration or scar formation. A quick (approximately two-week-long) resolution to this chronic inflammation with immune cell presence often indicates acceptance of the implant, whereas the persistence of immune infiltration for longer periods is often associated with infections, fibrous encapsulation and/or rejection of the implant.

6.3.1 Immune Response to Biodegradable Biomaterials

Biodegradation is described as a gradual degradation of a biomaterial driven by biological activities (such as enzymatic degradation, degradation via chemical secreted by cells, or erosion of the material in the presence of biological fluids). Physicochemical properties of a material may change upon exposure to body fluids (such as saliva, blood, mucus) due to mechanical, biophysical and biochemical interactions between the biomaterial and its microenvironment. The biodegradation of polymers depends on the polymer characteristics and where they are implanted in the body. Several mechanisms such as oxidation, hydrolytic and enzymatic dissociation are implicated in the biodegradation process of polymers. In the case of natural polymers such as hyaluronic acid, gelatin, chondroitin sulfate etc. there can be specific enzymes that are able to actively degrade the biomaterial. In the biodegradation of polymers, the activation of macrophages and their subsequent activities such as cytokine and ROS secretion and phagocytosis are the basic factors influencing their rate of biodegradation [11]. Once macrophages adhere onto the surface of biomaterials (and also later when they become foreign body giant cells), they release degradation mediators such as ROSs, lytic enzymes and acidic substances; then, the biomaterials' surface becomes susceptible to biodegradation. Degradation products are released and the surface of the biomaterial becomes altered, which has additional impact on immune responses [12]. Depending on the structure of the implanted material, the initial degradation can further facilitate the degradation and can even result in abrupt failure of the structure.

Inflammatory cells, especially macrophages, have the ability to secrete reactive oxygen species such as nitric oxide (NO), superoxide (O_2^-), hydrogen peroxide (H_2O_2) and hypochlorous acid (HOCl) as a part of the inflammatory response to the presence of foreign materials which may cause oxidative degradation. In the hydrolytic degradation of polymers, chemical bonds in the polymer chain are broken by water molecules, resulting in the decrease of molecular weight of polymer. Hydrolytic degradation may be induced by the presence of salts, acids and bases. Moreover, enzymes such as proteases, esterases, glycosidases and phosphatases may catalyse hydrolysis reactions. Due to the presence of a large number of enzymes and active degradation by the cells, the *in vivo* degradation rates of polymers could be faster than *in vitro* degradation [13]. However, in certain contexts, fast degradation rates can be advantageous to avoid a permanent and chronic immune response, provided that the integrity of the implanted material was secure during the planned activity period.

When biomaterial is implanted and exposed to body fluids, it immediately comes into contact with proteins, termed opsonins, that form an identifiable coating around the material for phagocytic cells. Recognition of opsonins through specific membrane receptors (for example, Fc, complement and mannose receptors) is one of the major pathways to induce and activate phagocytes and in general inflammatory response. Phagocytic cells are members of innate immunity, which mediates a non-specific first-line response against foreign materials. Polymorphonuclear (i.e., PMNs) and mononuclear cells (i.e., monocytes, macrophages and DCs) recognise the opsonised substance and engulf it [14].

Neutrophils and macrophages ingest foreign materials with a diameter smaller than 10 μm while larger substances (10–100 μm) are phagocytosed by multinucleated giant cells. When materials are large enough to prevent phagocytosis, a phenomenon called "frustrated phagocytosis" is observed, characterised by the secretion of additional proteases, radicals and acids to help the degradation without avail [15]. Size of the materials affects the amount of released ROS and enzymes. Enzymes affect the degradation of biomaterials by different rates depending on chemical composition, homogeneity and porosity. While enzymes degrade foreign materials, they may also be harmful to the surrounding tissue, generating an irreversible collateral damage in the chronic inflammatory stage. The release of enzymes by neutrophils and macrophages is highly dependent on the surface characteristics of polymeric materials. Hydrophilic surfaces promote interaction with fibronectin, fibrin and albumin in the blood, stimulating adhesion of neutrophils to the proteins and inducing the degranulation behaviour – or it can induce granule delivery (which contains high amounts of enzymes).

Chemical modification of a polymer structure or functionalisation of polymer by immobilisation of degradable molecules can affect degradability of polymer-based biomaterials in the presence of biological fluids and immune cells. Degradable polymeric systems may be used in a way where the degradation rate can be controlled to match the designed use, taking into consideration the potential immune response (such as in the case of controlled delivery systems based on degradable polymers).

For example, by adjusting the glycolic acid:lactic acid ratio of poly(lactic-glycolic) acid (PLGA) copolymer, it is possible to control the degradation rate of polymer. The higher the glycolic acid amount (up to 50%), the faster the rate of erosion. In the degradation of such polymers along with hydrolysis, the activity of phagocytes was implicated as the cause of degradation [16].

6.3.2 Immune Response to Cell-Grafted Biomaterials

In some tissue regeneration applications, cells are seeded on or encapsulated in the scaffolds for various reasons like production of therapeutic biomolecules, to facilitate the tissue regeneration or guiding the incoming host cells during tissue repair. The cells to be transplanted can originate from the host itself (autologous), from the same species but a different individual (allogeneic) or from a different species (xenogeneic). The presence of cells in implanted scaffolds can modulate both adaptive and innate immune response against the biomaterials. Especially in the case of allogeneic or xenogeneic cell implantation, not only the biomaterial becomes a target for the immune cells, but the donor cells of foreign origin also serve as a trigger for adaptive immunity. Under the influence of adaptive responses, the innate arm of immunity becomes more potent. Therefore, the reaction against the biomaterial and the embedded cells creates a loop where macrophages encapsulate part of the biomaterials (if the size and the chemistry of the biomaterial permit it) and digest and release digested fragments to stimulate adaptive immune cells, which results in more specific downstream immune responses. As mentioned previously, macrophages are of professional antigen-presenting cells (APCs) that efficiently engulf the materials they recognise and process them to present to T-cells and induce T-cell activation. In cases where cells are present (i.e., allogeneic or xenogeneic cells) that are recognised as foreign (non-self), macrophages and potentially other APCs collect protein antigens and trigger the adaptive immune responses through molecules such as MHC, CD80 and CD86 [17]. Moreover, the foreign antigens directly presented by the implanted cells to the host T-cells can also prime immune reactions leading T-rejection. Eventually, destruction of the transplanted cells can happen through the immune response, which will render the overall system dysfunctional. Therefore, additional immune modulation or suppression is required prior to implantation of biomaterials engrafted with xenogeneic and allogeneic cells, similar to transplants. Alternatively, immune responses to cell-grafted biomaterials can be controlled by limiting the access of the host immune cells to them by encapsulating the cells within polymeric structures such as hydrogels that have large enough mesh sizes to enable nutrient and oxygen transfer but small enough pores to prevent cellular infiltration of immune cells. This method has been largely employed for encapsulation of pancreatic islets in polymeric hydrogels such as alginate and Poly vinyl alcohol (PVA) [18].

6.3.3 Modulation of Immune Response Against Biomaterials

When a biocompatible material is implanted, the outcome of the implantation is influenced by the surface chemistry charge, topography and surface area:volume ratio of the biomaterial. After implantation, acute response begins as an immune reaction against injury and foreign materials, and is then followed by a chronic immune response including specific recognition of antigens from the material component or, if present, the transplanted cells. Exertion of control on tissue responses at the implant site using the properties of the implanted material is expected to promote the wound healing process and acceptance of the implant. Therefore, strategies have been developed such as selection of material, alteration of surface topography and surface modification in order to modulate the local immune response so that tissue regeneration around or in the implanted biomaterial can be more effectively achieved.

6.3.3.1 Selection of Material

Selection of an inert material or modifying its properties may lessen the immune response to implanted biomaterial. The reason for using inert biomaterial is to reduce the host response by preventing cell-biomaterial interactions. Inert biomaterials are still recognised as foreign by the host immune system, but they are well tolerated due to the limited interaction with the host and they are encapsulated by a fibrous tissue. However, such bioinertness also implies a definitive separation between the biomaterial and the host, which is not suitable for many applications (such as organ regeneration). Hence, it has been noted that allowing and controlling specific immune cell responses may actually be advantageous for the integration of implants and improving their performance.

The chemistry of material affects the adsorbed proteins, which in turn mediates the interactions with immune cells and may cause their activation. Mostly, monocyte adhesion tends to increase when hydrophobic materials are implanted leading to a more pronounced local immune response. When hydrophilic or neutral materials are used, monocyte/macrophage adhesion and also FBGC formation are reduced *in vitro*. However, the adhered cells produce high levels of pro-inflammatory cytokines [9]. In order to increase stability of natural matrices like the extracellular matrix (ECM), generally chemical cross-linking is applied, though it can affect immune response. It was reported that acellular ECM scaffolds without any chemical modification usually lead to an increased M2 macrophage polarisation, while chemical cross-linking of scaffolds causes an M1 macrophage response [19]. Blends of biomaterials can induce specific immune responses; for example, silicone and blends of polydioxanone, elastin and collagen are stated to induce modulated immune responses. It has been reported that in response to all kinds of biomaterials, natural killer (NK) cells reduce their activity while macrophage functions remain unaffected [20–22]. Thus, a specific mixture of biomaterials, such as blends of polydioxanone and elastin and collagen, may possess specific immunosuppressive effects on adaptive or innate immunity.

When we look at more specific applications, for example, for cardiovascular stents, material type, stent configuration and surface properties critically affect stent restenosis and related inflammation [23]. In recent years, drug-eluting stents and biodegradable stents are widely used in clinical practice. In both stent types, biodegradable polymers are used as coating or base materials and their risk in increasing inflammation in the stent microenvironment has been mentioned in clinical case reports. According to the study of Hara and colleagues, polylactic acid, polycaprolactone, polyethylvinylacetate and polyorganophosphazene have the ability to cause inflammation as stent coatings. Polyurethane- and polytetrafluoroethane-based coatings are reported to be more biocompatible polymers compared to others. Totally biodegradable stents, mostly composed of poly-L-lactate, are expected to show better anti-thrombogenic potential with less stent restenosis and minimum inflammatory response. These clinical results show that, for cardiovascular stents, proper polymer selection is important and their safety and inflammatory properties must be evaluated in long-term models.

Ti implants and Ti surfaces have a wide range of application in the biomedical field and they are promising materials for the development of new-generation intelligent nano-biomaterials. Neacsua and colleagues focused on a lipopolysaccharide bacterial mimicking model and investigated the inflammatory responses of TiO_2 nanotube surfaces in different culture mediums. The finding of this study showed that TiO_2 nanotubes decreased inflammatory activity of macrophages. In the presence of LPS, RAW 264.7 macrophages responded less to the nanotube-modified surface, compared to flat non-modified surface. TiO_2 nanotubes provided macrophage modulation directed towards healing, rather than induction of a pro-inflammatory environment [24]. There are also examples of Ti surface modifications with natural compounds like flavonoids. Flavonoids are polyphenols of natural origin with known antimicrobial, antioxidant and anti-inflammatory properties. Surface modification was carried out by covalent immobilisation of flavonoids (taxifolin and quercitrin) on titanium substrates. Ti surfaces modified with flavonoids showed anti-inflammatory properties and anti-fibrotic potential [25].

6.3.3.2 Alteration of Surface Topography

Variation of surface topography and roughness can also affect the interaction of immune cells with biomaterials and modulate their activation. Cells adhere, proliferate, migrate and express genes as a response to the extracellular matrix components in nanometer scale. Introduction of micro or nano patterns on the surface of biomaterials may simulate the natural topographical features of ECM and such topographical patterns can in turn influence the behaviour of cells. For instance, fibrous scaffolds with aligned fibres had less capsule formation and more cellular in-growth compared to the fibrous scaffolds random fibre alignment [26]. Moreover, when the surface of a biomaterial was modified by introduction of micron-scale architectures, a specific macrophage phenotype different from M1 and M2 was observed showing the necessity for further studies on the characterisation of macrophages on micro/nanopatterned structures [27]. In another study, microarchitecture decreased capsule formation *in vivo* [28]. Parallel gratings with line width ranging from 250 nm to 2 μm had significantly affected the morphology of macrophages and their cytokine secretion profiles *in vitro* and also influenced macrophage adhesion *in vivo* [29]. Another generic effect of the presence of surface topographies is the increased ratio of macrophage and FBGC presence compared to smooth surfaces [7].

Surface topography and wettability properties of Ti surfaces were also studied in the context of macrophage activation. Smooth Ti surface induced increased secretion of TNF-α, IL-1β and IL-6, whereas hydrophilic and rough surfaces increased the secretion of anti-inflammatory cytokines IL-4 and IL-10 [30].

6.3.4 Steroidal and Non-Steroidal Anti-Inflammatory Drugs

Steroidal and non-steroidal anti-inflammatory drugs (NSAID) are a broad spectrum of drugs that are widely used to control inflammation and suppress the host response in the body. However, long-term use of NSAIDs has major side effects and systemic toxicity problems and therefore their systemic use is limited. As an alternative approach, the localised therapeutic modalities are reported to decrease NSAID side effects with effective control of inflammation and fibrosis [31]. NSAID-formulated biomaterial strategies were developed in order to prevent a foreign body reaction to medical devices. Implants capable of NSAIDs elution have been developed in order to provide local NSAID release to sustain long-term immunomodulation with fewer side effects [32].

The most widely used application of NSAID-formulated biomaterials are wound dressings because acute and chronic wounds are worldwide health complications. In the wound healing process, firstly the release of the histamine serotonin takes place. Phagocytes reach the wound site. The inflammation results in the formation of blood clotting, and this blood clot mostly acts as a protection layer for the wound. During inflammation, most patients suffer from pain [33]. In infected wounds, continuous pain and an augmented inflammatory response take place. The infecting microorganisms cause the release of inflammatory mediators, enzymes and free radicals. Also, foreign body reaction mediated by wound dressings can be observed and the development of foreign body reaction slows down the wound healing process [33]. In the literature, there are several antimicrobial and/or anti-inflammatory drug-containing wound dressing formulations. In order to obtain a rapid and local pain relief, anaesthetics or NSAIDs-eluting wound dressings have been developed [33]. These systems have the advantage of dose arrangement while avoiding systemic toxicity. In this manner, Arapoglou et al. developed an ibuprofen-releasing wound dressing foam. Ibuprofen was selected due to its excellent local effects and analgesic efficacy on wounds. Clinical study showed that a wound dressing formulated with ibuprofen had proper effects on pain relief [34]. Meloxicam is another example of NSAIDs and inhibits COX-2 (cyclooxgenease-2). Meloxicam mostly relieves the inflammatory symptoms of osteoarthritis, rheumatoid and arthritis, but at high doses or long-term treatments it was reported to have gastrointestinal side effects, peptic ulceration and bleeding, etc. [35,36]. Khurana et al. prepared meloxicam containing a nano-emulsion gel formulation for transdermal applications and obtained a local and effective anti-inflammatory therapy with low-dose treatment. For symptomatic therapy of pain and inflammation in osteoarthritis, a rheumatoid arthritis aceclofenac non-steroidal anti-inflammatory drug is also used. Todosijevi et al. worked on microemulsion formulations via natural or synthetic surfactants to obtain efficient skin absorption of aceclofenac while avoiding irritation [37].

As a model for drug-eluting medical device surfaces, surface modification of polypropylene was performed via temperature- and pH-responsive copolymer grafting [38]. These temperature- and pH-responsive copolymer-grafted polypropylene surfaces were studied for the controlled release of NSAIDs. The apolar and polar sites of modified polypropylene surfaces interacted with hydrophobic and ionic groups of diclofenac and ibuprofen, respectively. Promising results were obtained for the design of hemocompatible and cytocompatible drug-eluting medical devices [38].

Glucose sensors are important medical devices, and their read-out accuracy and sensitivity are critically needed for the management of diabetes. For implantable glucose sensors, loss of device function is a widely seen problem, because after implantation tissue trauma occurs and this causes inflammation and fibrosis, which in turn reduces the ability of the sensor to make accurate measurements. Hickey et al. worked on the effect of dexamethasone/PLGA microspheres for suppressing the inflammatory tissue response against these implantable sensors. The results showed the minimisation of acute inflammatory reaction with low-dose dexamethasone and suppression of the inflammatory response of implanted material for at least one month upon *in vivo* implantation [31]. Chandorkar et al. investigated the effect of salicylic acid release from a biodegradable, cross-linked polyester backbone, for the reduction of foreign body response in mice where the incorporation of an anti-inflammatory drug into the polymer backbone was carried out. Salicylic acid is a deacetylation product of aspirin, the most widely used NSAID. Both aspirin and salicylic acid act by inhibition of the cyclooxygenase enzyme, which is necessary in the biosynthesis of prostaglandins, and as a result causes an anti-inflammatory activity. Salicylic acid-incorporated new polyester showed surface type erosion and decreased inflammatory cell densities. There was also less pro-inflammatory cytokine secretion (TNF-α and IL-1β) with a vascularised, homogeneous encapsulating tissue around the implant [32].

Peptide fibre gels are potential drug carrier systems for local delivery applications with advantageous release profiles due to increased surface area. Webber et al. prepared dexamethasone-releasing peptide amphiphile nanofibres. Histological examinations showed dexamethasone conjugated peptide amphiphile nanofibres reduced inflammatory cells [39]. In another study, MSH (melanocyte stimulating hormone with known anti-inflammatory properties)-adsorbed PLGA microspheres resulted in at least three days of release of MSH and decreased the inflammatory responses by reduction of inflammatory cytokine expression [40].

In order to obtain local drug delivery from the biomaterial surface, polymer coatings via electrostatic or covalent binding or layer-by-layer technologies are widely used. Multi-drug-eluting biomaterial surfaces can be organised by layer-by-layer technologies. As an example, a multidrug delivery system for anionic therapeutic heparin and a hydrophobic drug was designed by layer-by-layer film deposition technique [41]. In layer-by-layer systems, the presence of biodegradable polymers provided the advantage of a surface type of erosion and extended the drug release profiles. The selection of proper biodegradable polymers either as a suitable biomaterial coating or as a drug delivery vesicle for drug properties (stability, solubility etc.) is important and needs careful optimisation.

6.3.5 Surface Modification Strategies

Surface treatments or coatings may alter the immune response to the biomaterial by providing a modified surface chemistry for controlling protein adsorption and as a consequence the level of recognition and response by the immune system. Surface properties may be altered either passively by altering the physicochemical features (e.g., chemistry or topography) or actively by targeting cell behaviour systematically with specially designed molecules or matrices.

The purpose of passive modulation of biomaterial surface properties is to decrease the innate response targeting the adhesion of macrophages and their activation and eventual FBGC formation. Surface chemistry affects the conformation of the adsorbed proteins [12]. The most commonly adsorbed proteins include complement components, serum albumin, fibronectin, fibrinogen, vitronectin. Therefore, the composition of the adsorbed protein layer determines the binding and signalling by the immune cells. By altering the surface chemistry of biomaterial, different cellular responses will be observed. Studies have shown that surface modification of polymers by altering their hydrophobic, hydrophilic or ionic properties changes protein expression profiles and the cytokine/chemokine responses of macrophages [42]. Generally, protein adsorption takes place through hydrophobic interactions. Hydrophilicity of a biomaterial can change the level of water on the surface. The presence of water molecules on a biomaterial surface decreases the tendency of proteins to adsorb. When macrophages were cultured on hydrophilic and anionic surfaces, less macrophage spreading and eventual apoptosis were observed [43]. The presence of plasma proteins like fibronectin and vitronectin on the implant surface disrupts the FBGC formation. In order to reduce dendritic cell maturation, hydrophilicity of the biomaterial can be increased [15]. Likewise, surface coatings have been applied to control protein adsorption and decrease immune response. Coatings may provide a certain amount of steric hindrance due to their chain length and conformation and this can form a barrier to prevent protein adsorption. Cell mediators of the immune system cannot identify materials when protein adsorption is limited by coating and material is detected as immunologically inert. Several natural materials like chitosan, hyaluronan, alginate collagen, dextran and synthetic materials like PVA, PLGA and PEG have been used as coatings for biomaterials. The grafting of hydrogels onto polymeric surfaces led to diminished adsorption of proteins, less monocyte adhesion and pro-inflammatory cytokine secretion after implantation [44]. It was reported that capsule thickness around the positively charged polymer surfaces was reduced after osteopontin coating [45]. Surfactant-based treatments reduced biofouling and also adhesion of platelets [46]. It can be concluded that surface modification of biomaterials is an alternative approach in order to produce desired polymorphonuclear leukocyte (PMN) and macrophage activities.

6.3.6 Development of Multifunctional Surfaces

Multifunctional surfaces are expected to achieve multiple biological activities, either simultaneously or successively. Several strategies have been proposed in order to develop multifunctional surfaces. Muszanska et al. designed a model composed of anti-adhesive polymer brushes that prevents bacterial attachment, loaded with a contact-killing antimicrobial peptide, and arginine-glycine-aspartate (RGD) peptides that enhance cell adhesion [47]. In another study, antibiotic (rifampicin)-containing osteogenic polymeric (blends of PCL and chitosan) nanofibre meshes were prepared to create a multifunctional surface that kills bacteria while providing a proper microenvironment for tissue cells [48]. In order to improve surface properties, electrophoretic deposition (EPD) was used to deposit biopolymers, bioactive glass particles and antibiotics on metallic orthopaedic prostheses. Positive effects of improved composite coating on cell attachment, proliferation and antibacterial properties were reported [49]. The incorporation of bioactive molecules such as RGD sequences, cytokines, growth factor and drugs is one of the methods used for biomaterial functionalisation. For this purpose, polyelectrolyte multilayer coatings have been widely used. They are formed by sequential deposition of polyanions and polycations in order to obtain specific surface properties. For example, Ozcelik et al. developed a surface coating system composed of polyarginine (PAR) and HA polyelectrolyte multilayer films. Then film was modified by the incorporation of catestatin (CAT), which is a natural host defence peptide. Antimicrobial peptides secreted against pathogens are promising alternatives to conventional antibiotics as there is less risk of resistance development. Moreover, these peptides also demonstrate antiviral and antifungal activities and thus can provide an additional level of protection during wound healing. They have antimicrobial activity against both Gram-positive and Gram-negative bacteria and they are also known to be antifungal and antiviral. Such biomimetic coatings, which are simultaneously anti-inflammatory and antimicrobial, can be used to have more positive outcomes for implant application by decreasing infection risk and increasing implant integration at the same time [50].

The incorporation of specific integrin binding sites on biomaterial surfaces is another modification in order to direct responses of inflammatory cells. Immune cell adhesion and activation can be controlled by the presentation of adhesive oligopeptide sequences such as RGD. Besides RGD, proline-histidine-serine-arginine-asparagine (PHSRN) domain was reported to mediate macrophage adhesion and polarisation via integrins and controlled FBGC formation [51]. In addition to integrin ligand incorporation, biomaterial surface is also modified with PEG coatings, which is also known as PEGylation, to make non-interactive surfaces. Surface modification of biomaterials with both integrin ligands and PEG is advantageous since nonspecific cell-material interaction is prevented by PEGylation while controlled cell adhesion is achieved by integrin adhesion sites [52]. PVA, Dextran, poly(ethylene oxide) (PEO) and alginate are other coatings that can be used in a similar manner [12].

Glucocorticoids are another group of strong anti-inflammatory agents which decrease cytokine, PGE, ROS and chemokine secretion and contribute to the resolution of inflammation. They achieve this by suppressing Th1 response in favour of Th2 responses and tolerance [12]. However, as they have widespread effects, their presence must be tightly controlled. For example, delivery of dexamethasone *in vivo* decreased the inflammation around the implants but also decreased the levels of VEGF and resulted in delayed wound healing [53].

In the wound healing process, secretions (growth factors and cytokines) of monocytes/macrophages and fibroblasts and endothelial cells have reciprocal effects. Thus the incorporation of growth factors can be also used to control immune response; such as incorporation of TGF-β and PDGF.

6.4 CONCLUSIONS

Biomaterial surface properties have a profound effect on their recognition and processing by the immune system. The future designs for biomedical devices should incorporate the optimal surface properties harnessing the available knowledge on the mode and extent of immune reactions for a given surface chemistry to control the host reactions for better clinical outcomes. Currently, available surface modification technologies together with the development of smart, multifunctional surfaces can yield implantable structures with longer life time, better functionality and less complications.

REFERENCES

1. O'Brien F.J. (2011) Biomaterials & scaffolds for tissue engineering. *Materials Today* 14 (3), 88–95.
2. Guney A., Kara F., Ozgen O., Aksoy E.A., Hasirci V., Hasirci, N. (2013) Surface modification of polymeric biomaterials, in *Biomaterials Surface Science* (eds A. Taubert, J.F. Mano and J.C. Rodríguez-Cabello), Wiley-VCH Verlag GmbH & Co. KGaA, Weinheim, Germany.
3. Keselowsky B.G., Collard D.M., García A.J. (2003) Surface chemistry modulates fibronectin conformation and directs integrin binding and specificity to control cell adhesion. *J Biomed Mater Res A* 66, 247–259.
4. Wang Y.X., Robertson J.L., Spillman W.B., Claus R.O. (2004) Effects of chemical structure and surface properties of polymeric biomaterials on their biocompatibility. *Pharm Res* 21 (8), 1326–1373.
5. Sethuraman A., Han M., Kane R.S., Belfort G. (2004) Effect of surface wettability on the adhesion of proteins. *Langmuir* 20 (18), 7779–7788.
6. Ma Z., Mao Z., Gao G. (2007) Surface modification and property analysis of biomedical polymers used for tissue engineering. *Colloids and Surfaces B: Biointerfaces* 60, 137–157.
7. Anderson J.M., Rodriguez A., Chang D.T. (2008) Foreign body reaction to biomaterials. *Semin Immunol* 20, 86–100.
8. Anderson J.M. (1993) Mechanisms of inflammation and infection with implanted devices. *Cardiovasc Pathol* 2, 33S–41S.
9. Boehler R.M., Graham J.G., Shea L.D. (2011) Tissue engineering tools for modulation of the immune response. *Biotechniques* 51, 239–254.
10. Rostam H.M., Singh S., Vrana N.E., Alexander M.R., Ghaemmaghami A.M. (2015) Impact of surface chemistry and topography on the function of antigen presenting cells. *Biomater Sci* 3, 424–441.
11. Tamariz E., Rios-Ramírez A. (2013) Biodegradation of medical purpose polymeric materials and their impact on biocompatibility, in *Biodegradation – Life of Science*, Dr Rolando Chamy (Ed.), InTech.
12. Franz S., Rammelt S., Scharnweber D., Simon J.C. (2011) Immune response to implants – A review of the implications for the design of immunomodulatory biomaterials. *Biomaterials* 32, 6692–6709.
13. Jiang H.L., Tang G.P., Weng L.H., Zhu K.J. (2001) In vivo degradation and biocompatibility of a new class of alternate poly(ester-anhydrides) based on aliphatic and aromatic diacids. *J Biomater Sci Polym Ed* 12 (12), 1281–1292.
14. Aderem A., Underhill D.M. (1999) Mechanisms of phagocytosis in macrophages. *Annu Rev Immunol* 17, 593–623.

15. Kou P.M., Babensee J.E. (2011) Macrophage and dendritic cell phenotypic diversity in the context of biomaterials. *J Biomed Mater Res A* 96 (1), 239–260.
16. van der Giessen W.J., Lincoff A.M., Schwartz R.S., van Beusekom H.M., Serruys P.W., Holmes D.R., Ellis S.G., Topol E.J. (1996) Marked inflammatory sequelae to implantation of biodegradable and nonbiodegradable polymers in porcine coronary arteries. *Circulation* 94, 1690–1697.
17. Thiele L., Merkle H.P., Walter E.P. (2003) Phagocytosis and phagosomal fate of surface-modified microparticles in dendritic cells and macrophages. *Pharm Res* 20, 221–228.
18. Gozalez-Simon A.L., Eniola-Adefeso O. (2011) *Host Response to Biomaterials. Engineering Biomaterials for Regenerative Medicine Novel Technologies for Clinical Applications.* 1st Edition, XIV, 400, p. 76.
19. Brown B.N., Valentin J.E., Stewart-Akers A.M., McCabe G.P., Badylak S.F. (2009) Macrophage phenotype and remodeling outcomes in response to biologic scaffolds with and without a cellular component. *Biomaterials* 30, 1482–1491.
20. Bradley S.G., White K.L., McCay J.A., Brown R.D., Musgrove D.L., Wilson S. (1994) Immunotoxicity of 180-day exposure to polydimethylsiloxane (silicone) fluid, gel and elastomer and polyurethane disks in female B6C3F1 mice. *Drug Chem Toxicol* 17, 221–269.
21. Smith M.J., White K.L., Smith D.C., Bowlin G.L. (2009) In vitro evaluations of innate and acquired immune responses to electrospun polydioxanone-elastin blends. *Biomaterials* 30, 149–159.
22. Smith M.J., Smith D.C., Bowlin G.L., White K.L. (2010) Modulation of murine innate and acquired immune responses following in vitro exposure to electrospun blends of collagen and polydioxanone. *J Biomed Mater Res A* 93, 793–806.
23. Hara H., Nakamura M., Palmaz J.C., Schwartz R.S. (2006) Role of stent design and coatings on restenosis and thrombosis. *Advanced Drug Delivery Reviews* 58, 377–386.
24. Neacsua P., Mazareb A., Cimpeana A., Park J., Costachea M., Schmukib P., Demetrescud I. (2014) Reduced inflammatory activity of RAW 264.7 macrophages on titania nanotube modified Ti surface. *The International Journal of Biochemistry & Cell Biology* 55, 187–195.
25. Córdoba A., Satué M., Gómez-Florit M., Hierro-Oliva M., Petzold C., Lyngstadaas S.P., González-Martín M.L., Monjo M., Ramis J.M. (2015) Flavonoid-modified surfaces: Multifunctional bioactive biomaterials with osteopromotive, anti-inflammatory, and anti-fibrotic potential. *Adv Healthcare Mater* 4, 540–549.
26. Zdolsek J., Eaton J.W., Tang L. (2007) Histamine release and fibrinogen adsorption mediate acute inflammatory responses to biomaterial implants in humans. *J Transl Med* 5, 31.
27. Nimeri G., Ohman L., Elwing H., Wettero J., Bengtsson T. (2002) The influence of plasma proteins and platelets on oxygen radical production and F-actin distribution in neutrophils adhering to polymer surfaces. *Biomaterials* 23, 1785–1795.
28. Bota P.C., Collie A.M., Puolakkainen P., Vernon R.B., Sage E.H., Ratner B.D., Stayton P.S. (2010) Biomaterial topography alters healing in vivo and monocyte/macrophage activation in vitro. *J Biomed Mater Res A* 95, 649–657.
29. Chen S., Jones J.A., Xu Y., Low H.Y., Anderson J.M., Leong K.W. (2010) Characterization of topographical effects on macrophage behavior in a foreign body response model. *Biomaterials* 31, 3479–3491.
30. Hotchkiss K.M., Reddy G.B., Hyzy S.L., Schwartz Z., Boyan B.D., Olivares-Navarrete R. (2016) Titanium surface characteristics, including topography and wettability, alter macrophage activation. *Acta Biomaterialia* 31, 425–434.
31. Hickey T., Kreutzer D., Burgess D.J., Moussy, F. (2002) In vivo evaluation of a dexamethasone/PLGA microsphere system designed to suppress the inflammatory tissue response to implantable medical devices. *J Biomed Mater Res* 61, 180–187.

32. Chandorkar Y., Bhaskar N., Madras G., Basu B. (2015) Long-term sustained release of salicylic acid from cross-linked biodegradable polyester induces a reduced foreign body response in mice. *Biomacromolecules* 16 (2), 636–649.
33. Boateng J., Catanzano O. (2015) Advanced therapeutic dressings for effective wound healing – A review american pharmacists association. *J Pharm Sci* 104, 3653–3680.
34. Arapoglou V., Katsenis K., Syrigos K.N., Dimakakos E.P., Zakopoulou N., Gjodsbol K., Glynn C., Schafer E., Petersen B., Tsoutos D. (2011) Analgesic efficacy of an ibuprofen-releasing foam dressing compared with local best practice for painful exuding wounds. *J Wound Care* 20 (7), 319–320, 322–325.
35. Villegas I., Alarcon de la Lastra C., La Casa C., Motilva V., Martın M.J. (2001) Effects of food intake and oxidative stress on intestinal lesions caused by meloxicam and piroxicam in rats. *Eur J Pharmacol* 414, 79–86.
36. Khurana S., Jain N.K., Bed P.M.S. (2013) Nanoemulsion based gel for transdermal delivery of meloxicam: Physico-chemical, mechanistic investigation. *Life Sciences* 92, 383–392.
37. Todosijevi M.N., Savi M.M., Batini B.B., Markovi B.D., Gašperlin M., Ranpelovi D.V., Luki M.Ž., Snežana D., Savi S.D. (2015) Biocompatible microemulsions of a model NSAID for skin delivery: A decisive role of surfactants in skin penetration/irritation profiles and pharmacokinetic performance. *International Journal of Pharmaceutics* 496, 931–941.
38. Melendez-Ortiz H.I., Diaz-RodriIguez P., Alvarez-Lorenzo C., Concheiro A., Emilio Bucio E. (2014) Binary graft modification of polypropylene for anti-inflammatory drug–device combo products. *The American Pharmacists Association J Pharm Sci* 103, 1269–1277.
39. Webber M.J., Matson J.B., Tamboli V.K., Stupp S.I. (2012) Controlled release of dexamethasone from peptide nanofiber gels to modulate inflammatory response. *Biomaterials* 33, 6823–6832.
40. Go D.P., Palmer J.A., Gras S.L., Andrea J., O'Connor A.J. (2012) Coating and release of an anti-inflammatory hormone from PLGA microspheres for tissue engineering. *J Biomed Mater Res Part A*, 100A, 507–517.
41. Avouching S., Sukhishvili S. (2011) Polymer assemblies for controlled delivery of bioactive molecules from surfaces. *Advanced Drug Delivery Reviews* 63, 822–836.
42. Jones J.A., Chang D.T., Meyerson H., Colton E., Kwon I.K., Matsuda T. et al. (2007) Proteomic analysis and quantification of cytokines and chemokines from biomaterial surface-adherent macrophages and foreign body giant cells. *J Biomed Mater Res A* 83, 585–596.
43. Brodbeck W.G., Patel J., Voskerician G., Christenson E., Shive M.S., Nakayama Y. et al. (2002) Biomaterial adherent macrophage apoptosis is increased by hydrophilic and anionic substrates in vivo. *Proc Natl Acad Sci USA* 99, 10287–10292.
44. Bridges A.W., Singh N., Burns K.L., Babensee J.E., Andrew Lyon L., Garcia A.J. (2008) Reduced acute inflammatory responses to microgel conformal coatings. *Biomaterials* 29, 4605–4615.
45. Liu L., Chen G., Chao T., Ratner B.D., Sage E.H., Jiang S. (2008) Reduced foreign body reaction to implanted biomaterials by surface treatment with oriented osteopontin. *J Biomater. Sci Polym Ed* 19, 821–835.
46. Wang S., Gupta A.S., Sagnella S., Barendt P.M., Kottke-Marchant K., Marchant R.E. (2009) Biomimetic fluorocarbon surfactant polymers reduce platelet adhesion on PTFE/ePTFE surfaces. *J Biomater Sci Polym Ed* 20, 619–635.
47. Muszanska A.K., Rochford E.T., Gruszka A., Bastian A.A., Busscher H.J., Norde W., van der Mei H.C., Herrmann A. (2014) Antiadhesive polymer brush coating functionalized with antimicrobial and rgd peptides to reduce biofilm formation and enhance tissue integration. *Biomacromolecules* 15, 2019–2026.

48. Chen X.N., Gu Y.X., Lee J.H., Lee W.Y., Wang H.J. (2012) Multifunctional surfaces with biomimetic nanofibres and drug-eluting micro-patterns for infection control and bone tissue formation. *Eur Cells Mater* 24, 237–248.
49. Pishbin F., Mourino V., Flor S., Kreppel S., Salih V., Ryan M.P., Boccaccini A.R. (2014) Electrophoretic deposition of gentamicin-loaded bioactive glass/chitosan composite coatings for orthopaedic implants. *ACS Appl Mater Interfaces* 6, 8796–8806.
50. Ozcelik H., Vrana N.E., Gudima A., Riabov V., Gratchev A., Haikel Y., Metz-Boutigue M.H., Carradò A., Faerber J., Roland T., Klüter H., Kzhyshkowska J., Schaaf P., Lavalle P. (2015) Harnessing the multifunctionality in nature: A bioactive agent release system with self-antimicrobial and immunomodulatory properties. *Advanced Healthcare Materials* 4, 2026–2036.
51. Kao W.J., Lee D. (2001) In vivo modulation of host response and macrophage behavior by polymer networks grafted with fibronectin-derived biomimetic oligopeptides: The role of RGD and PHSRN domains. *Biomaterials* 22, 2901–2909.
52. Vandevondele S., Voros J., Hubbell J.A. (2003) RGD-grafted poly-L-lysine-graft-(polyethylene glycol) copolymers block non-specific protein adsorption while promoting cell adhesion. *Biotechnol Bioeng* 82, 784–790.
53. Morais J.M., Papadimitrakopoulos F., Burgess D.J. (2010) Biomaterials/tissue interactions: Possible solutions to overcome foreign body response. *AAPS J* 12, 188–196.

7 Hyaluronic Acid as a Biomaterial and Its Role in the Immune System

Barbora Safrankova, Kristina Nesporova and Ivana Scigalkova

CONTENTS

7.1 INTRODUCTION

Hyaluronic acid or hyaluronan (HA), was first described by Karl Meyer in the 1930s as an extracellular glue; i.e., only as a physical filler. However, over the last two decades a wide variety of biological functions of HA have been discovered which have made it a focal point of both basic and applied research. HA can be found in vertebrate connective tissues. Moreover, it is also available in capsids of several bacteria. Because the chemical structure of HA is very simple there are no notable differences between HA of animal and bacterial origin.

7.1.1 HA Structure and Its Basic Properties

HA is a non-sulphated, linear glycosaminoglycan made of repeating disaccharides (D-glucuronic acid and N-acetyl-D-glucosamine), linked via alternating β-1,4 and β-1,3 glycosidic bonds (Figure 7.1). The average size of newly synthesised HA is close to 2 MDa in humans; however, the average MW of HA can be up to 12 MDa in other animals [1].

Under physiological conditions HA is a polyanion – a negatively charged polymer. *In vivo*, it is in the form of sodium salt (this is the reason for the wide use of hyaluronan as a synonym for HA).

7.1.2 HA Metabolism

Most of the HA in human body is in skin and the total average is around 15 g. The metabolism of HA is highly tissue-dependent; where its half-life in cartilage can be between two and three weeks; whereas in skin half-life is less than 24 hours. In blood, it can be processed within minutes. Around one-third of total HA in human body is turned over daily [2]. Enzymatic degradation of HA is carried out by hyaluronidases (HYAL).

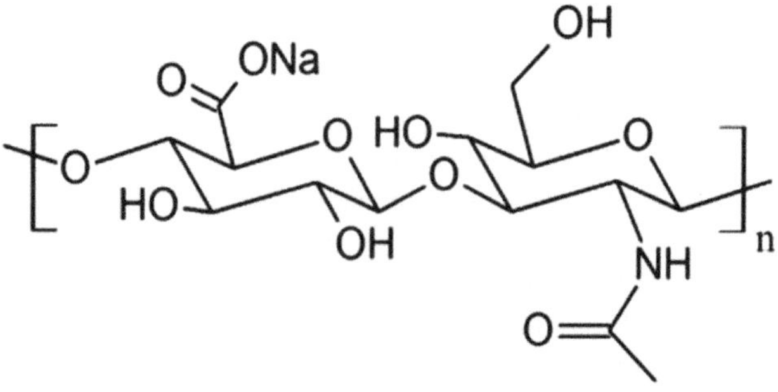

FIGURE 7.1 HA dimer molecular structure.

7.1.2.1 HA Synthesis

Main GAG synthesis takes place in the Golgi apparatus for sulphated proteoglycans, where they are also attached to core proteins. As distinguishing features, HA is not only non-sulphated but is not linked to any core proteins. Its enzymatic production takes place on the plasma membrane and synthesis starts on the cytoplasmic side of the membrane. The growing chain of HA is extruded to the pericellular space. There, the newly synthesised HA associates with proteins (HA-binding proteins). This results in a pericellular coat around the synthesising cell [3].

The synthesis is done in humans by three HA synthases: HAS1, HAS2 and HAS3, respectively. Although they are all able to produce long chains, they differ in their activity, the final length of HA and their regulation [4–6].

7.1.2.2 HA Degradation

HA chains are degraded either enzymatically or by non-specific reactive oxygen and nitrogen species (ROS/RNS)-based chain cutting [7]. Two main hyaluronidases, HYAL2 and HYAL1, process 2MDa chains into 20kDa fragments and tetramers (800 Da), respectively. These small oligosaccharides are then hydrolysed by other enzymes into monosaccharides.

Other proteins involved in HA degradation are SPAM1 and KIAA1199 [8]. SPAM1 (also called PH20) has a neutral optimum pH for enzymatic activity, whereas HYAL1 and HYAL2 have their maximum activity in acidic pH. SPAM1 is expressed mainly in testis and has a role in egg fertilisation as it helps the penetration of sperm through the mass surrounding the ovum via degradation. KIA1199 does not have any enzymatic activity alone but it has been shown to be essential for HA degradation in skin [9].

7.1.3 HA Interaction with Other Biomolecules

Although HA has a very simple chemical structure, it has numerous biological functions. These functions can be of physical form (such as lubrication) or might be direct effects on cell behaviour (such as differentiation). These functions are both dependent on HA interaction with ECM components and HA-specific cellular receptors. HA binding partners, hyaladherins, are generally characterised by the presence of a HA-specific domain that enables the protein to bind to HA. The HA-specific link module can be found in most of the proteoglycans, including aggrecan, neurocan, brevican and versican. The presence of the link module in proteoglycans results in the formation of highly branched nets that contributes to ECM integrity [10] (Figure 7.2). The link module is also present in several surface receptors and non-glycan hyaladherins such as CD44, LYVE-1, HARE and TSG-6. However, some other hyaladherins (RHAMM, IαI) do not contain the link module [11].

Several of these hyaladherins are present on immune cells and their activation through the binding of HA is considered one of the major biological roles of HA in the immune system.

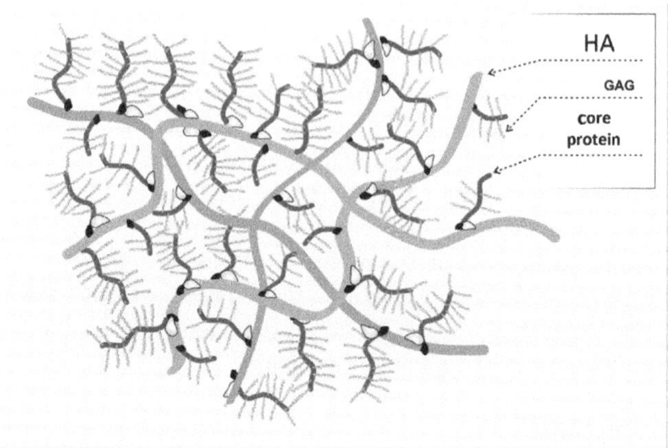

FIGURE 7.2 Glycosaminoglycan mesh in ECM.

7.2 HA USE IN BIOMEDICINE

HA is one of the most commonly used natural polymers in biomedical applications. Over the years, new HA derivatives with different physicochemical properties such as hydrophobicity, control over polyanionic properties, cross-linkability and improved stability have been successfully developed. The main aim in the development of the HA derivatives is to improve their biomechanical properties without compromising their important original characteristics such as low immunogenicity, specific interaction with cells and good water solubility. For examples of HA-based tissue engineering (TE) products, please see Figure 7.3 [12].

7.2.1 HA Preparation

7.2.1.1 Native HA

Nowadays, there are two major methods of obtaining HA on a large scale: extraction from HA-rich animal tissues (most commonly rooster combs) and biotechnological production utilising *Streptococcus* sp. Both approaches yield a high amount of high-molecular-weight (HMW) HA, but are also potential sources for contaminants, such as protein and viral particles from animal tissues and bacterial endotoxins from *Streptococcus*. Moreover, the isolation of HA from tissues requires harsh extraction conditions that can degrade HA to low molecular weight (LMW) fragments or unknown degradation products [13].

For these reasons, novel approaches to HA manufacturing are being developed, i.e., isolation from genetically modified bacteria that don't produce endotoxins (e.g., *B. subtilis* system employed by Novozymes) [14] or a cell-free *in vitro* synthesis [15].

7.2.1.2 Chemically Modified HA

HA can be modified by either cross-linking or conjugation [16]. The main difference is that, in the conjugation route, different groups/compounds are grafted on a single

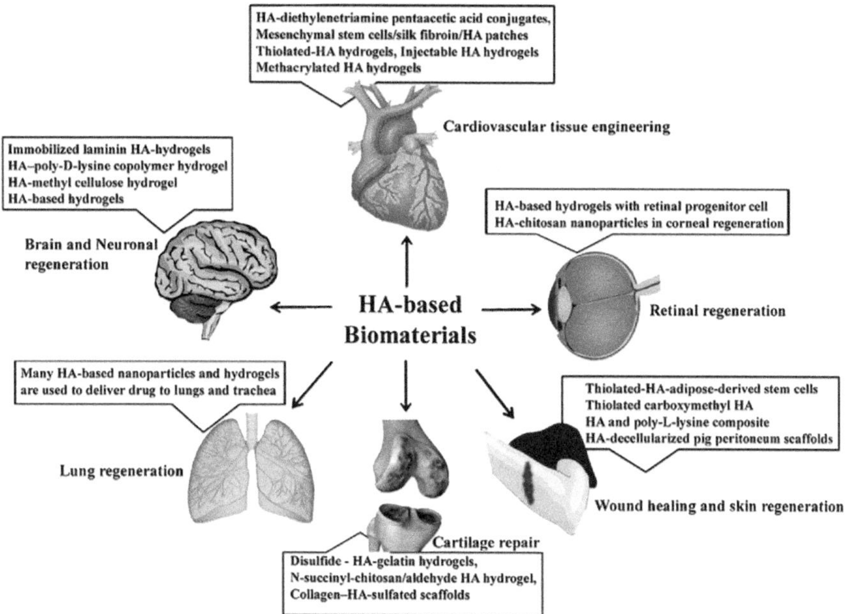

FIGURE 7.3 Use of HA-based biomaterials in vital organ treatment. (Adapted from Hemshekhar, M. et al., *Int J Biol Macromol*, 86, 917–928, 2016. With permission.)

HA chain by a single bond, whereas in cross-linking, different HA chains are cross-linked together through two or more bonds. For chemical modification of HA, two available functional sites of HA are regularly used: the hydroxyl and carboxylic acid groups. The amino group can also be used for modification following the deacetylation of the N-acetyl group of N-acetyl-D-glucosamine. The main problem with HA modification methods is HA degradation during the process and also the formation of potentially toxic degradation products. Currently, several synthetic approaches for the preparation of HA derivatives are under investigation. Such synthetic approaches would provide derivatives with a high level of control over MW and degree of substitution [17].

7.2.1.3 Cross-Linked HA

Cross-linking is primarily used in hydrogel preparation, creating a product more stable than native, highly soluble HA. For a direct cross-linking of HA, several agents like butanediol diglycidyl ether (BDDE), divinylsulfone (DVS) or glutaraldehyde are employed [18,19]. For a specific application, *in situ* cross-linking is preferable. In these cases, chemically modified HA must be applied together with the cross-linking agent by double-channel catheters. One potential *in situ* cross-linkable system is tyramine-grafted HA (HA-tyramine) that can be cross-linked by horseradish peroxidase in the presence of minute amounts of hydrogen peroxide [20]. Alternatively, two different HA derivatives can be developed that have reciprocal reactivity with one another. One example of such a system is the use of HA–aminoethyl methacrylate or

HA–aminopropyl methacrylamide with HA–cysteamine. The reaction requires no additional reagent. Another advantage of this reaction is the absence of toxic byproducts, making it a highly suitable for *in vivo* use of HA hydrogels that can be formed in-situ. Another potential way to cross-link HA is by development of photocross-linkable derivatives such as Methacrylated HA, which can form hydrogels in the presence of UV light and a photoinitiator [21].

7.2.1.4 HA Conjugates

HA derivatives where different functional groups attach to the HA chain are called HA conjugates. This refers to the cases where drugs such as paclitaxel, hydrocortisone, ibuprofen etc. [22–25] are attached to the HA directly. There are also derivatives with no direct biological activity (no toxicity, without specific response of immune system) however provides the ability to form various complexes, micelles and liposomes. The derivatives can also attach to surfaces of nanoparticles or larger objects like titanium implants with both anti-adhesive and pro-adhesive properties, depending on the type of HA derivative.

For tissue engineering purposes, HA sulphation is explored as a method for mimicking functions of native ECM in a reproducible manner. Sulphated HA is able to bind cytokines and growth factors similarly to native sulphated GAGs and thus influences the growth and differentiation of various cells [26].

7.2.2 HA Applications in Biomedicine

7.2.2.1 Dermal Fillers and Viscosupplementation

One common application of HA is as a filler in cosmetic surgeries. It is also widely used in orthopaedics as a viscosupplementation means for the repair of joint damage. Current dermal fillers in use are based on chemically cross-linked HA for improved stability as unmodified HA can be eliminated from the site of application in few days. A commonly used modification is the cross-linking of hydroxyl groups on native HA using BDDE and DVS [27]. Resulting hydrogels are more resistant to degradation, both enzymatically or ROS/RNS activity.

HA used for viscosupplementation, on the other hand, is mostly native HA (the few exceptions are those such as Hylan GF-20 (Genzyme)), where a HA derivative (HA amidated with palmitic acid) is used for additional stability [28,29]).

HA-based products do not have a high frequency of adverse effects. This can be related to HA's natural origin and its fast metabolism. More side effects were reported for a chemically modified filler and viscosupplementation in comparison to products based on native HA [30].

7.2.2.2 Wound Healing

Another common area of use of HA-based products is wound healing. This stems from the fact that HA is an important mediator of wound healing processes *in vivo*. Together with its advantageous physical properties, it is a strong candidate for the development of advanced wound healing products where it provides a stable structure with inherent cell migration and proliferation induction capacity. Another advantageous property of HA is its hydrophilicity as it provides an optimal microenvironment for moist healing process. Moreover, HA and polysaccharides in general also protect newly formed tissue against potential negative effects of antimicrobials within the dressings, which are included as a security measure [31]. This is due to ROS scavenging by polysaccharides.

7.2.2.3 Other Uses

Other common biomedical applications of HA are lubricant in eye drops, nasal sprays etc. [32,33], cross-linkable, chemically modified HA derivatives for tissue engineering scaffold development, implant coatings and amphiphilic HA derivatives for drug-delivery systems.

Novel biomaterials are often multifunctional and besides their primary purpose (i.e., drug or cell delivery), their composition should provide an addition of functions, including detectability, (non-)adhesion and regulation of immune response.

7.3 THE ROLE OF HA IN THE IMMUNE SYSTEM

Damage to tissue integrity results in the activation of processes that ensure tissue homeostasis. While the immune cells are essential for maintenance of this homeostasis as well as for host defence and inflammation required during tissue healing, cells from the damaged and surrounding tissues and the components of ECM are also involved in these actions. Thus, the interaction between them is necessary and the main HA receptor, CD44, is considered to be one of the molecules enabling this interaction and communication.

Nowadays, the generally accepted point of view on HA role within normal or damaged tissue is as follows: LMW HA is able to act as an endogenous signal of damage [34], because its native HMW molecule is fragmented during tissue damage or inflammation via the action of hyaluronidases or ROS/RNS produced by activated neutrophils and macrophages [35,36]. Thus, LMW HA represents one of several endogenous markers of inflammation, termed damage-associated molecular patterns (DAMPs), which is analogous to pathogen associated molecular patterns (PAMPs). It is assumed that members of both groups are recognised by their pattern recognition receptors (PRRs), which are expressed on a wide range of cells. The existence of DAMPs contributes to an explanation of how an alteration of ECM is able to potentiate the immune response without the presence of pathogens. The concept of sterile inflammation is useful for the description of injuries typically occurring in the absence of any microorganisms, which is similar to a situation after an implantation of sterile biomaterials.

7.3.1 Sterile Inflammation

Sterile inflammation, the inflammatory responses without an infection, is an important biological process for homeostasis. One example is the wound healing process, where controlled immune response is a requirement for proper recruitment of cells involved in wound healing. For this end, the recruitment of monocytes and their downstream control of wound healing via the secretion of cytokines, chemokines and growth factors is crucial [37].

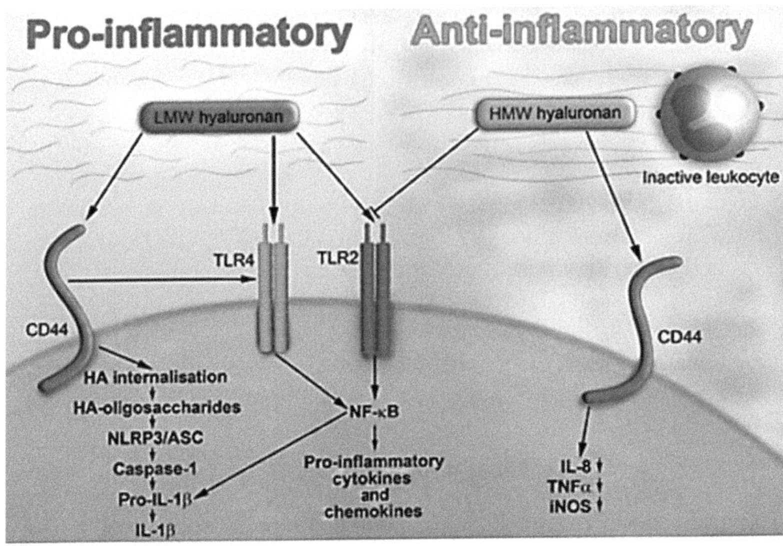

FIGURE 7.4 Role of MW HA in immune response. Low MW HA induces a pro-inflammatory effect mainly though TLR2 and TLR4. Also, CD44-dependent HA internalisation and subsequent fragmentation results in the activation of the NLRP3/ASC inflammasome. This leads to the secretion of IL-1β (pro-inflammatory). High MW HA induces anti-inflammatory effects via prevention of Low MW HA/TLR2 signalling and via downregulation of CD44-dependent expression of pro-inflammatory mediators. (Adapted from Frey, H. et al., *FEBS J*, 280, 2165–2179, 2013. With permission.)

In this sense the HA receptor-mediated interactions of HA with cells have been implicated in modulation of cellular behaviour in sterile inflammation conditions. One of the main receptors recognising HA fragments are members of TLR family. Both TLR2 and TLR4 recognise HA fragments as an endogenous damage signal and trigger pro-inflammatory responses (Figure 7.4) [38] necessary for injury repair and the establishment of homeostasis. The inhibition of TLR/HA interaction by peptide inhibitors, or as observed in transgenic mice, leads to worse injury repair in overall, while potentiation of this interaction (for example, by enhanced expression of HAS2) has protective effects against injury [39].

7.3.2 Major HA-Binding Proteins Involved in Immune Response

TLR2 and TLR4 are considered the most important HA-binding receptors involved in immune regulations. But the complex network of HA signalling and interactions contains other hyaladherins involved in inflammation and immunity. The main ones are cellular receptor CD44 and two soluble proteins secreted extracellularly, SHAP and TSG-6.

7.3.2.1 CD44

The increased expression of CD44 is linked with elevated monocyte [40], neutrophil [41] and T-cell [42] recruitment at the site of the inflammation because CD44 serves as a primary adhesion molecule that mediates the cell rolling along vascular endothelial cells. Experiments using transgenic mice showed that the CD44 expression is important both in leukocytes and endothelium for optimal leukocyte recruitment into tissues, but not for migration within tissues [43]. Several models of sterile inflammation in CD44 knockout mice (i.e., bleomycin-induced lung injury, infarcted myocardium) proved that a lack of CD44 leads to aggravated inflammation, prolonged neutrophil and macrophage infiltration, increased expression of pro-inflammatory cytokines, slower clearance of apoptotic neutrophils, accumulation of HA fragments at the site of injury and impaired activation of TGF β1 leading to decreased fibroblast proliferation and collagen deposition [44–46].

7.3.2.2 SHAP (HC)/TSG-6

The extracellular proteins SHAP (HC) and TSG-6 are responsible for modifying HA simple structure in more a biologically active molecular complex of HC-HA.

SHAP is identical to the heavy chains (HC) of inter-α (globulin) inhibitor (IαI), which belongs to the IαI family of structurally related plasma serine protease inhibitors involved in ECM stabilisation [47]. TSG-6, also known as TNF-α-induced protein 6, is involved in HC transfer to HA, where TSG-6 serves as a catalyst and a cofactor of HC transfer complex [48]. TSG-6 can also mediate native HA cross-linking [49].

Under pro-inflammatory conditions (such as in the presence of IL-1 and TNF-α), TSG-6 expression is up-regulated in many cell types including fibroblasts and monocytes. Moreover, it has been shown that in many inflammation-related chronic diseases such as rheumatoid arthritis, ECM remodelling is an important part of the inflammatory processes related to the disease [50].

TSG-6 inhibits neutrophil infiltration, whereas HA enhanced neutrophil infiltration in an air pouch model (murine) where the inflammation was induced by carrageenan/IL-1 [51]. In a model of bleomycin-induced injury of lungs in mice, inflammatory cell infiltration was decreased in the early stages with the intravenous administration of TSG-6. The treatment resulted in improved mice survival [52]. Interestingly, CD44-positive cells adhered preferentially to the immobilised HC-HA complex rather than to HA [53].

7.3.3 HA-Cell Interactions in Immune Response

Similarly to the molecular level of HA interactions, it is impossible to identify one or two main cell types responsible for HA functioning in immune response. HA involvement can be observed in various stages of inflammation and in various involved cells. Here, we focus on the cells important to the inflammation related to the biomaterial implantation or application.

7.3.3.1 Neutrophils/Granulocytes

Neutrophils, one of the first immune cells to be recruited to implantation sites, have been suggested to contribute to the establishment of the inflammatory microenvironment that initiates the fibrotic response [54]. CD44 is a key component in granulocyte-related inflammatory response. CD44 expression and its interactions with HA have direct effects on neutrophil polarisation and migration speed in mice. Blocking CD44 with an antibody (anti-CD44) blocked polarisation effect but did not have an effect on migration speed, which indicates that the chemotactic signalling and migration are mediated via different pathways [55].

Interestingly, the interaction of HA with CD44 on neutrophils might initiate cytotoxic response when these cells encounter high amounts of HA [56]. CD44 is also responsible for cytokine production as a CD44 antibody or HA binding on CD44 induced IL-6 secretion [57].

Interestingly, concerning HA of different MW, low MW HA stimulates neutrophils via TLR-dependent signals, which promotes lung allograft rejection through TLR-dependent signals stimulated neutrophils that promoted rejection [58]. HMW HA suppressed superoxide secretion by neutrophils. It also protected bovine corneal endothelial cells from activated neutrophils. However, the effect is more dose-dependent than MW-dependent and a similar effect was also seen with other viscoelastic substances like methylcellulose [59].

7.3.3.2 Dendritic Cells

In final combined TE products, the host response may consist of a nonspecific inflammatory response against the biomaterial component as well as a specific immune response directed against the biological component. The biomaterial component may boost the immune response against an immunogenic biological component by enhancing the recruitment of innate immune antigen-presenting cells (APCs) such as dendritic cells (DCs) or macrophages, and by supporting their activation [60].

In mice, the 135kDa HA fragments were shown to influence DCs maturation and initiate alloimmunity [61]. Activation of DCs by HA enhances expression of CD40, which in turn enhances their ability to stimulate T-cells [62]. Short HA fragments (tetra- and hexasaccharides) resulted in the maturation of human DCs with increased production of TNF-α and IL-1β [63].

7.3.3.3 T-Cells

T-cell activation in response to biomaterial presence can be modulated by APCs or by direct interaction with the biomaterial adherent macrophages and foreign body giant cells, leading to IFN-γ production [64]. Pre-activated T-cells are also able to bind to the HA by the surface CD44 receptor and this process is regulated by different cytokines and chemokines [65].

There are a few studies describing the effect of the HA on regulatory T-cells (Tregs), which have an important role in peripheral tolerance. It has been shown that Tregs selected by HMW HA binding were superior in suppressive function [66]. Also, it has been demonstrated that CD44 expression was directly correlated with the suppressive capacity of Tregs and had an effect on IL-10 secretion [67]. Moreover, HMW HA improves functional suppression of responder cell proliferation by human Tregs, whereas LMW HA does not have a similar effect [68].

7.3.3.4 Fibrocytes/Mast Cells

After implantation, almost all implants are covered by a fibrotic capsule, although the complete mechanism of biomaterial-mediated fibrotic reactions is still mostly under study. A study by Thevenot et al. suggested that mast cells are at least partially responsible for CD45+/Collagen I+ fibrocyte recruitment and subsequent fibrotic capsule formation [69]. Interestingly, HA is a component of mast cell granules together with other glycosaminoglycans [70]. Mast cells were shown to adhere to HA; the connection was mediated by CD44 [71]. In a model of interstitial cystitis in rats, HA inhibited mast cell activation [72].

7.3.3.5 Macrophages

Together with neutrophils, macrophages are the "first responder" to ECM fragments generated during implantation and potential contaminants present in the biomaterials. While TLR/HA interaction and subsequent signalling is considered the cornerstone of HA-mediated immune response to tissue damage, the exact mechanism is still debated and various models have been used to unveil the role of specific receptors and adaptor molecules.

For example, a study suggested that a complex formed by TLR4, CD44 and MD2 recognises HA under sterile inflammation conditions and induces MIP-2 secretion. In the absence of TLR4 or CD44, the response diminished significantly [73]. It was shown that CD44-deficient mice with zymosan-induced arthritis had more severe lesion in their joints. Moreover, bone marrow-derived macrophages isolated from the animals produced more IL-6 and TNF-α after zymosan stimulation compared to the control macrophages [74].

Another study suggested that HA degradation products initiate inflammatory responses through both TLR4 and TLR2. Stimulation of macrophages with HA fragments (MW 200 kDa) resulted in higher chemokine production which was TLR2- and TLR4-depentdent. TLR silencing in mice resulted in less inflammatory cell migration but also caused higher epithelial cell apoptosis following lung injury. It is also suggested that HMW HA presence on epithelial cell surface provided protection against apoptosis, in part, through TLRs-dependent basal activation of NFκB [75]. However, there are some studies indicating that HA is not recognised by TLRs [76] and thus the above-mentioned effect could be caused by HA contamination.

7.3.3.6 HA and Macrophage Polarisation

One of the most important properties of macrophages is their plasticity. The presence of the macrophages is important for the removal of apoptotic cells, pathogens, or different foreign materials. After the cause of inflammation is cleared away, the role of macrophages changes and so does their phenotype. M1 and M2 macrophages represent the opposite extremes, where M1 as pro-inflammatory phenotype is associated with a classical activation by microbial stimuli (LPS), IFN-γ, proinflammatory cytokines (TNF, IL-1β) or macrophage colony-stimulating factor. Typical stimuli for M2 macrophages are represented by IL-4 and IL-13 and these alternatively activated cells are characterised by low pro-inflammatory potential and, contrarily, they promote wound healing [77]. However, M1 and M2 macrophages portray two poles of continuous spectrum of functional states [78].

Mouse macrophage line J774A.1 was used for a confirmation of direct effect on different MW HA (digested HA without MW specification, low $\leq$ 5-kDa; intermediate 60–800-kDa, high > 800-kDa) on macrophage polarisation. The authors also explored whether the initial polarisation state of the cells played a role, specifically whether HA had a reprogramming potential. They observed that LMW HA, regardless of the initial macrophages state, promoted a classically activated-like state (M1), while HMW induced an alternatively activated-like state (M2). Digested HA usually shows the highest M1 polarisation potential [79], but it can be partially explained by the use of bovine testicular HYAL, in which there is a risk of a presence of endotoxin or other contaminant proteins [76]. The activation of human untreated macrophages as well as reprogramming of M2 macrophages to M1 phenotype after LMW HA (50–600 kDa) was observed [80]. Although the role of different MW HA on macrophage polarisation appears clear, the results indicate that this question is not so simple. LMW HA (30–60 kDa) pre-treated human monocytes lost the ability to produce TNF-α after repeated LMW HA exposure, but the production of IL-10 was maintained. The formation of both cytokines was significantly inhibited after CD44-HA blocking with anti CD44 antibody [81].

He and colleagues described the *in vitro* effect of a soluble HC-HA (MW > 3000 kDa) complex containing pentraxin 3 (PTX3), isolated from human amniotic membrane, which induced apoptosis of LPS-activated human neutrophils and mouse macrophages via the inhibition of cell adhesion and spreading on a plastic surface. Control cells were not affected in this way, but LPS-untreated macrophages exhibited enhanced phagocytosis of apoptotic neutrophils, whereas using immobilised HC-HA promoted phagocytosis in LPS-activated macrophages. This immobilised complex also polarised macrophages under LPS stimulation toward the M2 phenotype [82]. The same complex was tested *in vivo* in a model of mouse corneal allograft rejection. The subconjunctival application HC-HA with PTX3 significantly prolonged allografts survival [83].

HC-HA, chondroitin sulphate, proteoglycan versican, enzyme TSG6 and PTX3-containing matrix is important for the ability of human mesenchymal stem cells (MSC) from the umbilical cord to suppress host inflammation. Cell application into mouse cornea stroma after 24 hours after an alkali burn resulted in decreased inflammatory cell infiltration, inhibition of inflammatory cell adhesion and peritoneal macrophages polarisation from M1 towards normal or M2 type. The removal of the chondroitin sulphate/HA matrix, which was upregulated by MSCs in the presence of inflammatory cells, reduced the beneficial anti-inflammatory effect of MSCs [84]. It is also necessary to note that PTX3 itself exhibits the ability to regulate macrophage activity. Its effect on macrophages leads to reduced pro-inflammatory cytokine production (IL-1β, TNF-α, MCP-1) while TGF-β production is activated [85].

Notably, TSG-6-mediated formation of a covalent HC-HA complex is also important for the settlement and possibly for the differentiation of mouse MSCs within intact muscle as the injury increases the production of all above-mentioned components [86].

7.3.4 HA-Based Scaffolds and Immune Response

While we present HA as a potent active molecule able to modulate various biological processes, it is necessary to realise that most biomaterial and final tissue engineering products are intricate combinations of native and/or synthetic components sometimes enriched by recombinant proteins and living cells. To decipher which part of such complex products is responsible for immune response or other biological effects is often impossible. Here, we present several examples of biomaterial formulations containing HA and information about their behaviour post-implantation in relation to immune reaction.

The use of HMW HA as a component of scaffolds appears logical because of its physical and biological properties. For example, the addition of HMW HA (2500 kDa) to silk fibroin and polycaprolactone nanofibrous scaffolds leads to suppression of non-specific protein absorption and macrophage adhesion *in vivo* [87]. HA is also a component of the commercially available product Seprafilm, which is a bioresorbable membrane serving as an antiadhesive agent after postoperative abdominal adhesions. Application of this membrane did not induce inflammatory cytokine expression, nor did it modify the fibrosis process in the abdominal cavity of rats [88].

The positive effect of HMW HA hydrogels was shown on rat spinal dorsal hemisection injury, where the number of macrophages and microglia were significantly reduced as well as the deposition of chondroitin sulphate proteoglycan ten days after the injury. This suggests that HA is a promising biomaterial imitating scar formation, which prevents axonal growth [89].

The results from a porcine model of immune reaction to biomaterial based on a decellularised bladder indicates that addition of HA to a decellularised bladder may positively regulate host immune response, because gene expression of TGF-β1 was elevated, while IL-4, TLR2 and TLR4 expressions were decreased [90].

A hydrogel composed of chemically modified HA-gelatin (Carbylan-GSX) with encapsulated MSC showed the ability to reduce the expression of CD16 and the human leukocyte antigen HLA-DR and increased CD206 expression on human macrophages, which were directly cultured on the gel. Described changes are associated with the anti-inflammatory phenotype [91].

The beneficial role of HA, specifically highly sulfated HA, was confirmed *in vitro* with the use of a 2D structure composed of collagen I matrices and HMW HA (88–96% collagen and 4–12% HA). Human monocytes were seeded on the artificial ECM and M1 polarisation was induced. The production of proinflammatory cytokines (TNF-α and IL-12) was decreased through dampened activation of NFκB signalling pathway as well as GM-CSF-related activation of STAT1 and IRF5. On the other hand, the enhanced production of IL-10 was observed, suggesting that highly sulphated HA has a potential in the development of immunomodulatory biomaterial [92].

A study using a mouse model of endotoxemia showed that HA scaffolds protect embedded endothelial progenitor cells from LPS by reducing penetration into scaffolds, and thus provided a sheltered environment for cells, which revealed higher viability compared with cells delivered intravenously [93].

The positive effect of HA in a scaffold was not always confirmed. Chin and colleagues tested the expected positive contribution of HMW tyramine-substituted HA (TS-HA) after its application on decellularised human fascia in a rat abdominal wall defect model. Tyramine provides HA cross-linking and thus the hydrogel is not susceptible to hydrolysis. Surprisingly, the lymphocytes and plasma cell densities were comparable with water-treated fascia; moreover, the presence of macrophages and giant cells was enhanced. The fascia treated by HA or TS-HA exhibited a predominantly M2 macrophage profile similar to the water-treated control [94].

7.4 CONCLUSION

HA is being increasingly utilised in tissue augmentation, the development of TE and drug-delivery products and therapeutic and cosmetic topical applications. To date, there have been no indications that HA use in biomaterial is causing negative effects. For this reason, further use of HA has to be expected and, hopefully, it will bring much-needed information on its involvement in various biological processes, including inflammation.

REFERENCES

1. Tian, X., Azpurua, J., Hine, C., Vaidya, A., Myakishev-Rempel, M., Ablaeva, J. et al. (2013). High-molecular-mass hyaluronan mediates the cancer resistance of the naked mole rat, *Nature*, 499, pp. 346–349.
2. Stern, R. (2003). Devising a pathway for hyaluronan catabolism: Are we there yet?, *Glycobiology*, 13, pp. 105R–115R.
3. Rilla, K., Tiihonen, R., Kultti, A., Tammi, M., Tammi, R. (2008). Pericellular hyaluronan coat visualized in live cells with a fluorescent probe is scaffolded by plasma membrane protrusions, *J Histochem Cytochem*, 56, pp. 901–910.
4. Torronen, K., Nikunen, K., Karna, R., Tammi, M., Tammi, R., Rilla, K. (2014). Tissue distribution and subcellular localization of hyaluronan synthase isoenzymes, *Histochem Cell Biol*, 141, pp. 17–31.
5. Tien, J.Y., Spicer, A.P. (2005). Three vertebrate hyaluronan synthases are expressed during mouse development in distinct spatial and temporal patterns, *Dev Dyn*, 233, pp. 130–141.
6. Itano, N., Kimata, K. (2002). Mammalian hyaluronan synthases, *IUBMB Life*, 54, pp. 195–199.
7. Agren, U.M., Tammi, R.H., Tammi, M.I. (1997). Reactive oxygen species contribute to epidermal hyaluronan catabolism in human skin organ culture, *Free Radic Biol Med*, 23, pp. 996–1001.
8. Jiang, D., Liang, J., Noble, P.W. (2007). Hyaluronan in tissue injury and repair, *Annu Rev Cell Dev Biol*, 23, pp. 435–461.
9. Yoshida, H., Nagaoka, A., Nakamura, S., Tobiishi, M., Sugiyama, Y., Inoue, S. (2014). N-Terminal signal sequence is required for cellular trafficking and hyaluronan-depolymerization of KIAA1199, *FEBS Lett*, 588, pp. 111–116.
10. Wight, T.N., Toole, B.P., Hascall, V.C. (2011). Hyaluronan and the Aggregating Proteoglycans. In Mecham, P.R. (ed.), *The Extracellular Matrix: An Overview*. Berlin, Heidelberg: Springer; 2011, pp. 147–195.
11. Day, A.J., Prestwich, G.D. (2002). Hyaluronan-binding proteins: Tying up the giant, *J Biol Chem*, 277, pp. 4585–4588.
12. Hemshekhar, M., Thushara, R.M., Chandranayaka, S., Sherman, L.S., Kemparaju, K., Girish, K.S. (2016). Emerging roles of hyaluronic acid bioscaffolds in tissue engineering and regenerative medicine, *Int J Biol Macromol*, 86, pp. 917–928.
13. Sze, J.H., Brownlie, J.C., Love, C.A. (2016). Biotechnological production of hyaluronic acid: A mini review, *Biotech*, 6, pp. 67.

14. Widner, B., Behr, R., Von Dollen, S., Tang, M., Heu, T., Sloma, A. et al. (2005). Hyaluronic acid production in Bacillus subtilis, *Appl Environ Microbiol*, 71, pp. 3747–3752.
15. Yoshida, M., Itano, N., Yamada, Y., Kimata, K. (2000). In vitro synthesis of hyaluronan by a single protein derived from mouse has1 gene and characterization of amino acid residues essential for the activity, *J Biol Chem*, 275, pp. 497–506.
16. Schanté, C.E., Zuber, G., Herlin, C., Vandamme, T.F. (2011). Chemical modifications of hyaluronic acid for the synthesis of derivatives for a broad range of biomedical applications, *Carbohydr Polym*, 85, pp. 469–489.
17. Lu, Y., Park, K. (2013). Polymeric micelles and alternative nanonized delivery vehicles for poorly soluble drugs, *Int J Pharm*, 453, pp. 198–214.
18. Collins, M.N., Birkinshaw, C. (2007). Comparison of the effectiveness of four different crosslinking agents with hyaluronic acid hydrogel films for tissue-culture applications, *J Appl Polym Sci*, 104, pp. 3183–3191.
19. Collins, M.N., Birkinshaw, C. (2008). Investigation of the swelling behavior of cross-linked hyaluronic acid films and hydrogels produced using homogeneous reactions, *J Appl Polym Sci*, 109, pp. 923–931.
20. Kučera, L., Weinfurterová, R., Dvořákova, J., Kučera, J., Pravda, M., Foglarová, M. et al. (2015). Chondrocyte cultivation in hyaluronan-tyramine cross-linked hydrogel, *Int J Polym Mater Po*, 64, pp. 661–674.
21. Baier Leach, J., Bivens, K.A., Patrick, C.W., Jr., Schmidt, C.E. (2003). Photocrosslinked hyaluronic acid hydrogels: Natural, biodegradable tissue engineering scaffolds, *Biotechnol Bioeng*, 82, pp. 578–589.
22. Cai, S., Xie, Y., Bagby, T.R., Cohen, M.S., Forrest, M.L. (2008). Intralymphatic chemotherapy using a hyaluronan-cisplatin conjugate, *J Surg Res*, 147, pp. 247–252.
23. Homma, A., Sato, H., Tamura, T., Okamachi, A., Emura, T., Ishizawa, T. et al. (2010). Synthesis and optimization of hyaluronic acid-methotrexate conjugates to maximize benefit in the treatment of osteoarthritis, *Bioorg Med Chem*, 18, pp. 1062–1075.
24. Pouyani, T., Prestwich, G.D. (1994). Functionalized derivatives of hyaluronic acid oligosaccharides: Drug carriers and novel biomaterials, *Bioconjug Chem*, 5, pp. 339–347.
25. Xin, D., Wang, Y., Xiang, J. (2010). The use of amino acid linkers in the conjugation of paclitaxel with hyaluronic acid as drug delivery system: Synthesis, self-assembled property, drug release, and in vitro efficiency, *Pharm Res*, 27, pp. 380–389.
26. Scharnweber, D., Hubner, L., Rother, S., Hempel, U., Anderegg, U., Samsonov, S.A. et al. (2015). Glycosaminoglycan derivatives: Promising candidates for the design of functional biomaterials, *J Mater Sci Mater Med*, 26, pp. 232.
27. Tezel, A., Fredrickson, G.H. (2008). The science of hyaluronic acid dermal fillers, *J Cosmet Laser Ther*, 10, pp. 35–42.
28. Gigante, A., Callegari, L. (2011). The role of intra-articular hyaluronan (Sinovial) in the treatment of osteoarthritis, *Rheumatol Int*, 31, pp. 427–444.
29. Juni, P., Reichenbach, S., Trelle, S., Tschannen, B., Wandel, S., Jordi, B. et al. (2007). Efficacy and safety of intraarticular hylan or hyaluronic acids for osteoarthritis of the knee: A randomized controlled trial, *Arthritis Rheum*, 56, pp. 3610–3619.
30. Hunter, D.J. (2015). Viscosupplementation for osteoarthritis of the knee, *N Engl J Med*, 372, pp. 2570.
31. Voigt, J., Driver, V.R. (2012). Hyaluronic acid derivatives and their healing effect on burns, epithelial surgical wounds, and chronic wounds: A systematic review and meta-analysis of randomized controlled trials, *Wound Repair Regen*, 20, pp. 317–331.
32. Balazs, E.A. (2008). Hyaluronan as an ophthalmic viscoelastic device, *Curr Pharm Biotechnol*, 9, pp. 236–238.

33. Gelardi, M., Iannuzzi, L., Quaranta, N. (2013). Intranasal sodium hyaluronate on the nasal cytology of patients with allergic and nonallergic rhinitis, *Int Forum Allergy Rhinol*, pp. 108–813.
34. Ruppert, S.M., Hawn, T.R., Arrigoni, A., Wight, T.N., Bollyky, P.L. (2014). Tissue integrity signals communicated by high-molecular weight hyaluronan and the resolution of inflammation, *Immunol Res*, 58, pp. 186–192.
35. Moseley, R., Waddington, R.J., Embery, G. (1997). Degradation of glycosaminoglycans by reactive oxygen species derived from stimulated polymorphonuclear leukocytes, *Biochim Biophys Acta*, 1362, pp. 221–231.
36. Soltes, L., Mendichi, R., Kogan, G., Schiller, J., Stankovska, M., Arnhold, J. (2006). Degradative action of reactive oxygen species on hyaluronan, *Biomacromolecules*, 7, pp. 659–668.
37. Yamasaki, K., Muto, J., Taylor, K.R., Cogen, A.L., Audish, D., Bertin, J. et al. (2009). NLRP3/cryopyrin is necessary for interleukin-1beta (IL-1beta) release in response to hyaluronan, an endogenous trigger of inflammation in response to injury, *J Biol Chem*, 284, pp. 12762–12771.
38. Frey, H., Schroeder, N., Manon-Jensen, T., Iozzo, R.V., Schaefer, L. (2013). Biological interplay between proteoglycans and their innate immune receptors in inflammation, *FEBS J*, 280, pp. 2165–2179.
39. Jiang, D., Liang, J., Li, Y., Noble, P.W. (2006). The role of Toll-like receptors in non-infectious lung injury, *Cell Res*, 16, pp. 693–701.
40. Mun, G.I., Boo, Y.C. (2010). Identification of CD44 as a senescence-induced cell adhesion gene responsible for the enhanced monocyte recruitment to senescent endothelial cells, *Am J Physiol Heart Circ Physiol*, 298, pp. H2102–2111.
41. Katayama, Y., Hidalgo, A., Chang, J., Peired, A., Frenette, P.S. (2005). CD44 is a physiological E-selectin ligand on neutrophils, *J Exp Med*, 201, pp. 1183–1189.
42. DeGrendele, H.C., Estess, P., Siegelman, M.H. (1997). Requirement for CD44 in activated T cell extravasation into an inflammatory site, *Science*, 278, pp. 672–675.
43. Khan, A.I., Kerfoot, S.M., Heit, B., Liu, L., Andonegui, G., Ruffell, B. et al. (2004). Role of CD44 and hyaluronan in neutrophil recruitment, *J Immunol*, 173, pp. 7594–7601.
44. Jiang, D., Liang, J., Noble, P.W. (2011). Hyaluronan as an immune regulator in human diseases, *Physiol Rev*, 91, pp. 221–264.
45. Teder, P., Vandivier, R.W., Jiang, D., Liang, J., Cohn, L., Pure, E. et al. (2002). Resolution of lung inflammation by CD44, *Science*, 296, pp. 155–158.
46. Huebener, P., Abou-Khamis, T., Zymek, P., Bujak, M., Ying, X., Chatila, K. et al. (2008). CD44 is critically involved in infarct healing by regulating the inflammatory and fibrotic response, *J Immunol*, 180, pp. 2625–2633.
47. Zhao, M., Yoneda, M., Ohashi, Y., Kurono, S., Iwata, H., Ohnuki, Y. et al. (1995). Evidence for the covalent binding of SHAP, heavy chains of inter-alpha-trypsin inhibitor, to hyaluronan, *J Biol Chem*, 270, pp. 26657–26663.
48. Milner, C.M., Tongsoongnoen, W., Rugg, M.S., Day, A.J. (2007). The molecular basis of inter-alpha-inhibitor heavy chain transfer on to hyaluronan, *Biochem Soc Trans*, 35, pp. 672–676.
49. Baranova, N.S., Nileback, E., Haller, F.M., Briggs, D.C., Svedhem, S., Day, A.J. et al. (2011). The inflammation-associated protein TSG-6 cross-links hyaluronan via hyaluronan-induced TSG-6 oligomers, *J Biol Chem*, 286, pp. 25675–25686.
50. Milner, C.M., Day, A.J. (2003). TSG-6: A multifunctional protein associated with inflammation, *J Cell Sci*, 116, pp. 1863–1873.
51. Wisniewski, H.G., Naime, D., Hua, J.C., Vilcek, J., Cronstein, B.N. (1996). TSG-6, a glycoprotein associated with arthritis, and its ligand hyaluronan exert opposite effects in a murine model of inflammation, *Pflugers Arch*, 431, pp. R225–226.

52. Foskett, A.M., Bazhanov, N., Ti, X., Tiblow, A., Bartosh, T.J., Prockop, D.J. (2014). Phase-directed therapy: TSG-6 targeted to early inflammation improves bleomycin-injured lungs, *Am J Physiol Lung Cell Mol Physiol*, 306, pp. L120–131.
53. Zhuo, L., Kanamori, A., Kannagi, R., Itano, N., Wu, J., Hamaguchi, M. et al. (2006). SHAP potentiates the CD44-mediated leukocyte adhesion to the hyaluronan substratum, *J Biol Chem*, 281, pp. 20303–20314.
54. Jhunjhunwala, S., Aresta-DaSilva, S., Tang, K., Alvarez, D., Webber, M.J., Tang, B.C. et al. (2015). Neutrophil Responses to sterile implant materials, *PLOS One*, 10, pp. e0137550.
55. Alstergren, P., Zhu, B., Glogauer, M., Mak, T.W., Ellen, R.P., Sodek, J. (2004). Polarization and directed migration of murine neutrophils is dependent on cell surface expression of CD44, *Cell Immunol*, 231, pp. 146–157.
56. Pericle, F., Sconocchia, G., Titus, J.A., Segal, D.M. (1996). CD44 is a cytotoxic triggering molecule on human polymorphonuclear cells, *J Immunol*, 157, pp. 4657–4663.
57. Sconocchia, G., Campagnano, L., Adorno, D., Iacona, A., Cococcetta, N.Y., Boffo, V. et al. (2001). CD44 ligation on peripheral blood polymorphonuclear cells induces interleukin-6 production, *Blood*, 97, pp. 3621–3627.
58. Todd, J.L., Wang, X., Sugimoto, S., Kennedy, V.E., Zhang, H.L., Pavlisko, E.N. et al. (2014). Hyaluronan contributes to bronchiolitis obliterans syndrome and stimulates lung allograft rejection through activation of innate immunity, *Am J Respir Crit Care Med*, 189, pp. 556–566.
59. Lym, H.S., Suh, Y., Park, C.K. (2004). Effects of hyaluronic acid on the polymorphonuclear leukocyte (PMN) release of active oxygen and protection of bovine corneal endothelial cells from activated PMNs, *Korean J Ophthalmol*, 18, pp. 23–28.
60. Shankar, S.P., Babensee, J.E. (2010). Comparative characterization of cultures of primary human macrophages or dendritic cells relevant to biomaterial studies, *J Biomed Mater Res A*, 92, pp. 791–800.
61. Tesar, B.M., Jiang, D., Liang, J., Palmer, S.M., Noble, P.W., Goldstein, D.R. (2006). The role of hyaluronan degradation products as innate alloimmune agonists, *Am J Transplant*, 6, pp. 2622–2635.
62. Do, Y., Nagarkatti, P.S., Nagarkatti, M. (2004). Role of CD44 and hyaluronic acid (HA) in activation of alloreactive and antigen-specific T cells by bone marrow-derived dendritic cells, *J Immunother*, 27, pp. 1–12.
63. Termeer, C.C., Hennies, J., Voith, U., Ahrens, T., Weiss, J.M., Prehm, P. et al. (2000). Oligosaccharides of hyaluronan are potent activators of dendritic cells, *J Immunol*, 165, pp. 1863–1870.
64. Chang, D.T., Colton, E., Matsuda, T., Anderson, J.M. (2009). Lymphocyte adhesion and interactions with biomaterial adherent macrophages and foreign body giant cells, *J Biomed Mater Res A*, 91, pp. 1210–1220.
65. Ariel, A., Lider, O., Brill, A., Cahalon, L., Savion, N., Varon, D. et al. (2000). Induction of interactions between CD44 and hyaluronic acid by a short exposure of human T cells to diverse pro-inflammatory mediators, *Immunology*, 100, pp. 345–351.
66. Firan, M., Dhillon, S., Estess, P., Siegelman, M.H. (2006). Suppressor activity and potency among regulatory T cells is discriminated by functionally active CD44, *Blood*, 107, pp. 619–627.
67. Liu, T., Soong, L., Liu, G., Konig, R., Chopra, A.K. (2009). CD44 expression positively correlates with Foxp3 expression and suppressive function of CD4+ Treg cells, *Biol Direct*, 4, pp. 40.
68. Bollyky, P.L., Lord, J.D., Masewicz, S.A., Evanko, S.P., Buckner, J.H., Wight, T.N. et al. (2007). Cutting edge: High molecular weight hyaluronan promotes the suppressive effects of CD4+CD25+ regulatory T cells, *J Immunol*, 179, pp. 744–747.

69. Thevenot, P.T., Baker, D.W., Weng, H., Sun, M.-W., Tang, L. (2011). The pivotal role of fibrocytes and mast cells in mediating fibrotic reactions to biomaterials, *Biomaterials*, 32, pp. 8394–8403.
70. Eggli, P.S., Graber, W. (1993). Cytochemical localization of hyaluronan in rat and human skin mast cell granules, *J Invest Dermatol*, 100, pp. 121–125.
71. Fukui, M., Whittlesey, K., Metcalfe, D.D., Dastych, J. (2000). Human mast cells express the hyaluronic-acid-binding isoform of CD44 and adhere to hyaluronic acid, *Clin Immunol*, 94, pp. 173–178.
72. Boucher, W.S., Letourneau, R., Huang, M., Kempuraj, D., Green, M., Sant, G.R. et al. (2002). Intravesical sodium hyaluronate inhibits the rat urinary mast cell mediator increase triggered by acute immobilization stress, *J Urol*, 167, pp. 380–384.
73. Taylor, K.R., Yamasaki, K., Radek, K.A., Di Nardo, A., Goodarzi, H., Golenbock, D. et al. (2007). Recognition of hyaluronan released in sterile injury involves a unique receptor complex dependent on Toll-like receptor 4, CD44, and MD-2, *J Biol Chem*, 282, pp. 18265–18275.
74. Kawana, H., Karaki, H., Higashi, M., Miyazaki, M., Hilberg, F., Kitagawa, M. et al. (2008). CD44 suppresses TLR-mediated inflammation, *J Immunol*, 180, pp. 4235–4245.
75. Jiang, D., Liang, J., Fan, J., Yu, S., Chen, S., Luo, Y. et al. (2005). Regulation of lung injury and repair by Toll-like receptors and hyaluronan, *Nat Med*, 11, pp. 1173–1179.
76. Huang, Z., Zhao, C., Chen, Y., Cowell, J.A., Wei, G., Kultti, A. et al. (2014). Recombinant human hyaluronidase PH20 does not stimulate an acute inflammatory response and inhibits lipopolysaccharide-induced neutrophil recruitment in the air pouch model of inflammation, *J Immunol*, 192, pp. 5285–5295.
77. Galdiero, M.R., Mantovani, A. (2015). *Macrophage Plasticity and Polarization*, pp. 117–130.
78. Martinez, F.O., Gordon, S. (2014). The M1 and M2 paradigm of macrophage activation: Time for reassessment, *F1000Prime Rep*, 6, pp. 13.
79. Rayahin, J.E., Buhrman, J.S., Zhang, Y., Koh, T.J., Gemeinhart, R.A. (2015). High and low molecular weight hyaluronic acid differentially influence macrophage activation, *ACS Biomater Sci Eng*, 1, pp. 481–493.
80. Sokolowska, M., Chen, L.Y., Eberlein, M., Martinez-Anton, A., Liu, Y., Alsaaty, S. et al. (2014). Low molecular weight hyaluronan activates cytosolic phospholipase A2alpha and eicosanoid production in monocytes and macrophages, *J Biol Chem*, 289, pp. 4470–4488.
81. Kuang, D.M., Wu, Y., Chen, N., Cheng, J., Zhuang, S.M., Zheng, L. (2007). Tumor-derived hyaluronan induces formation of immunosuppressive macrophages through transient early activation of monocytes, *Blood*, 2, pp. 587–595.
82. He, H., Zhang, S., Tighe, S., Son, J., Tseng, S.C. (2013). Immobilized heavy chain-hyaluronic acid polarizes lipopolysaccharide-activated macrophages toward M2 phenotype, *J Biol Chem*, 288, pp. 25792–25803.
83. He, H., Tan, Y., Duffort, S., Perez, V.L., Tseng, S.C. (2014). In vivo downregulation of innate and adaptive immune responses in corneal allograft rejection by HC-HA/PTX3 complex purified from amniotic membrane, *Invest Ophthalmol Vis Sci*, 55, pp. 1647–1656.
84. Coulson-Thomas, V.J., Gesteira, T.F., Hascall, V., Kao, W. (2014). Umbilical cord mesenchymal stem cells suppress host rejection: The role of the glycocalyx, *J Biol Chem*, 289, pp. 23465–23481.
85. Shiraki, A., Kotooka, N., Komoda, H., Hirase, T., Oyama, J.-I., Node, K. (2016). Pentraxin-3 regulates the inflammatory activity of macrophages, *Biochem Biophys Rep*, 5, pp. 290–295.

86. Torihashi, S., Ho, M., Kawakubo, Y., Komatsu, K., Nagai, M., Hirayama, Y. et al. (2015). Acute and temporal expression of tumor necrosis factor (TNF)-alpha-stimulated gene 6 product, TSG6, in mesenchymal stem cells creates microenvironments required for their successful transplantation into muscle tissue, *J Biol Chem*, 290, pp. 22771–22781.
87. Li, L., Qian, Y., Jiang, C., Lv, Y., Liu, W., Zhong, L. et al. (2012). The use of hyaluronan to regulate protein adsorption and cell infiltration in nanofibrous scaffolds, *Biomaterials*, 33, pp. 3428–3445.
88. Nagata, M., Hoshi, N., Yoshinaka, H., Shiomi, H., Takenaka, M., Masuda, A. et al. (2016). Evaluation of the xenobiotic reaction against hyaluronate-based bioresorbable membrane in the abdominal cavity, *Prog Biomater*, 5, pp. 111–116.
89. Khaing, Z.Z., Milman, B.D., Vanscoy, J.E., Seidlits, S.K., Grill, R.J., Schmidt, C.E. (2011). High molecular weight hyaluronic acid limits astrocyte activation and scar formation after spinal cord injury, *J Neural Eng*, 8, pp. 046033.
90. Evren, S., Loai, Y., Antoon, R., Islam, S., Yeger, H., Moore, K. et al. (2010). Urinary bladder tissue engineering using natural scaffolds in a porcine model: Role of Toll-like receptors and impact of biomimetic molecules, *Cells Tissues Organs*, 192, pp. 250–261.
91. Hanson, S.E., King, S.N., Kim, J., Chen, X., Thibeault, S.L., Hematti, P. (2011). The effect of mesenchymal stromal cell-hyaluronic acid hydrogel constructs on immunophenotype of macrophages, *Tissue Eng Part A*, 17, pp. 2463–2471.
92. Franz, S., Allenstein, F., Kajahn, J., Forstreuter, I., Hintze, V., Moller, S. et al. (2013). Artificial extracellular matrices composed of collagen I and high-sulfated hyaluronan promote phenotypic and functional modulation of human pro-inflammatory M1 macrophages, *Acta Biomater*, 9, pp. 5621–5629.
93. Ghaly, T., Rabadi, M.M., Weber, M., Rabadi, S.M., Bank, M., Grom, J.M. et al. (2011). Hydrogel-embedded endothelial progenitor cells evade LPS and mitigate endotoxemia, *Am J Physiol Renal Physiol*, 301, pp. F802–812.
94. Chin, L., Calabro, A., Rodriguez, E.R., Tan, C.D., Walker, E., Derwin, K.A. (2011). Characterization of and host response to tyramine substituted-hyaluronan enriched fascia extracellular matrix, *J Mater Sci Mater Med*, 22, pp. 1465–1477.

8 Osteoimmunomodulation with Biomaterials

Bengü Aktaş, Bora Garipcan,
Zehra Betül Ahi, Kadriye Tuzlakoğlu,
Emre Ergene and Pınar Yılgör Huri

CONTENTS

8.1 INTRODUCTION

When a biomaterial is implanted, either within soft or hard tissues, the first response it receives from the body is the initiation of the inflammation cascade mediated by the innate immune system. This reaction eventually determines the fate of the biomaterial within the body: extrusion, resorption, integration or encapsulation. Therefore, although traditional biomaterial-based regenerative strategies focused primarily on the tissue-specific outcomes and hardly took immune response into consideration, the importance of the latter was later understood and is currently being considered an important component of therapy. It seems like a paradigm shift is happening in the field of biomaterials science; current therapeutic strategies incorporate methods to modulate the immune response within their approaches towards obtaining better regenerative outcomes.

The mutual interaction of bone and immune system is even more profound compared to the other tissues. Bone has an inherent importance for the immune system as it houses the bone marrow, where hematopoietic progenitors of the immune cells reside. The importance of immune cells in bone, however, was realised based on the clinical observations of bone loss in cases of autoimmune disorders and inflammatory diseases. Today, increasing evidence shows that the immune cells have important regulatory effects in modulating osteogenesis, osteoclastogenesis and bone metabolism as a whole.

8.1.1 Structure and Organisation of Bone

Bones serve for such important functions of the human body as providing shape, giving protection to internal organs, storing minerals and growth factors and the production of blood through the marrow. Bone has a high structural hierarchy made of collagen-based structures and hydroxyapatite minerals that are in association with mature and immature bone cells, osteoblasts, osteocytes and osteoclasts. Other than the mineralised tissue, organic parts and bone cells, bone tissue also contains blood vessels and nerves [1].

Bone is a complex, highly organised and mineralised connective tissue. Bone is stronger than steel in the sense that it can dissipate higher load and absorb a higher amount of shock before it breaks. On the other hand, bone is as light as wood, which makes the movement of the skeleton possible through the forces transmitted by the skeletal muscles. What makes these superior material properties possible is its structural hierarchy – the core-shell architecture. Structurally, the bones of the adult skeleton consist of cortical (compact) bone and cancellous (trabecular) bone, which make up 80% and 20% of the total bone mass, respectively. Cortical bone is found primarily in the shaft of the long bones that form the outer shell around the cancellous bone. Cortical bone is the load-carrying part of the tissue that provides its stiffness, and is much denser than cancellous bone, with a porosity ranging between 5 and 10% (Figure 8.1) [2,3]. Many osteons are bundled together in parallel along the axis of the cortical bone giving the tissue the capacity to withstand compressive and bending forces. Cancellous bone tissue fills the interior, which is composed of a network of rod- and plate-like elements that make the overall structure light and provide room for the blood vessels and the marrow. The osteons spread out and branch to form the meshwork of cancellous bone near the ends of the bones where the stresses become more multidirectional.

Microscopically bone has two distinct types: spongy and lamellar bone. Spongy bone is the immature and primitive type of bone. This structure can be observed in the embryonic stage, new-born and at the metaphysis during growth phase as well as in the fracture callus. The collagen bundles are arranged irregularly in the spongy bone and it contains a higher amount of cells for its unit volume compared to

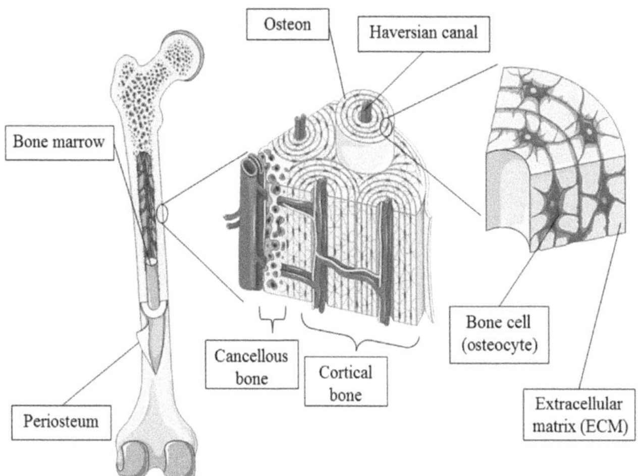

FIGURE 8.1 Schematic overview of the structure of bone (©2013 Bao CLM, Teo EY, Chong MSK, Liu Y, Choolani M, Chan KY. Published in *Regenerative Medicine and Tissue Engineering* under CC BY 3.0 license. Available from: http://dx.doi.org/10.5772/55916).

lamellar bone. Mechanically, spongy bone exerts isotropic character, i.e., mechanical response is not dependent on the stress applied. Lamellar bone, on the other hand, starts to form approximately one month after birth and by the age of 4 all bones in the body are lamellar. Lamellar bone exhibits anisotropic mechanical character and has a structural hierarchy as described previously.

In contrast to what is generally anticipated, bone is not a static tissue, but changes constantly. All of these activities are governed by bone cells: osteoblasts, osteoclasts and osteocytes.

8.1.2 Bone Cells and Bone Remodelling

We can start to investigate bone cells navigating from the outside in; all bones are covered with a dense membrane called periosteum, through which they receive nutrients and signals from the environment. Periosteum, which is connected to bone through strong collagenous fibres (Sharpey's fibres), is a double-layered membrane. The outer layer consists of collagen fibres and fibroblasts. We start to see bone cells at the inner layer of periosteum. This layer contains progenitor cells that give rise to osteoblasts – the "bone-making" cells.

8.1.2.1 Osteoblasts

Osteoblasts are single-nucleated cells that differentiate from mesenchymal stem cells (MSCs) residing in the stem cell niche within bone, following a well-established osteogenic differentiation pathway [4]. The crucial role of osteoblasts is to secrete osteoid, therefore they perform ossification (production of the new bone matrix). In this way, these cells are responsible for the growth of the width of long bones and the overall size of the other types of bone.

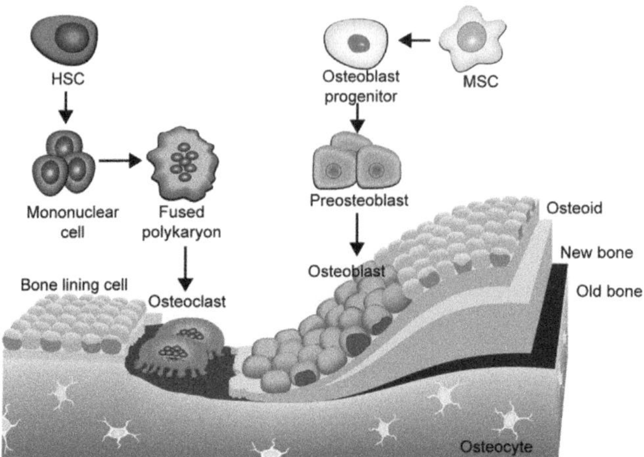

FIGURE 8.2 Diagram showing cellular distribution within bone and evolution of bone cells. (Reprinted from Rahman, M.S. et al., *Bone Res*, 3, 15005, 2015. With permission.)

Osteoblasts are arranged side-by-side at bone production sites (Figure 8.2) [5], like an epithelial layer without tight junctions. The connection and organisation between osteoblasts are very important for their activity, as disconnected cells cannot secrete matrix. Active osteoblasts have a cuboidal shape, are present superficially in bone and can be observed microscopically, neighbouring newly synthesised bone tissue. When bone synthesis is completed by active osteoblasts, surface osteoblasts become flattened and become "lining cells". Lining cells regulate the transition of minerals in and out of the bone tissue as well as secreting proteins for promoting the osteoclast cells [6].

8.1.2.2 Osteoclasts

Osteoclasts are multinucleated "bone-resorbing" cells [7]. The primary action of osteoclasts is to release acid and collagenase enzymes that resolve the mineral deposit within bone.

Osteoclasts stem from the hematopoietic stem cells (HSCs) that reside within the bone marrow. HSCs form mononuclear cells and eventually osteoclasts (Figure 8.2) [8]. It is worth noting that osteoclasts share the same maturation pathway as innate immune cells and macrophages and are considered to be resident macrophages specific to the bone microenvironment. In the bone microenvironment, localised multiple systemic hormones and cytokines are produced that promote osteoclast differentiation and function. These include receptor activator of nuclear factor κβ ligand (RANKL) and macrophage colony-stimulating factor (M-CSF) [9,10]. These membrane-bound proteins are produced by neighbouring stromal cells and osteoblasts. Therefore, osteoclastogenesis is regulated by osteoclast precursors together with osteoblasts, osteocytes and immune cells [9,10].

8.1.2.3 Osteocytes

Osteocytes are star-shaped mature bone cells that do not divide and are developed from osteoblasts. The main difference between osteocytes and osteoblasts is their area of settlement within bone (Figure 8.2). As osteoblasts continue synthesising the extracellular matrix, the mineralised tissue eventually grows over them and they remain embedded within the matrix, leading to reduced cellular activity and transformation into mature osteocytes. Osteocytes are arranged circumferentially around the central lumen of the osteons.

Bone remodelling is the process of coupled activity of osteoclasts and osteoblasts, in which the mineralised tissue is resorbed and then produced subsequently. Although declining with age, bone remodels itself continuously throughout life. During this remodelling, calcium homeostasis is regulated, micro-damages are repaired and the skeleton is shaped and sculpted. Bone also has the capacity of self-reconstruction and healing upon damage following similar coupled cellular activity.

8.2 BONE REGENERATION AND INTERACTIONS WITH THE IMMUNE SYSTEM

8.2.1 Bone Regeneration Cascade

Bone injury caused by reasons like trauma or tumour resection initiates the inherent regeneration cascade of bone, which occurs in three major steps; inflammation, repair and remodelling (Figure 8.3) [11]. Inflammatory reaction is initiated immediately following injury, during which a hematoma forms at the defect site, bridging the bone ends (day 0–3). Simultaneous vasodilatation facilitates the accumulation

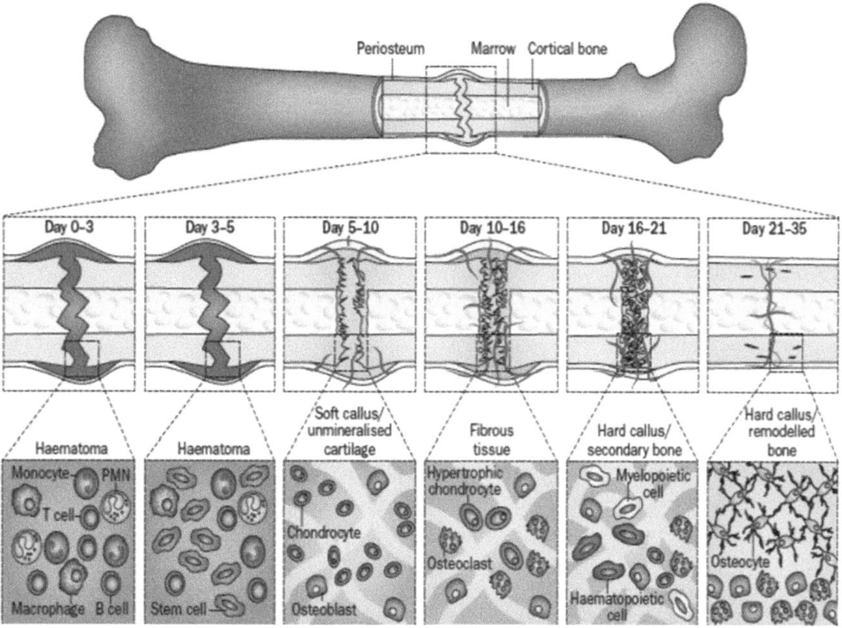

FIGURE 8.3 Schematic overview of bone regeneration cascade. (Reprinted from Einhorn, T.A. and Gerstenfeld, L.C., *Nat Rev Rheumatol*, 11, 45–54, 2015. With permission.)

of the plasma exudate and the recruitment of leucocytes, macrophages and lymphocytes in response to factors secreted by the platelets within (day 0–3). Locally produced cytokines and growth factors within the hematoma also promote the migration of fibroblasts and osteoprogenitor cells to the defect site (day 3–5). At this stage, angiogenesis is also initiated. By the end of this acute reaction to injury, inflammatory response resolves and necrotic tissue and plasma exudate starts to resorb. Osteoprogenitor cells within the hematoma differentiate in response to the local maxima of certain growth factors into specific lineages such as chondrocytes and osteoblasts responsible for hyaline cartilage and woven (fibrous) bone formation, respectively (day 5–10) [11,12].

In the reparative phase of bone repair, soft callus and non-mineralised cartilage bridges the defect as a result of local cellular activities and intramembranous ossification of the callus. In time, the cartilage is gradually replaced with lamellar bone, trabecular bone and finally with compact bone by endochondral ossification and mineralisation of the callus (day 10–35). The repair phase lasts until the bone site eventually duplicates the bone's original shape and strength.

Remodelling is the longest phase of bone regeneration and may last up to several years. During this phase, collagenous and other extracellular matrix components return to their normal levels and unnecessary callus tissue resorbs.

8.2.2 Inflammatory Response towards Biomaterials in the Bone Microenvironment

The implantation of a material causes an injury and homeostatic imbalance at the surgery site. The interface between the biomaterial and the tissue is highly dynamic, so that the healing cascade begins immediately as described for normal bone regeneration. Expectations from the healing process are based upon a series of molecular and cellular/extracellular interactions that result with the construction of new tissue. However, the initial interaction of the body with biomaterials accompanies multiple inflammatory responses that can interfere with the normal healing processes.

The first reaction of the host system after injury includes blood-material interaction. This interaction is consisted of a complex process of blood protein adsorption and desorption (Vroman effect), which further leads to initiation of a coagulation cascade, accumulation of platelets and formation of a conditioning film called provisional matrix [13–17]. Following this step, neutrophils (polymorphonuclear leukocytes), which represent acute inflammation, enter the injury site. Following acute inflammation, monocytes, lymphocytes, plasma cells and macrophages initiate a chronic inflammation phase.

All of these immune cells have distinct precursors and very specific roles in the inflammatory reaction. For example, monocytes are cells formed by precursor cells, called monoblasts, present in the bone marrow. These cells circulate via the bloodstream. During inflammation, monocytes leave the bloodstream and migrate to the tissues. Then, they differentiate into macrophages or dendritic cells under the influence of various growth factors and cytokines within tissues. Tissue macrophages are the first line of the body's defence mechanism and their primary action is to perform phagocytosis to digest any foreign substance to the body [18]. Granulocytes are a group of white blood cells with small granules in their cytoplasm. There are three different types of granulocytes: neutrophils, eosinophils and basophils. Neutrophils kill the invaders in three different ways: phagocytosis, secretion of soluble antimicrobials and neutrophil extracellular traps (NETs). Eosinophils are very important for fighting against parasitic infections as their granules contain cathepsin, which is a unique toxic protein. Basophils are responsible for immune response during the formation of acute and chronic allergic diseases [19].

Lymphocytes are a subclass of white blood cells implicated in adaptive immunity and there are different kinds of lymphocytes circulating in the bloodstream. The most commonly seen types of lymphocytes are B-lymphocytes (B-cells) and T-lymphocytes (T-cells). B-cells and T-cells are specific for a determined antigen, which can be considered one of their defining properties. In other words, each of them can bind to a particular molecular structure. They can recognise any antigen due to their specific surface receptor: the B-cell receptor (BCR) and the T-cell receptor (TCR) [20]. Bone marrow is the source of lymphocytes. However, the precursors of T-lymphocytes leave from bone marrow and migrate towards the thymus. After the migration, they acquire specific surface receptor molecules such as TCR and CD in the thymus. Through this process, they mature into T-lymphocytes with the ability to indicate a specific immune response [21].

B-cells are formed by HSCs in the bone marrow. They are responsible for producing antibodies. Firstly, BCRs bind the antigens, and antigens are engulfed into the B-cell and digested. Then cognate helper T-cells bind to B-cells and secrete lymphokines for mitosis and differentiation. Finally, B-cells differentiate into the plasma cell. Plasma cells are able to secrete large amounts of antibodies [22]. There are several kinds of T-cells. For example, T-helper cells (CD4+), the largest group of T-cells, stimulate the growth and proliferation of cytotoxic T-cells (CD8+). They also stimulate the growth and differentiation of B-cells and are responsible for activation of the macrophage system [23]. CD4+ T-cells might be infected by the human immunodeficiency virus (HIV). For this reason, the number of CD4+ T-cells decreases drastically and the ability of the immune response fails. Cytotoxic T-cells (CD8+), on the other hand, destroy virus-infected cells, tumour cells and cells that are transferred along with organ transplants.

As a highly vascularised organ, immune reaction in bone microenvironment is strong with both innate and adapted immunity systems, as described above, playing a role in the reactions to the implanted materials. The secreted molecules from activated immune cells (including pro-inflammatory cytokines secreted from macrophages) during acute response to bone injury have critical roles in the recruitment of osteoprogenitor and other cells that are important in bone healing and reassembling of vascularisation. [24–26]. For example, it has been shown that the exogenous admission of tumour necrosis factor-alpha (TNF-α), a pro-inflammatory cytokine, improves osteogenesis in both *in vitro* (osteogenic differentiation of mesenchymal stem cells from bone marrow and adipose tissue [27,28]) and *in vivo* conditions [29], as well as stimulation of angiogenesis [30]. However, there are also studies reporting the negative effect of TNF-α on angiogenesis [31]. These contradictory results indicate the importance of spatiotemporal control of dosing of factors released from immune cells on bone regeneration and re-vascularisation, and how the extent of immune reaction could affect the fate of implanted biomaterials within bone.

As another example, macrophages attack foreign substances (including biomaterials) as described above, in an effort to degrade them. Depending on the extent of macrophage activation and the inability of them to see off the target, macrophages coalesce to produce foreign body giant cells (FBGCs), which may eventually drive the formation of a fibrous capsule around the biomaterial. This capsule separates biomaterial from the surrounding tissues and restrains its integration with the bone. In the case of bone implants, this segregation might eventually lead to implant failure, because bone implant might not withstand the mechanical load without proper bone-implant integration [32]. Therefore, it is crucial to fine-tune the extent of immune response towards bone biomaterials in order to create an environment favourable to bone healing.

8.3 OSTEOIMMUNOLOGY

Bone has been a major target tissue for biomaterial-based therapeutic strategies for decades. One of the main reasons for that is the requirement of bone fillers in cases of large bone defects for tissue anchorage and growth. Based on this, there is a vast literature on the assessment of the interactions of bone cells and/or bone progenitors with biomaterials, and strategies to enhance bone formation on or within these materials. For example, osteogenic differentiation of mesenchymal stem cells (MSCs) on polymeric biomaterials is a common and well-studied strategy to develop 3D grafts for bone regeneration [33–35]. However, these biomaterial-based *in vitro* and *in vivo* studies incorporating bone cells and osteogenic progenitors have shown controversial results, implying poorly understood mechanisms of bone regeneration. Meanwhile, clinical observations have revealed the bilateral interactions of bone and immune cells specifically in cases of bone loss during inflammatory and auto-immune diseases. Nearly three decades after these observations, the discovery of the receptor activator of the NFkB ligand (RANKL) revealed the molecular-level coupling of the mutual interactions between bone cells and the immune system.

Based on these findings of crosstalk between bone and immune cells, the term “osteoimmunology” was derived [36]. Osteoimmunology is a field that studies the interactions of bone and immune cells in modulating osteogenesis and osteoclastogenesis. Osteoimmunology first studied the immune regulation of osteoclasts, since RANKL is expressed on activated T-cells, the main activator molecule for osteoclasts [37]. The area of focus, however, has been expanded since then to a sweeping range of cellular and molecular interactions, comprising those between osteoclasts and osteoblasts, osteoclasts and lymphocytes, and osteoblasts and HSCs. Thus, the osteoimmune system that is created by the integration of both systems is an exciting field not only for fundamental research but also for the development of novel treatments for diseases related with both systems [8].

8.3.1 Osteoimmunomodulatory Molecules

Since the first observations of significant bone loss in cases with malfunctioning immune systems in 1970s, the crosstalk between skeletal and immune systems is an area of interest for both researchers and clinicians. As mentioned above, the discovery of RANKL was the main cornerstone in the understanding of molecular-level interactions comprising bone and immune cells. RANKL is the main regulator of osteoclasts and is expressed on activated T-cells as well as on osteoblasts [36]. RANKL binds to RANK expressed on osteoclasts. By this way, activated T-cells enhance osteoclastic activity and triggers the process of bone remodelling. The excessive bone loss in cases of inflammatory and autoimmune diseases as well as cancer and even osteoporosis is associated with imbalances in the immune system response.

Current studies show that the interactions between these two interrelated systems go beyond the actions of RANKL, including the activity of osteoblasts in maintaining the HSC niche [38,39] and the functions of immune cells in osteoblast and osteoclast development. A number of molecules including cytokines, receptors and transcription factors have been identified as common regulators of both skeletal and immune systems [40,41]. As such, it is well established that M-CSF acts in the regulation of osteoclast differentiation together with RANKL, while a mutation in the corresponding gene for M-CSF negatively affects the development of osteoclasts and macrophages [42]. Insight into the roles of several other factors have been assessed by genetically modified animal models of inflammatory bone loss. For example, mutation in the interferon (IFN)γR1 receptor enhanced bone resorption mediated by osteoclasts [37]. This implies that IFN-γ produced by T-cells blocks osteoclast differentiation. In another study, it was shown that nuclear factor of activated T cells 1 (NFATcl) was essential for osteoclast differentiation both *in vitro* and *in vivo* [43]. Altering the levels of NFATcl has been stated as a promising way of decreasing the extent of osteoclast-mediated bone degradation [43]. Similarly, when mutations were made to the bone-related regulatory molecules, alterations in the immunological phenotype were observed in animal and clinical models [44]. For example, when the Sppl gene responsible for osteopontin production was knocked down, it was observed that fewer natural killer (NK) T-cells were produced by the animal [45]. Several other cytokines, including the interleukin (IL) group have been shown to affect bone metabolism. For example, osteoblast production was encouraged by IL-18 secreted by macrophages, where secretion of IL-1, IL-4 and IL-6 by the T-cells influenced osteoclast formation [46,47].

These studies have shed light on the interrelation and crosstalk between the skeletal and immune systems, which forms the basis of our understanding of the importance of their coupling in developing new bone regenerative strategies.

8.3.2 Cellular Interactions in the Osteoimmune System

The communication between bone cells and the immune system has an important impact on the regulation of bone formation and resorption. The process called hematopoiesis that occurs in the bone marrow enables the local and peripheral interactions of both cell types, since these cells have a common lineage origin and regulatory molecules. Besides, recent osteoimmunology studies have revealed the mechanism and crosstalk of these cells in inflammatory conditions such as rheumatoid arthritis and osteoporosis.

Osteoclasts (OCs) play a part in decalcification and degradation processes in bone remodelling. Moreover, they direct bone loss in pathological conditions. They are formed by the fusion of precursor cells of the monocyte-macrophage family. As a consequence, they have a multinucleated structure. On the other side, osteoblasts (OBs) come from mesenchymal stem cell origin and they have a single nucleus. They function at bone mineralisation [48–50]. The dynamic balance between bone formation and resorption is mediated by the complementary actions of osteoblasts and osteoclasts. Besides, dendritic cells, lymphocytes, macrophages etc. also participate in the regulation of bone remodelling processes, directly or indirectly. All the communications between these cells and their signalling molecules are carried out through specific interactions and pathways.

Osteoclast activation and differentiation deriving from osteoclast precursors (OCPs) is regulated by two cytokines, namely, macrophage-colony stimulating factor (M-CSF) and receptor activator of NF-κB ligand (RANKL) which are expressed by osteoblastic cells and stromal cells in the bone marrow [8,51]. The differentiation of osteoclasts is initiated by M-CSF binding to its specific receptor on OCPs [49]. RANKL binds to its receptor RANK on the surface of OCP and initiates maturation of osteoclast cells. RANK activation triggers several cascade mechanisms in osteoclast cells through TNF receptor-associated factor 6 (TRAF6), leading to the activation of c-Fos and NF-κB in connection with the nuclear factor of activated T-cells, cytoplasmic 1 (NFATc1), which is a master regulator of osteoclast differentiation [52]. The stimulation of osteoclastogenesis by osteoblasts is also achieved through immunoglobulin (Ig-like) receptors connected with immunoreceptor tyrosin-based activation motif (ITAM) co-stimulatory pathways such as Fc receptor common γ subunit (FcRγ) and DNAX-activating protein (DAP12) [8,53–56]. This pathway is essential for leading calcium-mediated signals associated with the synthesis of NFATc1 on the way to RANK/RANKL interaction [8,56].

These studies have revealed that cells such as T- and B-lymphocytes, macrophages, dendritic cells etc. may either support or inhibit osteoclast formation directly or indirectly [48,57,58]. Some natural killer cells (NK cells) and CD4+ T-helper subsets (Th1, Th2) secrete effector molecules and cytokines such as IFN-γ, IL-4 and IL-10 to reduce osteoclastogenic activity [48,52,59]. IFN-γ can both suppress the expression of RANK and induce the degradation of the TRAF6 molecule in order to prevent over-activation of osteoclasts under physiological conditions [37,52]. IFN-β also inhibits the induction of NFATc1 by preventing the translation of c-Fos transcription factor [52,60]. In a study by Moreno, it is found that IL-4 suppresses bone resorption through inhibiting the expression of RANK mRNA induced by M-CSF and RANKL in developing OCPs, and this suppression is mediated by a transcription factor, STAT6 [61]. A study by Mangashetti et al. showed that IL-4 inhibits the receptor activator of NF-κB and also Ca^{2+} signalling in mature osteoclast cells to inhibit bone resorption [62,63]. Evans and Fox show that IL-10 suppresses NFATc1 activity and inhibits osteoclastogenesis [59].

On the contrary, macrophages and Th1 cells secrete TNF-α for the activation of NF-κB to synthesise NFATc1 [64]. Th17 cells and memory T-cells secrete IL-17, which induces RANKL expression both on their membranes and also on synovial fibroblasts and triggers macrophages to produce pro-inflammatory cytokines such as

IL-1, IL-6 and TNF to activate osteoclastogenesis. IL-1 and IL-6 stimulate RANKL expression through fibroblasts and osteoblasts [48]. These cells also have the capacity to express RANKL on their surface membranes and interact with OCPs to target RANK directly.

Components such as 1,25-dihyroxyvitamin D_3 (1,25$(OH)_2D_3$), prostaglandin E2 (PGE2) and parathyroid hormone (PTH) regulate the expression of RANKL through osteoblasts. Their levels are considered important factors in terms of controlling bone resorption [8,49,65]. Vitamin D_3 and PTH are two significant components that participate in bone mineral metabolism since they regulate the balance of calcium and phosphorus. According to the studies, unremitting supply of PTH activates the expression of MCSF and RANKL [49,65]. Osteoclast cells do not have receptors for PTH on their cell walls; therefore, this action occurs through osteoblast cells. Along with the binding of PTH to osteoblasts, the cells increase their RANKL expression, thus ultimately increasing bone resorption. Osteoblasts and stromal cells further express a decoy receptor called osteoprotegerin (OPG) to reverse the effect of RANK/RANKL interaction. OPG binds to the RANKL receptors of osteoblasts in place of RANK to prevent the stimulation of osteoclastogenesis. PTH also has the property of inhibiting the secretion of OPG from osteoblasts. On the contrary, the intermittent supply of PTH causes an increase in bone formation due to the stimulation of several growth factors concomitantly [66]. Likewise, 1,25$(OH)_2$ vitamin D_3 or calcitriol indirectly regulates osteoclastogenesis through binding the receptors of osteoblasts and increasing the expression of RANKL and MCSF [49,65]. Another mediator that stimulates bone resorption is PGE2. PGE2 produced by osteoblasts may induce RANKL expression to stimulate bone resorption by binding one of the PGE receptor subtypes, EP4 [67]. In an indirect way, Udagawa et al. have showed that IL-17 that was secreted by T-cells effected on osteoblastic cells to stimulate PGE2 synthesis and induced RANKL expression [68]. As a solution, Lubberts et al. have showed that IL-4 inhibited the production of IL-17 in synovial tissues. They have indicated that local treatment with IL-4 cytokine prevented joint damage and bone resorption in mice with collagen-induced arthritis by downregulating IL-17 mRNA and RANKL expression [69]. There are also several types of hormones and metabolites that regulate bone metabolism by either directly or indirectly participating in the formation or resorption processes. For instance, oestrogen has dual effect on bone metabolism by acting through high-affinity receptors on both osteoblasts and osteoclasts. Oestrogen can increase the levels of OPG relating to a reduction in bone resorption while playing an important role in the increase of osteoblast cells in terms of number and function [65,70].

Apart from these, there is another pathway called Wnt signalling that is considered a key regulator for bone formation. According to studies, OPG expression is mediated by the Wnt signalling pathway [71,72]. The binding of Wnt signalling molecules activates two different signalling pathways, known as the β/catenin-dependent canonical and independent non-canonical pathway. The β/catenin-dependent canonical pathway has an essential role in promoting the differentiation of osteoblast precursor cells to mature osteoblasts. In a similar manner, this pathway has the property of suppressing bone resorption by changing the RANKL/OPG ratio [73]. In the study of Diarra et al., they indicate that TNF-mediated expression of Dickkopf-1 (DKK1) suppress Wnt signalling, thus this action hamper bone formation, meanwhile bone resorption is increased with the expression of RANKL in an inflammatory arthritis condition. Therefore, the blockade of DKK-1 induces bone formation since Wnt proteins are able to induce OPG expression [71]. On the other hand, Maeda et al. showed that Wnt5a, which is a non-canonical Wnt ligand, expressed by osteoblast-lineage cells, enhanced RANK expression through Ror-2 signalling in osteoclast precursors, thereby enhancing osteoclastogenesis, by effecting JNK and c-Jun pathways on the promoter of encoding RANK in both physiological and pathological conditions [74]. The above findings reveal that bone mass is commonly regulated by the combination of two signalling pathways; RANK/RANKL and Wnt/β-catenin.

Osteoimmunology is a dynamic field that studies the communication between bone systems and immune systems. All these recent findings about physiological and pathological conditions of skeletal systems are important advancements for leading to an understanding of cellular and molecular levels of interactions that will allow the development of new clinical insights for the treatment of bone diseases.

8.4 STRATEGIES TO MODULATE IMMUNE RESPONSES TOWARDS BONE BIOMATERIALS

Recent developments in biomaterials, regenerative medicine, tissue engineering and other related fields have provided a wide variety of options in the use of implantable devices for different medical purposes. However, complications remain due to the loss of functionality and durability of materials, which is caused by the failure of modulating host response at the earliest stage of the wound healing process that even leads to the requirement of a second operation.

Modulation of the inflammatory responses to a suitable state requires biomaterials to be equipped with various specific features. These features can be listed as follows: micro- and nanoscale architecture, mechanical strength and stiffness, surface properties (e.g., charge, roughness, topography and wettability), porosity etc. (Figure 8.4).

Tremendous progress has been made in the biomaterials field in a stepwise manner since the 1960s. First-generation biomaterials have only been developed to fulfil the mechanical needs of the specific bone region and materials should display inertness with a minimal toxicity [75,76]. Researchers started to focus on common materials such as metal, ceramic, polymers and composites. However, unspecific signal production associated with protein adsorption provoked fibrous capsule formation on the material surface, which isolates the interaction of materials with surrounding tissue and causes further scar formation and device failure [16,75]. From this point of view, second-generation biomaterials were designated as biocompatible biomaterials as they actively interact with the physiological environment [75,77]. The scaffolds were expected to support cell migration, differentiation and growth, and also to eliminate any toxic effect while inducing new bone formation. For inducing bioactivity, numerous types of scaffolds (such as bioactive glasses, glass-ceramics, HA etc.) have been synthesised by modifying their surface properties or adjusting porosity. These key factors pave the way for an ideal scaffold while providing *in vivo* tissue growth and controlling the degradation kinetics. Third-generation types are developed to stimulate cell responses at molecular level while being bioresorbable to

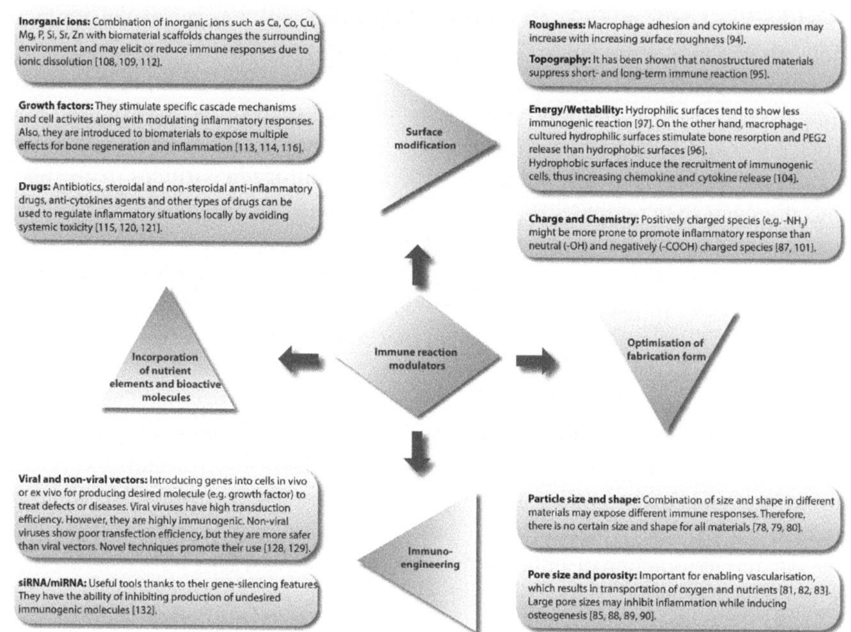

FIGURE 8.4 Biological, chemical and physical features of biomaterials to modulate the inflammatory response.

make room for new tissue formation by degrading in time. These molecular interactions are carried out by the interaction of specific molecules with integrin receptors, which are modified or loaded to the material beforehand.

In light of this information, current bone materials are expected to have the listed qualities to allow the formation of new bone structures: osteogenesis – the potential of proliferation and differentiation of osteoprogenitor cells on the material; osteoinduction – the stimulation of immature cells to bone-forming osteoblasts; osteoconduction – the ingrowth of vascularisation and infiltration of cells into the material. Besides, bone materials should definitely attain specific details to modulate immune responses at the osseointegration process. All properties mentioned here can be provided by changing material properties with strategies such as optimisation of the fabrication form (particle size, pore size and porosity), modification of material surface (chemistry/charge/hydrophilicity, coating, roughness/topology), incorporation of nutrient elements and bioactive molecules (anti-inflammatory drugs, growth factors, ions etc.) and application of immunoengineering (siRNA, gene therapy).

8.4.1 Optimisation of Fabrication Form

Immune response against an implant can be altered by changing the size of particles of foreign material. Macrophages engulf particles smaller than 10 μm by processes called phagocytosis and intracellular digestion. From 10- to 100-μm particle sizes, macrophages fuse together and form foreign body giant cells for ingestion.

Moreover, these cells release certain enzymes and pH-lowering molecules for facilitating extracellular degradation [78].

Numerous studies have shown the particle size effect over immune system. For example, Caicedo et al. has reported that the size and shape effect of CoCrMo-alloy particles (~1 and 6–7 μm) on phagocytosis, lysosomal destabilisation and inflammasome activation. They also have shown that 6–7 μm-sized particles in all shapes induced greater than tenfold pro-inflammatory cytokine IL-1β production compared to smaller-sized particles with similar shapes. Furthermore, larger/irregular-shaped particles (6 μm) that can be phagocytosed have showed the greatest lysosomal destabilisation and inflammatory reactivity compared to smaller/spherical (1 μm) particles *in vitro* [79]. Ward et al. have shown that solid polyurethane with silicone and polyethylene oxide (PU-S-PEO), respectively 300 μm (thin) and 2000 μm (thick) in size, has generated different foreign body capsule (FBC) formation. Their findings indicate that FBC on thin implants is thinner than on thick implants [80]. In a study by Veiseh et al., spheres with diameter of 1.5 mm and above, including ceramics, hydrogels, metals and plastic materials, were found to be biocompatible and mitigated the foreign body responses and fibrosis compared to small-sized counterparts in rodent and non-human primate animal models. However, they have also specified that simply increasing implant size might be insufficient, meaning that spherical shape was also integrated with size [81].

In sum, the parameters related to particle size and shape varying from different class of bone materials may reveal different amounts immune reaction; therefore, it's unlikely to say that a size or shape is appropriate for all materials.

Another major feature that should be primarily introduced to optimise bone biomaterials is creating a pore network and porosity on scaffolds. This process is especially important for prompting *in vivo* tissue growth or regeneration processes [82,83]. Scaffold porosity allows vascularisation, thus enables the transportation of fundamental nutrients and gases while clearing away metabolic wastes [83,84]. Liu et al. have demonstrated that introducing porosity to shape-memory alloys (e.g., Cu-Al-Ni or NiTi) increases ingrowth bone formation while making them suitable for load-bearing applications compared to smooth ones [85].

Small pore sizes may limit cell migration. This restricts the transportation of nutrients and oxygen as well as matrix elaboration within the scaffolds [84,86,87]. Oxygen deficiency gives rise to a hypoxic environment at the injury site, which in turn may enhance inflammation. However, moderate hypoxia also induces vascularisation by the effect of stabile hypoxia-inducible factors (HIFs) [88]. Several studies have reported that small pore sizes (75–100 μm) induces chondrogenesis due to the low oxygen tension, while large pore sizes (>300 μm) induce osteogenesis as a result of enhanced vascularisation, which result in the transportation of nutrients and a high degree of oxygen [86,89,90]. The second approach of large pore size takes cell adhesion into account. Cells may not adhere to the surface of large-pore-sized scaffolds. As a result, the subsequent events such as cell proliferation and differentiation will be hampered [86,87]. Moreover, the combination of higher porosity (around 80%) and macro-porosity is also believed to enhance osteogenesis due to successful nutrient delivery, vascularisation and tissue regeneration.

As indicated by Garg et al., bone marrow-derived macrophages cultured on polydioxane (PDO) electrospun scaffolds have yielded an increase in the expression of the M2 marker, which is an immunomodulatory phenotype of macrophages due to the increase in the fibre/pore size of the scaffold [91]. In another study, Chang et al. examined different-shaped pore types on hydroxyapatite (HA) scaffolds with a wide range of size. They observed that scaffolds were biocompatible and none of them showed any foreign body reactions [92].

Many researchers have focused on porous scaffolds made of ceramics, composites, polymers and metals. Studies on pore size and porosity show that immune system may give different responses to distinctive materials with varied pore sizes and porosity.

8.4.2 Surface Modification

It is also important to highlight that surface properties such as charge, chemistry, roughness, wettability and their implementation or alteration modulate immune responses while bringing bioactive characteristics to the scaffolds.

Surface topography and micro-/nanoscale architecture modulate cell adhesion, proliferation and spreading while directing immune cell interaction. For improving tissue remodelling rather than only supporting the injury site, the chosen scaffold should mimic the natural bone surface roughness. Each different cell response varies on different scales of roughnesses (e.g., macro, micro- and nanoscale roughness) [93]. Similarly, immune response also depends on the topographic structure of the surface even more than its chemical properties.

It has shown that polished titanium surfaces treated with a mixture of acidic solutions with different etched conditions exhibited higher roughness than smooth surfaces, in addition to their biocompatibility for MG63 osteoblast cells [94]. Takebe et al. (2002) investigated the macrophage adhesion and spreading on polished, machined and grit-blasted commercially pure Ti surfaces. They have showed that macrophage adhesion increased for all surfaces. Macrophage spreading enhanced with increasing surface roughness and the highest spreading observed on grit-blasted surfaces. Moreover, they concluded that surface roughness modulated the expression of cytokines [95]. A study by Smith et al. examined the short- and long-term immune reaction of titania nanotube arrays against biomedical-grade titanium by culturing white blood lysate. They concluded that there was a decrease in monocyte, macrophage and neutrophil functionality on titania nanotube arrays as compared to biomedical-grade titanium, which was evidence that nanoarchitecture has high potential for biomedical applications [96].

Surface energy and wettability are also considerable properties that influence the adsorption kinetics and conformation characteristics of the proteins, eventually affecting inflammatory responses. Hydrophilic surfaces thermodynamically tend to adsorb lower amounts of protein in comparison to hydrophobic surfaces. Hence, the reduction in cell responses to hydrophilic surfaces evokes less immune reaction in the body. However, Murray et al. reported that hydrophilic surfaces stimulated more bone resorption and prostaglandin E2 (PGE2) release than hydrophobic surfaces. PGE2 is released in inflammatory situations by macrophages or foreign body giant cells. In this regard, they concluded that bone resorption with hydrophilic surfaces might evoke inflammatory responses [97]. A recent study by Dai et al. reports that the growth rate of RAW 264.7 macrophages was higher on a hydrophilic Ti surface than polished Ti. Additionally, a lower level of pro-inflammatory factor TNF-α and a higher level of anti-inflammatory factor IL-10 were observed on the Ti-H_2O_2 surface compared to polished Ti [98]. On the other part, hydrophobic surfaces cause an increase of fibrinogen, IgG and non-specific antibodies adsorption on the material surface, as well as an increase in coagulation factors [99]. In this scenario, the change in the conformation of fibrinogen initiates platelet adhesion, as well as the recruitment of macrophages and their fusion into foreign body giant cells by exposing their hidden domains (D domain) as a ligand for inflammatory cell receptors [100–102]. Macrophages that are gathered on the surface release larger amounts of cytokines and chemokines such as IL-1, IL8, MCP-1 etc., which in turn induces the recruitment of fibroblasts and leukocytes [88,100,103,104]. Hezi-Yamit et al. mention that hydrophobic polymers induce an increase in monocyte adhesion, whereas hydrophilic polymers do not [105].

Surface charge and chemistry have considerable influences on protein adsorption, denaturation and subsequent cellular responses. Surface functionality with hydrophilic or neutral groups is more favourable than hydrophobic functionality. In the case of charge properties, it has been proven that fibrinogen prefers hydrophobic and positively charged surfaces instead of hydrophilic and negatively charged surfaces [99,101]. In the same vein, Brodbeck highlighted the effect of surface chemistry on adherent human monocyte/macrophage cytokine expression *in vitro* by using a polyethylene terephthalate (PET)-base surface, which was modified with photograft co-polymerisation. Brodbeck also reported that hydrophilic and anionic surfaces showed an anti-inflammatory type of response by dictating selective cytokine production by adherent monocytes and macrophages [106]. It is a widespread expectation that positively charged species (e.g., NH_3) are more prone to promote inflammatory responses than neutral (-OH) and negatively (e.g., -COOH) charged species [88,102]. Contrary to these expectations, Rostam et al. showed that human monocytes can be cultured on untreated hydrophobic polystyrene (PS) and hydrophilic O_2 plasma-etched polystyrene (O_2-PS40) surfaces. O_2-PS40 surfaces are polarised M1-like phenotypes, whereas PS surfaces are polarised M2-like phenotypes together with the expressions of transcription factors and cytokines [107].

8.4.3 Incorporation of Nutrient Elements and Bioactive Molecules

Since the skeletal system is coordinated by a variety of regulatory elements and molecules such as growth factors, hormones, inorganic ions etc., recent studies are generally focused on the fabrication of biomaterials, which are equipped with these factors for creating a natural microenvironment. In the same manner, these elements and molecules can be manipulated to modulate immune responses.

Some inorganic ions, such as Ca, Co, Cu, Mg, P, Si, Sr and Zn, are common elements that are involved in bone metabolism. These elements are also incorporated into biomaterials as ionic dissolution products to affect the behaviour of cells, in addition to increase bioactivity. Calcium phosphates (e.g., tricalcium phosphates-TCPs, hydroxyapatite-HA), bioactive glasses, silica-based glasses and so forth are widely used materials for bone tissue applications as their nature is similar to bone tissue and they include some of the mentioned inorganic ions in their structure [90,108]. Thus, the solution of these materials in the physiological environment and the participation of dissolved ions to different pathways may stimulate new bone formation upon the activation of osteoblast cells and suppression of the immune system.

In a study by Toita et al., lipopolysaccharide-stimulated RAW 264.7 macrophages were cultured on Ca-modified poly(ether ether ketone)(PEEK). These macrophages produced lower levels of pro-inflammatory cytokines due to higher IL-10 production mediated by Ca-activated calmodulin signalling pathways and higher levels of anti-inflammatory cytokines compared to pristine PEEK [109]. Wu et al. used mesoporous bioactive glass (MGB) scaffolds with controllable Co^{+2} ion release to induce osteogenesis and angiogenesis by mimicking a hypoxic condition. They showed that Co-MGB scaffolds enhanced VEGF secretion, HIF-1a expression and bone-related gene expression of BMSCs. Moreover, well-ordered mesopore channel structures of the scaffold have succeeded at controllable antibiotic release. In conclusion, they combined angiogenesis with osteogenesis, as well as an anti-bacterial function with Co-MGB scaffolds [110].

Si intake has a strong effect on bone mineral density. Although it also has a role on collagen synthesis and matrix mineralisation, the biological reaction of Si is not yet fully understood [111]. Zinc is another essential trace element that plays an important role in the metabolic pathways of bone and the immune system [112]. Day and Boccaccini have put an emphasis on the ionic dissolution of silicate- and zinc phosphate-based bioactive glasses and, as associated with this, cytokine release from human macrophages and monocytes. However, they have showed that TNF-α and IL-6 secretion from stimulated cells was lower in the presence of the silicate glasses than with the zinc phosphate glasses [113].

The degradation of scaffolds accompanying ion dissolution changes the surrounding environment and may elicit or reduce immune response. Therefore, optimisation and refined fabrication of scaffolds that are combined with ions in appropriate concentration is of great importance.

8.4.4 Growth Factors

Growth factors act as signal molecules that stimulate specific cascade mechanisms and cell activities. Most recent biomaterial studies have been focused on introducing growth factors to biomaterials to realise these molecular and cellular activities, along with the modulation of inflammatory reactions. Among growth factors, bone morphogenetic protein family (BMPs), fibroblast growth factor (FGF), insulin-like growth factor (IGF), platelet-derived growth factor (PDGF), transforming growth factor (TGF) and vascular endothelial growth factor (VEGF) are the most relevant constituents for bone formation and regeneration.

BMPs have an important role in inducing bone formation and repair, and osteoblast differentiation, ultimately for bone and cartilage development. BMP-2 through BMP-7 constitute a subgroup of molecules that belong to the TGF-β superfamily. TGF-βs that have mitogenic and chemotactic effects regulate the increase in type-I collagen and osteoblast matrix production while inducing mature osteoclast apoptosis. Furthermore, TGF-βs, together with IL-4 and IL-10, are among macrophage-deactivators. A study by Brandes et al. reported that TGF-β1 suppresses the evolution of acute and chronic-phase arthritis in streptococcal cell wall (SCW)-injected rats [114].

VEGF is a signal protein that is secreted by endothelial and osteoblast cells. This protein plays an important role in the formation of blood vessels and endothelial cell activity. VEGF stimulates vasculogenesis and angiogenesis during endochondral ossification in the bone formation process. Apart from these, it also plays a role in chondrocyte and osteoblast differentiation and osteoclast recruitment [115]. Localised delivery of dexamethasone and VEGF with the use of PLGA microsphere/PVA hydrogel composites has been investigated at the tissue implant interface and it has been observed that inflammation and fibrosis were suppressed while neo-angiogenesis was stimulated in a rat model [116].

PDGF is a potent mitogen molecule for mesenchymal origin cells, and also a chemoattractant molecule for fibroblasts, neutrophils and monocytes. It is released from platelets after tissue injury and it accelerates the wound healing process by interacting with TGF. In addition, macrophages can also release PDGFs.

IGF prolongs the effect of BMPs and TGF-βs and contributes to skeletal growth and bone formation. It has been shown that the administration of IGF-1 in poly(lactide-co-glycolide) microspheres on ovine long bones resulted in new bone formation and inflammation reduction. It was concluded that the administration of the IGF-1 delivery system downregulates inflammatory marker gene expression [117].

8.4.5 Drugs

Modulating the inflammatory response at the injury site or treating bone disorders by drug scaffold incorporation has been a pivotal therapeutic method in recent years for avoiding systemic toxicity. Especially, 3D bioactive bone scaffolds that are fabricated from bioceramics, biodegradable polymers and composites enhance the effectiveness of drug locally, enabling drug release control. Nevertheless, the mechanical properties of material should also be considered with regard to the physiological environment and pharmacokinetics of the drug.

One of the main problems affecting the life-span of implants and hampering the wound healing process is bacterial infection, which is originated from the homeostatic imbalance at the tissue site or contamination from other sources. It is worth noting that bacterial infection should be stopped with antibiotics before it prevents the wound healing process. This is because specific bacteria types may form a biofilm layer on the implant surface and these biofilms are highly resistant to immune reaction, making them difficult to destroy. To overcome this, antibiotics can be introduced to the implantation site as quickly as possible. Ciproflozacin, gentamicin and vancomycin exemplify antibiotics that can be introduced with scaffolds. Chang et al. (2013) have searched after an optimal antibiotic-loaded bone cement (ALBC) for infection prophylaxis in total joint arthroplasty (TJA) [118]. In that study, they investigated the antibacterial effects of PMMA bone cements loaded with ceftazidime, imipenem, piperacillin, teicoplanin, tobramycin and vancomycin against methicillin-sensitive *S. aureus* (MSSA), methicillin-resistant *S. aureus* (MRSA), coagulase-negative *staphylococci* (CoNS), *E. coli*, *Pseudomonas aeruginosa* and *Klebsiella pneumonia*. Their conclusion was that ALBC with gentamicin showed longer duration of antibiotic release than other samples and had a broad antibacterial spectrum against all organisms that were used in the experiment. In addition to this, imipenem-loaded cement had a negative effect on the compressive strength of scaffold, but all antiobiotics maintained their properties after being mixed with PMMA.

Anti-inflammatory agents including steroids (glucorticoids) or non-steroids are other drugs that are used in bone tissue engineering applications to suppress immune reaction. Glucocorticoids are especially known to promote the differentiation of cells and tissues such as bone, cartilage and muscle by exhibiting inhibitory effects for inflammatory factors (IL-1, IL-4, IL-8, TNF-α etc.) [26,119,120]. Non-steroidal anti-inflammatory drugs (NSAIDs) are the most commonly used drugs against inflammation. This is because they inhibit the activity of cyclooxygenase (COX-I and COX-II) enzymes, which in turn inhibits the synthesis of prostaglandins. COXs are responsible for the conversion of arachidonic acid to prostaglandin H2 (PGH2). PGH2 is then catalysed into other types of prostaglandins, such as PGI2, PGD2 and PEG2. An essential function of PEG2 is to regulate the cytokine production by activated macrophages. It also plays a central role in the regulation of T- and B-cells [121,122]. However, there is some controversy about the use of NSAIDs, since these drugs inhibit fracture healing and reduce bone density. For example, Beck et al. observed that the oral administration of diclofenac to rats with short-term therapy and long-term therapy registered a delay in fracture healing [123].

Anti-cytokine agents are also important tools for the regulation of inflammatory responses. The introduction of several anti-cytokines such as adalimumab (monoclonal antibody; inhibits TNF-α), anakinra (IL-1 receptor antagonist), etanercept (fusion protein; inhibits TNF-α) and infliximab (chimeric monoclonal antibody; inhibits TNF-α) has been preferred for the treatment of diseases such as rheumatoid arthritis (RA) [124]. However, there are some adverse effects inflicting the application of these therapies, such as infections, injection site reactions, induction of autoimmunity etc. In addition, high cost and loss of efficacy cause a secondary problem [125,126].

8.4.6 Immunoengineering

Recombinant growth factors are introduced to the injury site directly or combined with graft substitutes to accelerate bone healing. Since the release of molecules in the body is hardly manageable, life spans are very low, and cost is high; gene therapy may be an alternative for producing these proteins in the body. In its most general application, gene therapy is a technique to introduce genes into cells or tissues *in vivo* or *ex vivo* to treat or prevent a defect or disease. There are viral and non-viral delivery techniques for both *in vivo* and *ex vivo* gene therapy strategies. The *in vivo* delivery technique aims for local production of the desired molecule by the administration of viral or non-viral vectors to the damaged site. In *ex vivo* delivery technique, cells (bone marrow and adipose tissue mesenchymal stem cells; embryonic stem cells (ESCs) and mesenchymal stem cells (MSCs) derived from bone marrow, muscle and adipose tissue) are harvested for the transduction or transfection process. Following this, transduced cells are transplanted to the injury site.

Viral vectors used in gene therapy generally include adenovirus, adeno-associated virus (AAV), baculovirus, modified bacteriophage, lentivirus and retrovirus. When these vectors permeate to body, they might be recognised as foreign material by immune system and innate immune response evolves rapidly. Moreover, they might cause another problem called insertional mutagenesis. Despite this, they have advantages such as high transduction efficiency and ease of production. Among a variety of viruses, adenovirus and retrovirus are the most common vectors used in bone tissue engineering. Adenovirus vectors also have the advantage of high transduction efficiency for both dividing and non-dividing cells. On the other hand, they are highly immunogenic. There are pre-existing antibodies in the human body that can fight against these vectors. Note that this counteraction may limit the effectiveness of the treatment. Researches of gene therapy for bone/cartilage defects or diseases are extensively focused on BMP loading. For articular cartilage repair, Zhang et al. have combined microfracture, perforated decalcified cortical bone matrix (DCBM) and gene therapy with adenovirus bone morphogenetic protein-4 (Ad-BMP4). In doing so, they have successfully induced native hyaline articular cartilage within a short period of six weeks [127]. In a study by Saito, biomineral coatings in bone regeneration were investigated by using SFF scaffolds made of PLLA and PCL in combination with *ex vivo* gene therapy. Human gingival fibroblasts (HGF) were transduced with adenovirus-encoded with BMP-7 or green fluorescent protein (GFP). It was shown that only scaffolds with BMP-7-transduced HGFs exhibited mineralised tissue formation [128].

Non-viral gene therapy is based on the administration of nucleic acids such as small or larger DNA molecules (oligodeoxynucleotides, plasmid DNA etc.), and RNA (siRNA, mRNA) to host cells chemically or physically. The main advantage of non-viral vectors is that they are less immunogenic and can carry unrestricted genetic materials when compared to viral vectors. Poor transfection efficiency of non-viral vectors makes them less preferable over viral vectors. However, novel developments and safety concerns have promoted the use of these vectors. For example, Yue investigated the effect of *in vitro* gene delivery by using chitosan-g-PEI as a non-viral vector in bone marrow stem cells. Plasmid pIRES2-ZsGreen1-hBMP2 has been constructed for monitoring the transgene expression level. It has been shown that gene transfer showed 17.2% of transfection efficiency and more than 80% of cell viability in stem cells [129]. Polymer-based non-viral vectors are broadly classified into natural and synthetic polyplexes such as polyethylenimine (PEI), chitosan, poly(DL-lactide) (PLA) and poly(DL-lactide-co-glycolic acid) (PLGA), dendrimers and polymethacrylate. Chitosan is a widely used cationic polymer in gene therapy studies. However, its transfection efficiency is low. PEI, on the other hand, is a very strong candidate for *in vivo* and *in vitro* gene therapy applications. Nevertheless, it should be noted that it might exhibit highly toxic characteristics depending on its dose and molecular weight. For that reason, Yue et al. have used the combination of chitosan and PEI, since together they increase transfection efficiency and decrease cytotoxicity. In another study, Kawai constructed a vector carrying a double-gene expression cassette that incorporated the coding sequences for BMP-2 and BMP-7 into one expression vector (pCAGGS-BMP-2/7). As indicated in the paper, the expression of this vector induced osteogenic differentiation in various cell lines with the same efficiency as BMP-2 and BMP-7 co-expressed from separate vectors. Furthermore, this vector strongly induced bone formation in rat skeletal muscle when introduced by *in vivo* electroporation, compared with BMP-2 or BMP-7 alone [130].

Besides gene therapy, ribonucleic acid (RNA)-based approaches have become a novel therapeutic procedure for bone disorders. RNA interference (RNAi) is a cellular mechanism for gene silencing and is an umbrella term for small interfering RNA (siRNA) and micro RNA (miRNA). siRNA and miRNA are short duplex RNA molecules, which have different gene silencing effects. siRNA is highly specific to particular mRNA targets, while miRNA regulates multiple targets. The gene silencing effects of siRNA and miRNA make them useful tools for delivery systems. There are polymer-based and lipid-based vectors for delivering these RNAs [131,132]. In a study by Zhang, they have linked (AspSerSer)6, which is a targeting moiety *in vivo* for bone formation surfaces, with a DOTAP-based cationic liposome encapsulating an osteogenic siRNA, and these (AspSerSer)6-liposome have been targeted a negative regulator (Plekhol) of osteogenic lineage activity without modulating bone resorption. It was shown that the approach markedly promoted bone formation, enhanced the bone micro-architecture and increased the bone mass in both healthy and osteoporotic rats [133].

Current therapies might remain insufficient for many skeletal disorders, especially for those within the area of inadequate blood flow. Moreover, these adopted strategies might require several-step surgeries and cause donor site morbidity. As a solution to these problems, gene delivery technologies have the potential to heal disorders by transferring desired osteogenic molecules to the local site directly with a sustained expression for bone formation and regeneration therapies.

8.5 CONCLUSION

The interactions between bone and immune systems were first realised due to clinical observations of excessive bone loss in cases of autoimmune disorders. Then, the discovery of RANKL revealed the molecular-level tie in between the systems, leading to the birth of the term "osteoimmunology". Today, exponentially increasing scientific evidence tell us that in order to set proper regenerative therapies toward bone with using biomaterials, the immune system response should be taken into account as well as osteogenesis. The crosstalk between the systems as well as the spatiotemporal and dose-dependent nature of the effect of immunomodulatory molecules on bone metabolism suggest that further studies are needed to set the ground for optimised recipes of bone regeneration using biomaterials.

REFERENCES

1. Berendsen, A.D. and Olsen, B.R. (2015). Bone development. *Bone*, 80, pp. 14–18.
2. Buckwalter, J.A., Glimcher, M.J., Cooper, R.R. and Recker, R. (1996). Bone biology. II: Formation, form, modeling, remodeling, and regulation of cell function. *Instr Course Lect*, 45, pp. 387–399.

3. Bao, C.L.M., Teo, E.Y., Chong, M.S.K., Liu, Y., Choolani, M. and Chan, K.Y. Published in *Regenerative Medicine and Tissue Engineering* under CC BY 3.0 license. Available from: http://dx.doi.org/10.5772/55916.
4. Birmingham, E., Niebur, G.L., McHugh, P.E., Shaw, G., Barry, F.P. and McNamara, L.M. (2012). Osteogenic differentiation of mesenchymal stem cells is regulated by osteocyte and osteoblast cells in a simplified bone niche. *Eur Cell Mater*, 23, pp. 13–27.
5. Rahman, M.S., Akhtar, N., Jamil, H.M., Banik, R.S. and Asaduzzaman, S.M. (2015). TGF-beta/BMP signaling and other molecular events: Regulation of osteoblastogenesis and bone formation. *Bone Res*, 3, pp. 15005.
6. Saad, M. (2015). Specialized cells in the skeletal system, www.livestrong.com /article/72443-specialized-cells-skeletal-system.
7. Vaananen, H.K., Zhao, H., Mulari, M. and Halleen, J.M. (2000). The cell biology of osteoclast function. *J Cell Sci*, 113, pp. 377–381.
8. Takayanagi, H. (2007). Osteoimmunology: Shared mechanisms and crosstalk between the immune and bone systems. *Nat Rev Immunol*, 7, pp. 292–304.
9. Teitelbaum, S.L. (2000). Bone resorption by osteoclasts. *Science*, 289, pp. 1504–1508.
10. Yavropoulou, M.P. and Yovos, J.G. (2008). Osteoclastogenesis – current knowledge and future perspectives. *J Musculoskelet Neuronal Interact*, 8, pp. 204–216.
11. Einhorn, T.A. and Gerstenfeld, L.C. (2015). Fracture healing: Mechanisms and interventions. *Nat Rev Rheumatol*, 11, pp. 45–54.
12. Rahman, M.S., Akhtar, N., Jamil, H.M., Banik, R.S. and Asaduzzaman, S.M. (2015). TGF-β/BMP signaling and other molecular events: Regulation of osteoblastogenesis and bone formation. *Bone Res*, 3, pp. 15005.
13. Schmidt, D.R., Waldeck, H. and Kao, W.J. (2009). Protein adsorption to biomaterials, in *Biological Interactions on Materials Surfaces: Understanding and Controlling Protein, Cell, and Tissue Responses*, eds Puleo, D.A. and Bizios, R. (New York, Springer), pp. 1–18.
14. Raffaini, G. and Ganazzoli, F. 2010. Protein adsorption on biomaterial and nanomaterial surfaces: A molecular modeling approach to study non-covalent interactions. *J Appl Biomater Biomech*, 8, pp. 135.
15. Amini, A.R., Wallace, J.S. and Nukavarapu, S.P. (2011). Short-term and long-term effects of orthopedic biodegradable implants. *J Long Term Eff Med Implants*, 21, pp. 93–122.
16. Anderson, J.M., Rodriguez, A. and Chang, D.T. (2008). Foreign body reaction to biomaterials. *Sem Immunol*, 20, pp. 86–100.
17. Chester, D. and Brown, A.C. (2016). The role of biophysical properties of provisional matrix proteins in wound repair. *Matrix Biol*. 60–61, pp. 124–140.
18. Elhelu, M.A. (1983). The role of macrophages in immunology. *J Natl Med Assoc*, 75, pp. 314–317.
19. Mukai, K. and Galli, S.J. (2001). *Basophils* (John Wiley & Sons, Ltd). https://doi .org/10.1002/9780470015902.a0001120.pub3.
20. Cooper, M.D. (2015). The early history of B cells. *Nat Rev Immunol*, 15, pp. 191–197.
21. Schwarz, B.A. and Bhandoola, A. (2006). Trafficking from the bone marrow to the thymus: A prerequisite for thymopoiesis. *Immunol Rev*, 209, pp. 47–57.
22. Yuseff, M.I., Pierobon, P., Reversat, A. and Lennon-Dumenil, A.M. (2013). How B cells capture, process and present antigens: A crucial role for cell polarity. *Nat Rev Immunol*, 13, pp. 475–486.
23. Gutcher, I. and Becher, B. (2007). APC-derived cytokines and T cell polarization in autoimmune inflammation. *J Clin Invest*, 117, pp. 1119–1127.
24. Ai-Aql, Z.S., Alagl, A.S., Graves, D.T., Gerstenfeld, L.C. and Einhorn, T.A. (2008). Molecular mechanisms controlling bone formation during fracture healing and distraction osteogenesis. *J Dent Res*, 87, pp. 107–118.

25. Kolar, P., Schmidt-Bleek, K., Schell, H., Gaber, T., Toben, D., Schmidmaier, G., Perka, C., Buttgereit, F. and Duda, G.N. (2010). The early fracture hematoma and its potential role in fracture healing. *Tissue Eng Part B Rev*, 16, pp. 427–434.
26. Mountziaris, P.M. and Mikos, A.G. (2008). Modulation of the inflammatory response for enhanced bone tissue regeneration. *Tissue Eng Part B Rev*, 14, pp. 179–186.
27. Hess, K., Ushmorov, A., Fiedler, J., Brenner, R.E. and Wirth, T. (2009). TNFalpha promotes osteogenic differentiation of human mesenchymal stem cells by triggering the NF-kappaB signaling pathway. *Bone*, 45, pp. 367–376.
28. Lu, Z.F., Wang, G.C., Dunstan, C.R. and Zreiqat, H. (2012). Short-term exposure to tumor necrosis factor-alpha enables human osteoblasts to direct adipose tissue-derived mesenchymal stem cells into osteogenic differentiation. *Stem Cells Dev*, 21, pp. 2420–2429.
29. Glass, G.E., Chan, J.K., Freidin, A., Feldmann, M., Horwood, N.J. and Nanchahal, J. (2011). TNF-alpha promotes fracture repair by augmenting the recruitment and differentiation of muscle-derived stromal cells. *Proc Natl Acad Sci USA*, 108, pp. 1585–1590.
30. Hutton, D.L., Kondragunta, R., Moore, E.M., Hung, B.P., Jia, X. and Grayson, W.L. (2014). Tumor necrosis factor improves vascularization in osteogenic grafts engineered with human adipose-derived stem/stromal cells. *PLoS One*, 9, pp. e107199.
31. Nakagami, H., Cui, T.X., Iwai, M., Shiuchi, T., Takeda-Matsubara, Y., Wu, L. and Horiuchi, M. (2002). Tumor necrosis factor-alpha inhibits growth factor-mediated cell proliferation through SHP-1 activation in endothelial cells. *Arterioscler Thromb Vasc Biol*, 22, pp. 238–242.
32. Nuss, K.M. and von Rechenberg, B. (2008). Biocompatibility issues with modern implants in bone – a review for clinical orthopedics. *Open Orthop J*, 2, pp. 66–78.
33. Yilgor, P., Tuzlakoglu, K., Reis, R.L., Hasirci, N. and Hasirci, V. (2009). Incorporation of a sequential BMP-2/BMP-7 delivery system into chitosan-based scaffolds for bone tissue engineering. *Biomaterials*, 30, pp. 3551–3559.
34. Yilgor, P., Yilmaz, G., Onal, M.B., Solmaz, I., Gundogdu, S., Keskil, S., Sousa, R.A., Reis, R.L., Hasirci, N. and Hasirci, V. (2013). An in vivo study on the effect of scaffold geometry and growth factor release on the healing of bone defects. *J Tissue Eng Regen Med*, 7, pp. 687–696.
35. Yilgor, P., Sousa, R.A., Reis, R.L., Hasirci, N. and Hasirci, V. (2010). Effect of scaffold architecture and BMP-2/BMP-7 delivery on in vitro bone regeneration. *J Mater Sci Mater Med*, 21, pp. 2999–3008.
36. Arron, J.R. and Choi, Y. (2000). Bone versus immune system. *Nature*, 408, pp. 535–536.
37. Takayanagi, H., Ogasawara, K., Hida, S., Chiba, T., Murata, S., Sato, K., Takaoka, A., Yokochi, T., Oda, H., Tanaka, K., Nakamura, K. and Taniguchi, T. (2000). T-cell-mediated regulation of osteoclastogenesis by signalling cross-talk between RANKL and IFN-gamma. *Nature*, 408, pp. 600–605.
38. Dazzi, F., Ramasamy, R., Glennie, S., Jones, S.P. and Roberts, I. (2006). The role of mesenchymal stem cells in haemopoiesis. *Blood Reviews*, 20, pp. 161–171.
39. Jung, Y., Wang, J.H., Aaron, H.A., Sun, Y.X., Wang, J.C., Jin, T.C. and Taichman, R.S. (2005). Cell-to-cell contact is critical for the survival of hematopoietic progenitor cells on osteoblasts. *Cytokine*, 32, pp. 155–162.
40. Takayanagi, H. (2005). Mechanistic insight into osteoclast differentiation in osteoimmunology. *J Mol Med*, 83, pp. 170–179.
41. Walsh, M.C., Kim, N., Kadono, Y., Rho, J., Lee, S.Y., Lorenzo, J. and Choi, Y. (2006). Osteoimmunology: Interplay between the immune system and bone metabolism. *Annu Rev Immunol*, 24, pp. 33–63.
42. Yoshida, H., Hayashi, S.I., Kunisada, T., Ogawa, M., Nishikawa, S., Okamura, H., Sudo, T., Shultz, L.D. and Nishikawa, S.I. (1990). The murine mutation osteopetrosis is in the coding region of the macrophage colony stimulating factor gene. *Nature*, 345, pp. 442–444.

43. Asagiri, M., Sato, K., Usami, T., Ochi, S., Nishina, H., Yoshida, H., Morita, I., Wagner, E.F., Mak, T.W., Serfling, E. and Takayanagi, H. (2005). Autoamplification of NFATc1 expression determines its essential role in bone homeostasis. *J Exp Med*, 202, pp. 1261–1269.
44. Takayanagi, H. (2012). New developments in osteoimmunology. *Nat Rev Rheumatol*, 8, pp. 684–689.
45. Diao, H., Iwabuchi, K., Li, L., Onoe, K., Van Kaer, L., Kon, S., Saito, Y., Morimoto, J., Denhardt, D.T., Rittling, S. and Uede, T. (2008). Osteopontin regulates development and function of invariant natural killer T cells. *Proc Natl Acad Sci USA*, 105, pp. 15884–15889.
46. Mirosavljevic, D., Quinn, J.M.W., Elliott, J., Horwood, N.J., Martin, T.J. and Gillespie, M.T. (2003). T-cells mediate an inhibitory effect of interleukin-4 on osteoclastogenesis. *J Bone Miner Res*, 18, pp. 984–993.
47. Takayanagi, H., Ogasawara, K., Hida, S., Chiba, T., Murata, S., Sato, K., Takaoka, A., Yokochi, T., Oda, H., Tanaka, K., Nakamura, K. and Taniguchi, T. (2000). T-cell-mediated regulation of osteoclastogenesis by signalling cross-talk between RANKL and IFN-gamma. *Nature*, 408, pp. 600–605.
48. Arboleya, L. and Castaneda, S. (2013). Osteoimmunology: The study of the relationship between the immune system and bone tissue. *Reumatol Clin*, 9, pp. 303–315.
49. Crockett, J.C., Rogers, M.J., Coxon, F.P., Hocking, L.J. and Helfrich, M.H. (2011). Bone remodelling at a glance. *J Cell Sci*, 124, pp. 991–998.
50. Phan, T.C.A., Xu, J. and Zheng, M.H. (2004). Interaction between osteoblast and osteoclast: Impact in bone disease. *Histol Histopathol*, 19, pp. 1325–1344.
51. Suda, K., Udagawa, N., Sato, N., Takami, M., Itoh, K., Woo, J.T., Takahashi, N. and Nagai, K. (2004). Suppression of osteoprotegerin expression by prostaglandin E-2 is crucially involved in lipopolysaccharide-induced osteoclast formation. *J Immunol*, 172, pp. 2504–2510.
52. Hu, X.Y. and Ivashkiv, L.B. (2009). Cross-regulation of signaling pathways by interferon-gamma: Implications for immune responses and autoimmune diseases. *Immunity*, 31, pp. 539–550.
53. Inui, M., Kikuchi, Y., Aoki, N., Endo, S., Maeda, T. Sugahara-Tobinai, A., Fujimura, S., Nakamura, A., Kumanogoh, A., Colonna, M. and Takai, T. (2009). Signal adaptor DAP10 associates with MDL-1 and triggers osteoclastogenesis in cooperation with DAP12. *Proc Natl Acad Sci USA*, 106, pp. 4816–4821.
54. Yamashita, T., Takahashi, N. and Udagawa, N. (2012). New roles of osteoblasts involved in osteoclast differentiation. *World J Orthop*, 3, pp. 175–181.
55. Karsten, C.M. and Kohl, J. (2015). A bone to pick with Fc gamma receptors. *Ann Transl Med*, 3, pp. 218.
56. Koga, T., Inui, M., Inoue, K., Kim, S., Suematsu, A., Kobayashi, E., Iwata, T., Ohnishi, H., Matozaki, T., Kodama, T., Taniguchi, T., Takayanagi, H. and Takai, T. (2004). Costimulatory signals mediated by the ITAM motif cooperate with RANKL for bone homeostasis. *Nature*, 428, pp. 758–763.
57. Kawai, T., Matsuyama, T., Hosokawa, Y., Makihira, S., Seki, M., Karimbux, N.Y., Goncalves, R.B., Valverde, P., Dibart, S., Li, Y.P., Miranda, L.A., Ernst, C.W., Izumi, Y. and Taubman, M.A. (2006). B and T lymphocytes are the primary sources of RANKL in the bone resorptive lesion of periodontal disease. *Am J Pathol*, 169, pp. 987–998.
58. Li, Y., Terauchi, M., Vikulina, T., Roser-Page, S. and Weitzmann, M.N. (2014). B cell production of both OPG and RANKL is significantly increased in aged mice. *Open Bone J*, 6, pp. 8–17.
59. Evans, K.E. and Fox, S.W. (2007). Interleukin-10 inhibits osteoclastogenesis by reducing NFATc1 expression and preventing its translocation to the nucleus. *BMC Cell Biol*, 8, pp. 4.

60. Takayanagi, H., Kim, S., Matsuo, K., Suzuki, H., Suzuki, T., Sato, K., Yokochi, T., Oda, H., Nakamura, K., Ida, N., Wagner, E.F. and Taniguchi, T. (2002). RANKL maintains bone homeostasis through c-Fos-dependent induction of interferon-beta. *Nature*, 416, pp. 744–749.
61. Moreno, J.L., Kaczmarek, M., Keegan, A.D. and Tondravi, M. (2003). IL-4 suppresses osteoclast development and mature osteoclast function by a STAT6-dependent mechanism: Irreversible inhibition of the differentiation program activated by RANKL. *Blood*, 102, pp. 1078–1086.
62. Palmqvist, P., Lundberg, P., Persson, E., Johansson, A., Lundgren, I., Lie, A., Conaway, H.H. and Lerner, U.H. (2006). Inhibition of hormone and cytokine-stimulated osteoclastogenesis and bone resorption by interleukin-4 and inter-leukin-13 is associated with increased osteoprotegerin and decreased RANKL and RANK in a STAT6-dependent pathway. *J Biol Chem*, 281, pp. 2414–2429.
63. Mangashetti, L.S., Khapli, S.M. and Wani, M.R. (2005). IL-4 inhibits bone-resorbing activity of mature osteoclasts by affecting NF-kappa B and Ca^{2+} signaling. *J Immunol*, 175, pp. 917–925.
64. Parameswaran, N. and Patial, S. (2010). Tumor necrosis factor-alpha signaling in macrophages. *Crit Rev Eukaryot Gene Expr*, 20, pp. 87–103.
65. Usha, K. and Nandeesh, B.N. (2012) Radionuclide and hybrid bone imaging, in *Physiology of Bone Formation, Remodeling, and Metabolism*, eds Fogelman, I., Gnanasegaran, G. and van der Wall, H. (Berlin, Springer), pp. 29–57.
66. Pacifici, R. (2010). T cells: Critical bone regulators in health and disease. *Bone*, 47, pp. 461–471.
67. Ohshiba, T., Miyaura, C. and Ito, A. (2003). Role of prostaglandin E produced by osteoblasts in osteolysis due to bone metastasis. *Biochem Biophy Res Commun*, 300, pp. 957–964.
68. Udagawa, N. (2003). The mechanism of osteoclast differentiation from macrophages: Possible roles of T lymphocytes in osteoclastogenesis. *J Bone Miner Metab*, 21, pp. 337–343.
69. Lubberts, E., Joosten, L.A.B., Chabaud, M., van den Bersselaar, L., Oppers, B., Coenen-de Roo, C.J.J., Richards, C.D., Miossec, P. and van den Berg, W.B. (2000). IL-4 gene therapy for collagen arthritis suppresses synovial IL-17 and osteoprotegerin ligand and prevents bone erosion. *Eur J Clin Invest*, 105, pp. 1697–1710.
70. Hofbauer, L.C., Khosla, S., Dunstan, C.R., Lacey, D.L., Spelsberg, T.C. and Riggs, B.L. (1999). Estrogen stimulates gene expression and protein production of osteoprotegerin in human osteoblastic cells. *Endocrinology*, 140, pp. 4367–4370.
71. Diarra, D., Stolina, M., Polzer, K., Zwerina, J., Ominsky, M.S., Dwyer, D., Korb, A., Smolen, J., Hoffmann, M., Scheinecker, C., van der Heide, D., Landewe, R., Lacey, D., Richards, W.G. and Schett, G. (2007). Dickkopf-1 is a master regulator of joint remodeling. *Nat Med*, 13, pp. 156–163.
72. Boyce, B.F. and Xing, L.P. (2007). Biology of RANK, RANKL, and osteoprotegerin. *Arthritis Res Ther*, 9(Suppl 1), p. S1.
73. Kobayashi, Y., Maeda, K. and Takahashi, N. (2008). Roles of Wnt signaling in bone formation and resorption. *Jpn Dent Sci Rev*, 44, pp. 76–82.
74. Maeda, K., Kobayashi, Y., Udagawa, N., Uehara, S., Ishihara, A., Mizoguchi, T., Kikuchi, Y., Takada, I., Kato, S., Kani, S., Nishita, M., Marumo, K., Martin, T.J., Minami, Y. and Takahashi, N. (2012). Wnt5a-Ror2 signaling between osteoblast-lineage cells and osteoclast precursors enhances osteoclastogenesis. *Nat Med*, 18, pp. 405–U166.
75. Navarro, M., Michiardi, A., Castano, O. and Planell, J.A. (2008). Biomaterials in orthopaedics. *J R Soc Interface*, 5, pp. 1137–1158.

76. Hench, L.L. and Polak, J.M. (2002). Third-generation biomedical materials. *Science*, 295, pp. 1014–7.
77. Ning, C.Y., Zhou, L. and Tan, G.X. (2016). Fourth-generation biomedical materials. *Mater Today*, 19, pp. 2–3.
78. Sheikh, Z., Brooks, P.J., Barzilay, O., Fine, N. and Glogauer, M. (2015). Macrophages, foreign body giant cells and their response to implantable biomaterials. *Materials*, 8, pp. 5671–5701.
79. Caicedo, M.S., Samelko, L., McAllister, K., Jacobs, J.J. and Hallab, N.J. (2013). Increasing both CoCrMo-alloy particle size and surface irregularity induces increased macrophage inflammasome activation in vitro potentially through lysosomal destabilization mechanisms. *J Orthop Res*, 31, pp. 1633–1642.
80. Ward, W.K., Slobodzian, E.P., Tiekotter, K.L. and Wood, M.D. (2002). The effect of microgeometry, implant thick-ness and polyurethane chemistry on the foreign body response to subcutaneous implants. *Biomaterials*, 23, pp. 4185–4192.
81. Veiseh, O., Doloff, J.C., Ma, M.L., Vegas, A.J., Tam, H.H., Bader, A.R., Li, J., Langan, E., Wyckoff, J., Loo, W.S., Jhun-jhunwala, S., Chiu, A., Siebert, S., Tang, K., Hollister-Lock, J., Aresta-Dasilva, S., Bochenek, M., Mendoza-Elias, J., Wang, Y., Qi, M., Lavin, D.M., Chen, M., Dholakia, N., Thakrar, R., Lacik, I., Weir, G.C., Oberholzer, J., Greiner, D.L., Langer, R. and Anderson, D.G. (2015). Size- and shape-dependent foreign body immune response to materials implanted in rodents and non-human primates. *Nat Mater*, 14, pp. 643–U125.
82. Hutmacher, D.W., Schantz, J.T., Lam, C.X.F., Tan, K.C. and Lim, T.C. (2007). State of the art and future directions of scaffold-based bone engineering from a biomaterials perspective. *J Tissue Eng Regen Med*, 1, pp. 245–260.
83. Bose, S., Roy, M. and Bandyopadhyay, A. (2012). Recent advances in bone tissue engineering scaffolds. *Trends Biotechnol*, 30, pp. 546–554.
84. Leong, K.F., Cheah, C.M. and Chua, C.K. (2003). Solid freeform fabrication of three-dimensional scaffolds for engineering replacement tissues and organs. *Biomaterials*, 24, pp. 2363–2378.
85. Liu, X.M., Wu, S.L., Yeung, K.W.K., Chan, Y.L., Hu, T., Xu, Z.S., Liu, X.Y., Chung, J.C.Y., Cheung, K.M.C. and Chu, P.K. (2011). Relationship between osseointegration and superelastic biomechanics in porous NiTi scaffolds. *Biomaterials*, 32, pp. 330–338.
86. Murphy, C.M. and O'Brien, F.J. (2010). Understanding the effect of mean pore size on cell activity in collagen-glycosaminoglycan scaffolds. *Cell Adh Migr*, 4, pp. 377–381.
87. Murphy, C.M., Haugh, M.G. and O'Brien, F.J. (2010). The effect of mean pore size on cell attachment, proliferation and migration in collagen-glycosaminoglycan scaffolds for bone tissue engineering. *Biomaterials*, 31, pp. 461–466.
88. Chen, Z.T., Klein, T., Murray, R.Z., Crawford, R., Chang, J., Wu, C.T. and Xiao, Y. (2016). Osteoimmunomodulation for the development of advanced bone biomaterials. *Mater Today*, 19, pp. 304–321.
89. Jin, Q.M., Takita, H., Kohgo, T., Atsumi, K., Itoh, H. and Kuboki, Y. (2000). Effects of geometry of hydroxyapatite as a cell substratum in BMP-induced ectopic bone. *J Biomed Mater Res*, 51, pp. 491–499.
90. Hannink, G. and Arts, J.J. (2011). Bioresorbability, porosity and mechanical strength of bone substitutes: What is optimal for bone regeneration? *Injury*, 42 Suppl 2, pp. S22–5.
91. Garg, K., Pullen, N.A., Oskeritzian, C.A., Ryan, J.J. and Bowlin, G.L. (2013). Macrophage functional polarization (M1/M2) in response to varying fiber and pore dimensions of electrospun scaffolds. *Biomaterials*, 34, pp. 4439–4451.
92. Chang, B.S., Lee, C.K., Hong, K.S., Youn, H.J., Ryu, H.S., Chung, S.S. and Park, K.W. (2000). Osteoconduction at po-rous hydroxyapatite with various pore configurations. *Biomaterials*, 21, pp. 1291–1298.

93. Chang, H. and Wang, Y. (2011). Cell responses to surface and architecture of tissue engineering scaffolds, in *Regenerative Medicine and Tissue Engineering – Cells and Biomaterials*, ed. Eberli, D. (InTech), www.intechopen.com/books/export/citation/EndNote/regenerative-medicine-and-tissue-engineering-cells-and-biomaterials/cell-responses-to-surface-and-architecture-of-tissue-engineering-scaffolds.
94. Zareidoost, A., Yousefpour, M., Ghaseme, B. and Amanzadeh, A. (2012). The relationship of surface roughness and cell response of chemical surface modification of titanium. *J Mater Sci Mater Med*, 23, pp. 1479–1488.
95. Takebe, J., Champagne, C.M., Offenbacher, S., Ishibashi, K. and Cooper, L.F. (2003). Titanium surface topography alters cell shape and modulates bone morphogenetic protein 2 expression in the J774A.1 macrophage cell line. *J Biomed Mater Res A*, 64A, pp. 207–216.
96. Smith, B.S., Capellato, P., Kelley, S., Gonzalez-Juarrero, M. and Popat, K.C. (2013). Reduced in vitro immune response on titania nanotube arrays compared to titanium surface. *Biomaterials Science*, 1, pp. 322–332.
97. Murray, D.W., Rae, T. and Rushton, N. (1989). The influence of the surface-energy and roughness of implants on bone-resorption. *J Bone Joint Surg Br*, 71, pp. 632–637.
98. Dai, X.H., Wei, Y., Zhang, X.H., Meng, S., Mo, X.J., Liu, X., Deng, X.L., Zhang, L. and Deng, X.M. (2015). Attenuating immune response of macrophage by enhancing hydrophilicity of ti surface. *J Nanomater.*
99. Sit, P.S. and Marchant, R.E. (1999). Surface-dependent conformations of human fibrinogen observed by atomic force microscopy under aqueous conditions. *Thromb Haemost*, 82, pp. 1053–1060.
100. Amini, A.R., Wallace, J.S. and Nukavarapu, S.P. (2011). Short-term and long-term effects of orthopedic biodegradable implants. *J Long Term Eff Med Implants*, 21, pp. 93–122.
101. Evans-Nguyen, K.M., Fuierer, R.R., Fitchett, B.D., Tolles, L.R., Conboy, J.C. and Schoenfisch, M.H. (2006). Changes in adsorbed fibrinogen upon conversion to fibrin. *Langmuir*, 22, pp. 5115–5121.
102. Thevenot, P., Hu, W.J. and Tang, L.P. (2008). Surface chemistry influences implant biocompatibility. *Current Topics in Medicinal Chemistry*, 8, pp. 270–280.
103. Jones, J.A., Chang, D.T., Meyerson, H., Colton, E., Kwon, I.K., Matsuda, T. and Anderson, J.M. (2007). Proteomic analysis and quantification of cytokines and chemokines from biomaterial surface-adherent macrophages and foreign body giant cells. *J Biomed Mater Res A*, 83A, pp. 585–596.
104. Boehler, R.M., Graham, J.G. and Shea, L.D. (2011). Tissue engineering tools for modulation of the immune response. *Biotechniques*, 51(4), passim.
105. Hezi-Yamit, A., Sullivan, C., Wong, J., David, L., Chen, M., Cheng, P., Shumaker, D., Wilcox, J.N. and Udipi, K. (2009). Impact of polymer hydrophilicity on biocompatibility: Implication for DES polymer design. *J Biomed Mater Res A*, 90, pp. 133–141.
106. Brodbeck, W.G., Nakayama, Y., Matsuda, T., Colton, E., Ziats, N.P. and Anderson, J.M. (2002). Biomaterial surface chemistry dictates adherent monocyte/macrophage cytokine expression in vitro. *Cytokine*, 18, pp. 311–319.
107. Rostam, H.M., Singh, S., Salazar, F., Magennis, P., Hook, A., Singh, T., Vrana, N.E., Alexander, M.R. and Ghaemmaghami, A.M. (2016). The impact of surface chemistry modification on macrophage polarisation. *Immunobiology*, 221, pp. 1237–1246.
108. Khang, G. (2012). *Handbook of intelligent scaffolds for tissue engineering and regenerative medicine.* 1st Ed. (Pan Stanford Publishing, USA).
109. Toita, R., Rashid, S.A.N., Tsuru, K. and Ishikawa, K. (2015). Modulation of the osteoconductive property and immune response of poly(ether ether ketone) by modification with calcium ions. *J Mater Chem B*, 3, pp. 8738–8746.

110. Wu, C.T., Zhou, Y.H., Fan, W., Han, P.P., Chang, J., Yuen, J., Zhang, M.L. and Xiao, Y. (2012). Hypoxia-mimicking mesoporous bioactive glass scaffolds with controllable cobalt ion release for bone tissue engineering. *Biomaterials*, 33, pp. 2076–2085.
111. Jugdaohsingh, R. (2007). Silicon and bone health. *J Nutr Health Aging*, 11, pp. 99–110.
112. Dibner, J.J., Richards, J.D., Kitchell, M.L. and Quiroz, M.A. (2007). Metabolic challenges and early bone development. *J Appl Poult Res*, 16, pp. 126–137.
113. Day, R.M. and Boccaccini, A.R. (2005). Effect of particulate bioactive glasses on human macrophages and monocytes in vitro. *J Biomed Mater Res A*, 73A, pp. 73–79.
114. Brandes, M.E., Allen, J.B., Ogawa, Y. and Wahl, S.M. (1991). Transforming growth factor beta 1 suppresses acute and chronic arthritis in experimental animals. *J Clin Invest*, 87, pp. 1108–1113.
115. Yang, Y.Q., Tan, Y.Y., Wong, R., Wenden, A., Zhang, L.K. and Rabie, A.B.M. (2012). The role of vascular endothelial growth factor in ossification. *Int J Dent Oral Sci*, 4, pp. 64–68.
116. Patil, S.D., Papadmitrakopoulos, F. and Burgess, D.J. (2007). Concurrent delivery of dexamethasone and VEGF for localized inflammation control and angiogenesis. *J Control Release*, 117, pp. 68–79.
117. Meinel, L., Zoidis, E., Zapf, J., Hassa, P., Hottiger, M.O., Auer, J.A., Schneider, R., Gander, B., Luginbuehl, V., Bettschart-Wolfisberger, R., Illi, O.E., Merkle, H.P. and von Rechenberg, B. (2003). Localized insulin-like growth factor I delivery to enhance new bone formation. *Bone*, 33, pp. 660–672.
118. Chang, Y., Tai, C.L., Hsieh, P.H. and Ueng, S.W. (2013). Gentamicin in bone cement: A potentially more effective prophylactic measure of infection in joint arthroplasty. *Bone Joint Res*, 2, pp. 220–226.
119. Hardy, R. and Cooper, M.S. (2011). Glucocorticoid-induced osteoporosis - a disorder of mesenchymal stromal cells? *Front Endocrinol (Lausanne)*, 2, pp. 24.
120. Mourino, V. and Boccaccini, A.R. (2010). Bone tissue engineering therapeutics: Controlled drug delivery in three-dimensional scaffolds. *J R Soc Interface*, 7, pp. 209–227.
121. Cho, J.Y. (2007). Immunomodulatory effect of nonsteroidal anti-inflammatory drugs (NSAIDs) at the clinically available doses. *Arch Pharm Res*, 30, pp. 64–74.
122. Harris, S.G., Padilla, J., Koumas, L., Ray, D. and Phipps, R.P. (2002). Prostaglandins as modulators of immunity. *Trends Immunol*, 23, pp. 144–150.
123. Beck, A., Krischak, G., Sorg, T., Augat, P., Farker, K., Merkel, U., Kinzl, L. and Claes, L. (2003). Influence of diclofenac (group of nonsteroidal anti-inflammatory drugs) on fracture healing. *Arch Orthop Trauma Surg*, 123, pp. 327–332.
124. Wagner, G. and Laufer, S. (2006). Small molecular anti-cytokine agents. *Med Res Rev*, 26, pp. 1–62.
125. Taylor, P.C. and Feldmann, M. (2009). Anti-TNF biologic agents: Still the therapy of choice for rheumatoid arthritis. Nature Reviews Rheumatology, 5, pp. 578–582.
126. Raychaudhuri, S.P. and Raychaudhuri, S.K. (2009). Biologics: Target-specific treatment of systemic and cutaneous autoimmune diseases. *Indian J Dermatol*, 54, pp. 100–109.
127. Zhang, X., Zheng, Z., Liu, P., Ma, Y., Lin, L., Lang, N., Fu, X., Zhang, J., Ma, K., Chen, P., Zhou, C. and Ao, Y. (2008). The synergistic effects of microfracture, perforated decalcified cortical bone matrix and adenovirus-bone morphogenetic protein-4 in cartilage defect repair. *Biomaterials*, 29, pp. 4616–4629.
128. Saito, E., Suarez-Gonzalez, D., Murphy, W.L. and Hollister, S.J. (2015). Biomineral coating increases bone formation by ex vivo BMP-7 gene therapy in rapid prototyped poly(L-lactic acid) (PLLA) and poly(epsilon-caprolactone) (PCL) porous scaffolds. *Adv Healthc Mater*, 4, pp. 621–632.

129. Yue, J., Wu, J., Liu, D., Zhao, X. and Lu, W.W. (2015). BMP2 gene delivery to bone mesenchymal stem cell by chitosan-g-PEI nonviral vector. *Nanoscale Res Lett*, 10, pp. 203.
130. Kawai, M., Maruyama, H., Bessho, K., Yamamoto, H., Miyazaki, J. and Yamamoto, T. (2009). Simple strategy for bone regeneration with a BMP-2/7 gene expression cassette vector. *Biochem Biophys Res Commun*, 390, pp. 1012–1017.
131. Lam, J.K.W., Chow, M.Y.T., Zhang, Y. and Leung, S.W.S. (2015). siRNA versus miRNA as therapeutics for gene silencing. *Mol Ther Nucleic Acids*, 4, p. e252.
132. Carthew, R.W. and Sontheimer, E.J. (2009). Origins and mechanisms of miRNAs and siRNAs. *Cell*, 136, pp. 642–655.
133. Zhang, G., Guo, B., Wu, H., Tang, T., Zhang, B.T., Zheng, L., He, Y., Yang, Z., Pan, X., Chow, H., To, K., Li, Y., Li, D., Wang, X., Wang, Y., Lee, K., Hou, Z., Dong, N., Li, G., Leung, K., Hung, L., He, F., Zhang, L. and Qin, L. (2012). A de-livery system targeting bone formation surfaces to facilitate RNAi-based anabolic therapy. *Nat Med*, 18, pp. 307–314.

9 Macrophage-Based Immunomodulation for Biomaterial Applications

Helena Knopf-Marques, Lilian Paiva, Flavie Prévot and Julien Barthès

CONTENTS

9.1 INTRODUCTION

Nowadays, despite the fact that implants are used for a myriad of applications (tooth, knee, hip, shoulder, spine, larynx, skin etc.), the adverse host immune response known as foreign body response (FBR) still remains an important issue since it can lead to excessive inflammation with tissue fibrosis, thrombogenic responses and reactive gliosis [1–3]. Despite the upsurge of bioengineering research to define how to modulate immune reactions in favour of implantable devices, no fully acceptable technology has yet been invented.

The human body possesses a defence mechanism to eliminate any foreign body. Upon penetration of the foreign substance (such as implantation), an acute inflammation commences after protein adsorption on the surface. This leads to recruitment of immune cells (such as neutrophils and monocytes/macrophages) and secretion of soluble factors (chemokines and cytokines). When the inflammation is not rapidly resolved, there is a risk of implant failure due to fibrous encapsulation and foreign body giant cell formation-directed chronic inflammation [4]. The degree of the inflammation reaction is linked to two principal parameters: the nature of the implant's base material and its chemical or physical properties.

Firstly, the choice of implant material is crucial to control the macrophage response, avoid long-term adverse immune responses and consequently resolve the inflammation. Currently, there are implants in regular clinical use made of metal alloys, ceramics, polymers or composites, depending on the application and implantation location. Secondly, to enhance implantation success, intensive research effort has been focused on the physical and chemical properties of each material and their importance on the implant's fate *in vivo*. Indeed, the selection of the adapted strategy for each type of implant would have an important benefit for the patient such as the limitation of side effects (implant rejection, chronic inflammation and additional surgery) and the increase of quality of life after implantation.

Following recent studies, implant integration has been shown to be significantly correlated with the polarisation of the macrophages (within the spectrum of M1/M2 polarisation). M1 phenotypes classically induce the secretion of pro-inflammatory cytokines (TNFα, interleukin IL-1β, IL-6 and chemokines). It has been highlighted that modulation of the degree of immune response is a better solution than strictly preventing inflammation, as the initial phase of inflammation (cell recruitment, clearance of microbial presence, elimination of cell debris etc.) is essential for the healing of the wound [5,6]. In other words, the most promising strategy would be to reach an early resolution of the initial phase of the immune response, characterised by the presence of pro-inflammatory macrophages (M1), and to facilitate the second phase, characterised by the conversion of M1 macrophages to anti-inflammatory macrophages (M2), which are responsible for the orchestration of the healing phase and tissue remodelling leading to the success of implantation. Recent studies have shown that the polarisation of macrophages can be directly linked to the chemical properties of biomaterials, such as surface chemistry and hydrophilicity, and physical properties such as surface topography, roughness, stiffness or porosity. Control over the chemical and the physical features of biomaterials would then allow orientation, modulation and control over the severity of inflammation after implantation [7].

9.2 MACROPHAGE RESPONSE TO BIOMATERIALS

9.2.1 Polymers

Polymeric materials are widely used in the implant field as they possess innate advantageous qualities in terms of biocompatibility with the human body (as a significant portion of the human body is also composed of polymers by definition). A wide range of studies have been carried out on this class of material to improve their functions in the medical field. Different classes of polymers are investigated for different types of applications. In a general manner, natural polymers are preferential candidates to improve the biocompatibility of the implant since they can be made of ECM components or naturally occurring structures with low immunogenicity. This class of polymers are particularly well suited for applications like tissue regeneration and wound healing. Indeed, biopolymers are physiologically comparable to existing active proteins and polysaccharides present in the human body and consequently thanks to their structural similarity to native ECM they can support cell adhesion and enhance cell proliferation [8]. For these reasons, the use of natural polymers is commonly known to improve implant/host tissue interactions even if they could occasionally induce adverse effects (as there is a certain level of immune recognition due to the sourcing of these polymers from other animal species and plants and also ease of contamination of such proteins/polysaccharides with endotoxins). The two main undesirable effects are a potential strong immune reaction generally due to xenogeneic/allogenic properties of natural materials (well tolerated by the human body, but species-specific sequences in molecules such as collagen, elastin, fibronectin etc. can be recognised by the adaptive immune component of the immune system) and a limited stability *in vivo*, essentially due to hydrolytic and enzymatic degradation [8,9]. Numerous natural polymers (collagen, silk, chitosan alginate, gelatin etc.) are under investigation on order to understand their immunomodulation behaviour. As an example, silk-based materials are being studied for potential use as scaffold in the tissue engineering field and already present a low inflammatory potential as they do not induce significant macrophage activation once the sericin component is removed [10].

Synthetic polymers are also widely used since it is much easier to control their physico-chemical properties during synthesis and so they can offer a greater range of properties in comparison to natural materials. Their interactions with the immune system depends on their structure but many synthetic polymers are well tolerated. Moreover, they can be chemically modulated with a high degree of control over their properties to approach the goal desired (for example, attaining a degradation rate that is suitable for the implantation site without having excessive byproducts that would provoke additional inflammation). A large variety of these polymers are currently utilised in the implant field (PLLA, PLGA, PCL, PLA, PET, PTFE, PU) as they can easily be engineered to fit specific needs [11]. Synthetic polymers can be divided into two subgroups: biodegradable and non-biodegradable. Indeed, one of the adverse effects known for synthetic polymers is related to the possible partial degradation of the material resulting in a local pH decrease and the release of potentially toxic byproducts which can induce severe inflammatory reactions. As an example, the synthetic polymer poly (ethylene terephthalate) (PET) is used in a myriad of medical applications like sutures or vascular grafts and is equally known to stimulate fibrous encapsulation as a consequence of adverse immune responses [12].

Polymers can be used as bulk materials or as surface coatings. In fact, they are often used to coat implant biomaterial surfaces in order to reduce the immune response by isolating the implant from the surrounding microenvironment. Polymer materials (bulk and surface coating) are often presented under hydrogel or scaffold forms. Hydrogels are attractive matrices thanks to their three-dimensional structure (composed of cross-linked hydrophilic polymer chains) close to native soft tissue and their high water content [13]. Hydrogels possess hydrophilic properties due to the presence of hydrophilic moieties (carboxyl, amide, amino and hydroxyl groups). The hydrophilic properties responsible for hydrogel popularity will be discussed further later in the chapter. In scaffold form, hydrogels are equally widespread in tissue engineering as they provide advantageous properties for creating an amenable environment for proper cell function, 3D cell adhesion and survival after transplantation due to the potential to encapsulate live cells for *in vivo* delivery.

Recently, numerous studies have focused on the design of hydrogel scaffolds as their morphological properties (shape, porosity and topography design) can be engineered with ease and thus provide new possibilities to improve applications in tissue engineering like vascularisation and tissue/organ replacement [14]. When a polymer material is used, for example, as a coating in order to decrease the immune response of another biomaterial, different methods of coating have been developed depending on the kind of polymer and other parameters, such as the required thickness, and surface aspects that can be controlled (such as topography/chemistry) [6].

As mentioned previously, foreign body reaction is directly linked to the chemical and physical properties of a biomaterial's surface. Through various examples of polymers, the influence of physicochemical properties like molecular weight, surface topography or non-fouling coating will be discussed to illustrate their impact on the pro-inflammatory or anti-inflammatory responses on the human body when it comes into contact with the polymeric implant. These properties, allowing the alteration of material properties to modulate the immune response, belong to the passive approach. A second approach (bioactive coatings) is equally currently investigated and essentially concerns the material functionalisation with drugs/bioactive molecule release. Due to our main focus on the direct effect of biomaterials, this chapter will only address the passive approach. It is essential to note that even if the modulation of biomaterial physicochemical properties always has an impact on the material-host interaction, it is difficult to elaborate a general trend as each polymer generates a singular response. Consequently, modification has not yet been identified to reach the optimal immune response to an implant. However, the properties discussed below have allowed the partial identification of key factors that can be used to induce desired responses.

9.2.1.1 Polymers' Chemical Properties/Surface Chemistry

Chemical properties are a main factor that can influence monocyte differentiation, macrophage polarisation and cytokine secretion profiles towards a pro-inflammatory or an anti-inflammatory response. Each polymer possesses its own chemical properties. A study has highlighted that chitosan (a derivative of a natural polysaccharide, chitin, obtained from crustacean carapaces) induces with time a phenotypic switch on the macrophage close to the M2 polarisation state. Indeed, it has been established that after ten days, TNF-α (tumour necrosis factor alpha, a pro-inflammatory cytokine) production decreased while IL-10 (an anti-inflammatory cytokine member of interleukin family) increased. Furthermore, the study reveals that chitosan materials generate a pro-inflammatory activation of dendritic cells without inducing a T-cell proliferation [15].

Some studies have highlighted the importance of the molecular weight of the polymer used to modulate the immune response. For example, a study that was led on polyethylene polymers to investigate the effect of several properties on macrophage response showed that production of TNF-α (pro-inflammatory factor) was directly linked to the molecular weight (MW), the degree of cross-linking and the roughness [16]. Another study showed that hyaluronic acid polymers show different immune behaviour depending on their molecular weight. Indeed, macrophage polarisation and cytokine production could be affected as a function of HA MW. Low MW HA induced a pro-inflammatory response while high MW HA induced an inflammation resolving response, notably thanks to the activation of IL-10 production [17].

Another important property for the modulation of the immune response is the hydrophilicity of the material. Hydrophilic polymers are of first interest since they can induce limited adverse effects. They limit protein adsorption (and consequently diminish monocyte adhesion), preventing foreign body giant cell formation and as a result decreasing adverse immune reaction [18,19]. Recent studies show that hydrophilic surfaces such as PVA and PEG are an interesting choice as they are associated with cytokine expression including an increase of anti-inflammatory interleukin (IL)-10 and a decrease of pro-inflammatory interleukin (IL-8) productions indicating an alternatively activated anti-inflammatory macrophage phenotype. Some hydrophilic polymers can be designed to possess a wide range of mechanical properties; they can also be easily attached to the implant surfaces with good stability [20]. Nevertheless, hydrophilicity cannot fully explain the immunomodulation properties of these materials. Surface chemistry also needs to be considered. A recent study about the artificial modification of polystyrene (PS) surface chemistry through plasma treatment showed that hydrophobic surfaces could also promote the polarisation of macrophages into M2 phenotype. It demonstrated that protein adsorption on polystyrene surfaces could be modified by O_2 plasma treatment. Untreated hydrophobic PS material influences M2 macrophage polarisation, which is a sign of anti-inflammatory response, while highly hydrophilic O_2-PS40 stimulates the opposite reaction with the expression of M1 associated markers [21]. As cited previously and in regards to other studies promoting hydrophilic materials for decreasing the monocyte adhesion instead of hydrophobic materials, it is important to emphasise that each polymer could induce its own response depending on the interplay of several factors in regards to immune response [22].

Many biomaterials (metals, polymers, ceramics) are used as bulk structures despite the adverse immune response they could cause. To overcome these undesirable effects, polymeric coatings can be engineered to modulate the immune response of the bulk material. For example, poly(N-isopropylacrylamide)-co-acrylic acid microgel particles cross-linked with poly(ethylene glycol) (PEG) diacrylate were engineered as a hydrogel-based coating for PET substrate to control cell adhesion, protein adsorption and consequently minimise chronic inflammation [12]. In general, hydrophilic hydrogel coatings such as PEG-based hydrogels are used as a non-fouling surface treatment (also called "non-interactive" surface) [23–25]. Dextran-based gels, poly(ethylene oxide) (PEO) and alginate are equally recognised as non-fouling coatings [26–28]. Researchers have identified other hydrophilic polymers resisting to protein adsorption like poly(2-hydroxyethyl methacrylate), poly(N-isopropyl acrylamide), poly(acrylamide) and phosphoryl choline-based polymers [29–32].

Another example is the immunomodulatory coating based on polyelectrolyte multilayer films formed by self-cross-linked of poly-L-lysine (PLL) and hyaluronic acid aldehyde derivative (HA-Ald), recently developed by Knopf-Marques et al. (2016) [33]. The release of immunomodulatory cytokines (IL-4) from the films induces the production of anti-inflammatory cytokines (IL1-RA and CCL18) from primary human monocytes seeded on the films. These monocytes also significantly reduce the release of pro-inflammatory cytokines (TNF-α, IL-1β and IL-12) (Figure 9.1). Moreover, even without IL-4 cytokine, PLL/HA-Ald film is efficient in limiting inflammatory processes.

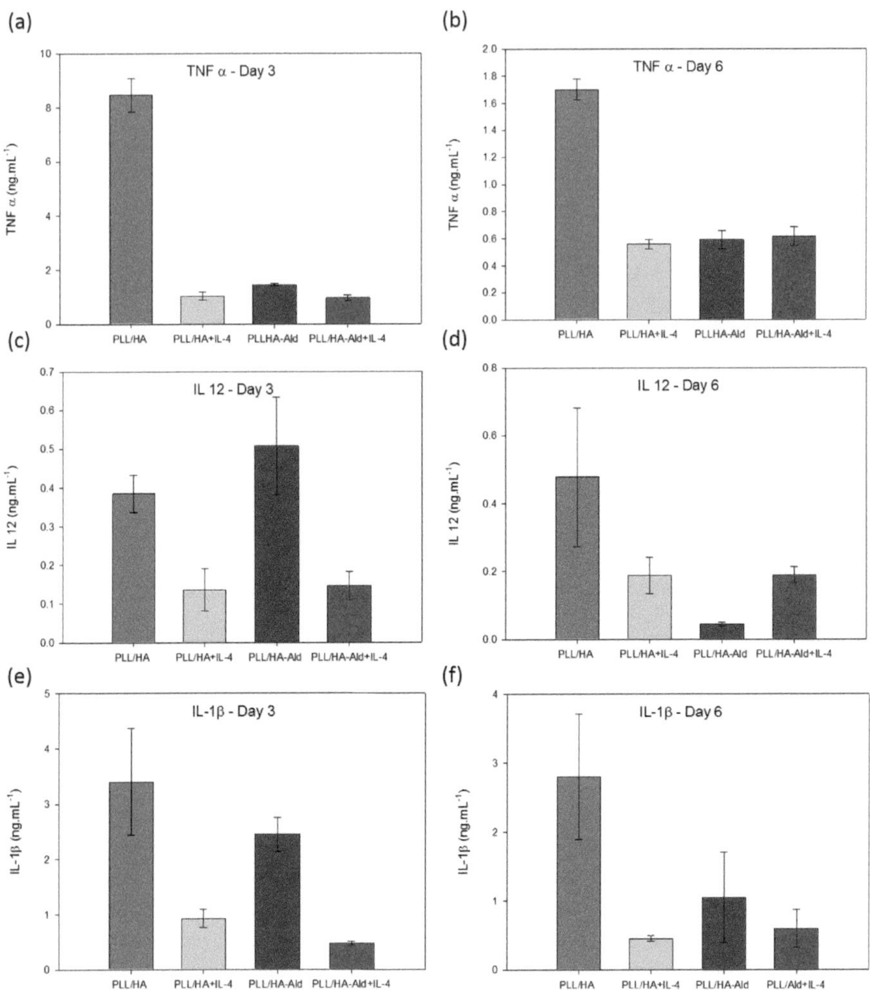

FIGURE 9.1 Pro-inflammatory cytokines produced from monocytes seeded on PLL/HA, PLL/HA-Ald with or without IL-4: TNF-α after three (a) and six days (b); IL-12 after three (c) and six days (d), IL-1β after three (e) and six days (f). (Reprinted from Knopf-Marques, H. et al., *Biomacromolecules*, 17(6), 2189–2198, 2016. With permission.)

9.2.1.2 Physical Properties

The modification of polymer's physical properties represents the second main factor for immunomodulation. Modulation of polymer surface topography encompasses numerous surface factors like surface roughness, microscale/nanoscale topography and the dimension and nature of surface features (pore size, fibre diameter). As a polymeric bulk/polymeric coating implant already represents a wide range of potential properties, the level of modulation that can be achieved by physical modifications is considerable. Recent researches agree that the modification of the surface topography may induce different macrophage phenotypes [34,35]. As an example, a study has been conducted to investigate the effect on the immune response of PTFE (Teflon) implants possessing the same surface chemistry but a different surface topography. A modulation of cytokine production and a decrease in fibrous capsule thickness have been observed in regards to the different topographic surfaces and expanded PTFE surfaces have shown a more favourable *in vivo* response [36]. In the following part, some biomaterial physical properties important for immunomodulation, such as micro/nano topography, pore size and fibre diameter, will be discussed.

First, we will explain the influence of micro/nano topography. The modulation of immune response through surface pattern size has been investigated for PCL, PDMS and PLA. The results show that cytokine secretion and cell adhesion are directly affected by the topography of the surface, in particular for larger size patterns compared to planar surface. In this study, it has been highlighted that surface topography with pattern sizes comprised between 500 nm to 2 μm allow limitation of macrophage activation and consequently control of inflammatory response. On the contrary, surface topography with smaller pattern sizes has a behaviour close to that of a planar surface, enhancing cell adhesion [37]. Some studies suggest that surfaces with micron-scale architecture could beneficially affect interactions between the biomaterial and the immune system by inducing a possible control of macrophage phenotype (M1 vs M2) [23]. Polyvinylidene fluoride microstructured and nanostructured surfaces with the same surface chemistry have been studied to see the effect of topography on the activation of human macrophages. They have demonstrated that only the microstructured topography induces a specific activation of macrophages with a specific cytokine profile and gene expression. This activation was mainly pro-inflammatory but did not completely fit into the pre-defined macrophage polarisation profiles. These results show the importance of surface topography to influence the response of the biomaterial toward the immune system and as a consequence the biocompatibility [38].

Porous surfaces have been established to influence better implant integration in comparison to non-porous form. Pore size is a determinant physical cue to orientate the polarisation of macrophages and consequently decrease the formation of foreign body giant cells [5]. A study has been led on polydioxanone (PDO) scaffolds to compare the influence of fibres diameter and pore size on the ratio of M1:M2 macrophages [39]. The results show that M2 macrophage phenotype is better represented on scaffolds with larger fibres and pore dimensions. It has equally been highlighted that the pore size of a scaffold plays a more significant role influencing M2 macrophage phenotype than fibre size. A study dedicated to the effect of pore size on angiogenesis and fibrotic capsule formation was performed on porous poly(hydroxyethyl methacrylate-co-methacrylic acid) materials. The authors have shown that materials possessing pores between 30–40 μm in size induce the minimal fibrosis and the highest vascularity, with a shift in macrophage polarisation towards the M2 state [40].

Some other studies have also investigated the influence of fibre diameter and fibre alignment in minimizing immune response. A study focusing on the elaboration of a PCL scaffold using the electrospinning technique demonstrated that aligned fibre topography (500 nm) contributes to the reduction of adverse host response in comparison to random electrospun nanofibers (310 nm) [41]. Another study performed with PLLA electrospun fibres comes to the conclusion that fibre diameter is more relevant than fibre alignment in modulating inflammatory response. In their study they have cultivated macrophages on four different PLLA scaffolds (aligned microfibres, aligned nanofibres, random nanofibres and random microfibres) and they demonstrated a minimal inflammatory response on nanofibrous scaffolds. These data have shown for this polymer that nanofibres are more efficient in modulating immune response than microfibres. They have also demonstrated that fibre diameter is a more crucial parameter than fibre aligment since they minimise the immune response for nanofibrous scaffolds with fibres in both aligned and non-aligned configurations [42].

9.2.2 Metallic

Adverse immune reactions to implanted materials is of crucial importance once medical devices require biological integration and vascularisation [6]. In this part we are going to describe the immunomodulatory macrophage behaviour in the function of metallic implants. Metals are present in almost all orthopaedic devices and some problems can be found due to the risk of adverse biological reactions by generation of metallic particles and ions [43–45]. Moreover, currently used metals (such as titanium and its alloys) are non-biodegradable, which induces frustrated phagocytosis by phagocytic cells such as macrophages. The role of macrophages in hip prosthesis and dental implant failure are described in this section.

Among the metallic implantable medical devices, metal-on-metal (MoM) has promoted the most number of studies about excessive and prolonged exposure to prosthetic debris due to the higher rate of complications linked to these implants [46]. The loosening of hip implants (MoM) can be related to the biological response that is the cause of long-term failure for about 65% of hip prostheses [47]. Hip prostheses are widely composed of metallic alloy, such as cobalt-chromium-molybdenum and titanium-aluminium-vanadium [46]. Metallic ions released upon implantation are generated by wear and corrosion of the metallic prosthesis. The biological response to this prosthetic debris depends on the size of the release particles; diameters up to a few micrometres are phagocytosed by macrophages, while bigger particles can induce a foreign-body response [48,49].

The microenvironment around the implant, where particles are deposited, can lead to adverse local tissue responses. Those responses are related to adverse reactions to metal debris, for example, pseudotumours and aseptic lymphocyte-dominated vasculitis-associated lesions (ALVAL). Pseudotumours may grow at the implant periphery, thus the patient will suffer from pain provoked by the compression caused by these masses. Macrophage infiltration is induced by the continuous release of metallic particles, which will induce apoptosis after phagocytosis of excess toxic particles. This can induce tissue necrosis; consequently, the presence of pseudotumours can lead to implant failure by preventing proper integration [50]. The origin of the ALVAL is related to the swelling of the vascular endothelium, to extensive necrosis and to suspected hypersensitivity involving T-cells [51,52]. The pain suffered by patients with pseudotumours and ALVAL is correlated to tissue necrosis and compression of the femoral nerve. Pseudotumours and ALVAL are not directly related and may occur independently [53].

The advantages of titanium (Ti) alloys for biomedical applications are related to their lower modulus, superior biocompatibility and enhanced corrosion resistance when compared to cobalt-based alloys or stainless steels [54]. The interactions of metallic particles with immune cells are described in this chapter, focusing on Ti alloys, as they are commonly used to manufacture hip and other orthopaedic prostheses. The immune system is influenced by Ti debris. Regarding macrophage response, the production of pro-inflammatory cytokines (TNF-α, IL-12, IL-1β and IL-6) is increased in the presence of Ti ions [55]. Moreover, Ti ions are also responsible for activating T-cells, which play a central role in cell-mediated immunity [56]. *In vivo* experiments reported Ti particle-induced immune response. It was demonstrated that intraperitoneal injection of Ti particles in mice caused IL-1β secretion and activation of a NALP3 complex [57]. Additionally, studies concerning femoral osteolysis (a pathological deterioration of bone tissue) demonstrated that patients with focal osteolysis had a higher number of macrophages that phagocytised small particles, whereas those without osteolysis had more fibroblasts. At that point, the pro-inflammatory cytokines produced by the macrophages may contribute to focal osteolysis, which can lead to implant failure [58].

The role of macrophages in dental implant failure has been widely studied [6,59,60]. The released particles from the prostheses are apparently phagocytosed by macrophages. Those particles behave as haptens (small molecules that elicit an immune response when conjugated to a larger molecule), which are responsible for the macrophage presence [61]. As it happens with hip prostheses, macrophages loaded with metallic particles composed of Ti release pro-inflammatory cytokines toward the bone surface, contributing to its resorption by osteoclast activation. The presence of metallic particles that results from the process of corrosion may directly inhibit osteoblast function, and the lack of integration can cause opportunistic infections resulting in peri-implantitis, which is a destructive process that affects the soft and hard tissues surrounding dental implants [60].

A study developed by Tomas and colleagues suggested that patients with oral implants also suffer with problems related to marginal bone loss (MBL) [62]. Marginal bone loss around oral implants is primarily dependent on an immunologic reaction to the bacteria infection around the implant. Bone resorption is commonly a result of complication to treatment in the first year of the implantation. A series of factors will work together to activate the immune system. Those factors can be related to several problems: adverse implant loading, microbe presence, cement excess, released ions from the implant, broken/damaged components and so on, ultimately shifting the delicate balance between the osteoblast and the osteoclast towards osteoclasts, which results in bone resorption (Figure 9.2). A tightly regulated balance of osteoclastic and osteoblastic activity maintains a steady state of total bone mass in healthy adults. However, a disturbed balance will lead to a disease: loss (such as in the case of osteoporosis) and gain of bone tissue (such as in the case of osteopetrosis). It usually starts with the accumulation of wear particles at the implant-tissue interface. These induce a cellular response through phagocytosis. Host cells, primarily resident macrophages and fibroblasts, start to produce a wide range of pro-inflammatory cytokines. These inflammatory factors induce osteoclast formation, which stimulates bone loss [6].

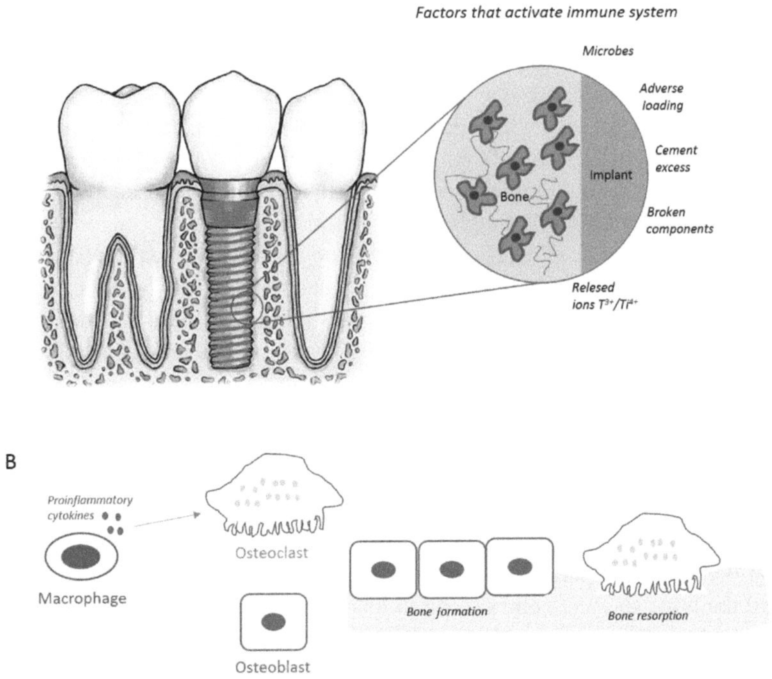

FIGURE 9.2 (A) A series of factors will work together to activate the immune system, ultimately shifting the delicate balance between the osteoblast and the osteoclast, resulting in bone resorption. (B) Macrophages release pro inflammatory cytokines toward the bone surface, contributing to its resorption by osteoclast activation.

9.2.3 Ceramic

Both the study of cell-material interactions and immunochemistry approaches have contributed to the concept of engineered ceramics as biomaterials over the years. New ceramic biomaterials ranged from bioinert to bioactive materials for the coating of replacement and regenerative materials in orthopaedic, maxillofacial and dental surgery. The high failure rates of bone grafts and the lack of osteoinductive properties of alloplastic implants on bone healing over large defects have triggered the quest for new designed bioactive materials, such as bioglasses and calcium phosphate-based ceramics. Bioactive ceramics interact with body fluids by inorganic chemical and biochemical processes, stimulating network dissolution into calcium and phosphate ions followed by the precipitation of biological apatite on their surfaces. This process contributes to the biodegradation of implanted material and induction of bone regeneration to succeed simultaneously. Being similar to the mineral composition of bone and teeth makes sintered hydroxyapatite (HA), which is osteoconductive, the perfect choice for fabrication of bone substitutes. The diversity of chemical composition, crystallographic structure and water solubility of calcium orthophosphates give this family of ceramics favourable biological properties such as biocompatibility, tissue conductivity and biodegradability. Amongst calcium phosphates, non-stoichiometric apatites, such as beta-tricalcium phosphate (β-TCP), which is bioresorbable, have been proved in recent decades to be excellent biomimetic compounds [63]. Also, bioactive silica-based glasses undergo five inorganic reaction phases at the glass surface in contact with physiological fluids. These dissolution products deposit a calcium hydroxyl-carbonate apatite (HCA) layer, which induces the adsorption of biological moieties and further macrophage activation. These biochemical changes result in gene regulation necessary for bone growth and development [64].

Appropriate morphogenic and physicochemical cues are a key step in achieving tailored temporal and immune responses upon implantation. This is because the modulation of microenvironmental cues in the interfaces of biomaterials induces macrophage phenotype polarisation, dictating a favourable immune response. Therefore, the properties inherent to biomaterials have influence on the control of the M2:M1 ratio. Surface properties, particle size and geometry, porosity and biodegradability are mainly involved in these responses to bioceramics.

Physical characteristics, such as size and shape, of HA particles are an important factor in the modulation of the immune response, because they can trigger cytokine production by human monocytes and affect the activation of macrophages [65]. Laquerriere et al. demonstrated that shape and the size of the particles were the most important characteristics influencing the production of cytokines. HA particles (1–30 μm) stimulate the production of greater amounts of pro-inflammatory cytokines (TNF-α, IL-1b, IL-6) compared to large particles, whereas needle-shaped particles induced the production of anti-inflammatory cytokines (TNF-α, IL-6 and IL-10) by cells [66]. Also, needle-shaped and small particles were found to induce an increase of IL-1, IL-6, IL-8 and IL-10 production as a function of surface area ratio. Needle-shaped particles augment the production of pro-inflammatory IL-18 by monocytes/macrophages, which works antagonistically to osteoclastogenesis activated by IL-6 [67,68]. The small size (1–2 μm) of HA crystals stimulates macrophage TNF-α secretion, a vascular calcifying agent, and depends on NF-κB activation [69]. In contrast, the largest β-TCP particles increased IL-1, IL-8 and TNF production on human peripheral blood mononuclear cells *in vitro,* suggesting a less inflammatory and cytotoxic profile with a smaller primary particle size when compared to larger particles [70]. Nevertheless, in an *in vivo* study, due to high biodegradation rates, small biphasic CaP particles (10–20 μm) appeared to promote a brief and strong inflammatory reaction, positively modulating the interaction with the immune system and favouring the osteoconduction process [71].

In a network resulting from alpha-TCP degradation into HA crystal subproducts, micrometric plate-like or nanometric needle-like substrates present distinct behaviours in terms of macrophage proliferation and activation, the first releasing higher reactive oxygen species (ROS) compared to the almost non-existent release on needle-like nanosized crystals [72]. Accordingly, cytotoxicity and oxidative stress through ROS formation in rat NR8383 and primary alveolar macrophages showed no significant responses for HA nanoparticles (NPs) with different shapes (nano/needle-shaped, nano/rod-like, nano/plate-like, fine/dull needle-shaped), supporting a good biocompatibility to both cell types [73]. Still, the toxicity of ceramic nanoparticles is a matter of debate. Some studies have tried to understand whether agglomeration induces NP uptake by different cells, or if it is basically influenced by other parameters such as the specific-surface area, Ca:P ratio and crystallinity of the particles [74]. Researchers discovered that the biological effect of the NPs do not only depend on their degree of uptake by cells, but also whether NP agglomeration prompts the mode of internalisation of the NPs into a surface-connected compartment (SCC), as a mechanism of particle degradation by human monocyte-derived macrophages. Dispersed NPs prevent the formation of SCC, but do not inhibit NP uptake by other mechanisms [75].

Notably, the degradability rate of ceramic nanoparticles is of major importance for immunomodulation and cytotoxicity. The inhalation of amorphous or crystalline silica particles is reported to cause an inflammatory reaction and chronic exposure leads to silicosis. This is attributed to the fact that silica particles cannot be dissolved after being phagocytosed by macrophages; they remain in the lung and cause further fibrosis [76]. Recently, IL-1β was found to play a critical role in switching on regulation of inflammation by micro-sized silica particles [77].

Biodegradation, i.e., the disintegration and fragmentation of the material via a solution-driven extracellular dissolution or cell-mediated resorption processes is closely related to the physicochemical cues of the CaP-based material. So the speed of degradability depends on particle size, crystallinity, surface area, porosity, Ca:P ratio and environmental cues, such as Ph, cells and H_20 presence [78]. Comparing both micron-sized HA and beta-TCP particles, which have different Ca:P ratios and degradability rates, the production of cytokines connected to osteoclast and dendritic cell differentiation (OPG, RANKL, M-CSF, GM-CSF) was investigated on human peripheral blood mononuclear cells *in vitro*. Both phases induce the production of pro-inflammatory cytokines.

However, beta-TCP caused no induction of RANKL, which is known as responsible for osteoclastogenesis, and a low inductive effect on the production of GM-CSF, known for promoting dendritic cells [79]. Also, *in vivo* biodegradation studies of sintered beta-TCP scaffolds and a CaP bone cement (CPC) evince differences on both the resorption processes [80,81]. Biodegradation is uniform in beta-TCP scaffolds, which present high crystallinity and solubility, and there is an absence of particle formation or visible phagocytosis, suggesting the occurrence of a solution-driven dissolution of the material. CPCs, which hydrolyse into brushite, present disintegration in smaller particles and numerous macrophages and multinucleated giant cells, suggesting the occurrence of a degradation process through dissolution associated with a cellular resorption.

The cell-induced process of resorption is mediated by macrophages and their fused morphologic variants, multinucleated giant cells or foreign body giant cells [82]. Macrophages internalise fragments and particles <10 μm in diameter via phagocytosis, while FBGCs take action via engulfment of larger particles. If particles are larger than 100 μm, surface dissolution is carried out via extracellular degradation by macrophages and FBGCs through the release of enzymes and/or the release of protons (Figure 9.3) [83,84]. Osteoclasts may also mediate the long-term resorption process by creating an acidic environment on mineral surfaces similar to the bone-remodelling process [85]. Nonetheless, a crucial fact that compromises the long-term

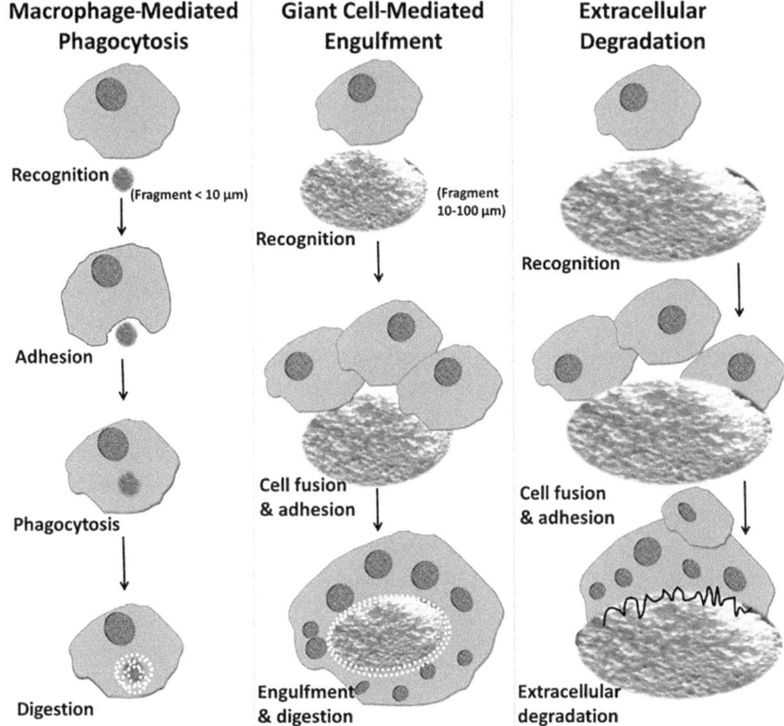

FIGURE 9.3 A schematic depiction of macrophage response to biomaterials depending on the size of the implanted materials. (Reprinted from Sheikh, Z. et al., *Materials*, 8(9), 2015. With permission.)

success of implants is the activation of phagocytic cells by particles originating from the wear of implanted bioceramic surfaces, leading to bone resorption and aseptic loosening of the implant.

The geometric characteristics, pore size and porosity of bioceramics play an important role in neovascularisation and osteoinduction, and enable mimicking of the bone microenvironment for bone tissue regeneration. For example, β-TCP scaffolds with hole diameter of 300 μm improve bone formation, specifically bone marrow-like tissue and patterns of bone tissue formation similar to the host bone [86–88]. Despite their high porosity compromising the mechanical integrity of the scaffolds, the presence of interconnected micropores (<5 μm) increases the surface area, promoting higher adsorption of proteins and facilitating the biodegradation of scaffolds. The absence of porosity hinders vascularisation in the centre of the implant, resulting in a local hypoxic microenvironment. In addition, macroporous (>100 μm) materials provide feasible structural factors for bone in-growth and vascularisation, improving mechanical interlocking of the implanted material. Pore sizes >300 μm enhance direct osteogenesis and the formation of capillaries. However, a moderate hypoxia environment avoids a significant inflammatory reaction but preserves the angiogenic effects, and pore sizes of 90–120 μm may lead to chondrogenesis [89]. Indeed, the cross-talk between inflammatory reaction and osteogenesis is crucial for the success of bioabsorbable scaffolds. Chen et al. [89] suggest that there might be a correlation between increasing pore size and macrophage polarisation, by the upregulation expression of the M2 markers, along with the downregulated expression of the M1 markers.

Mechanical cues are special keys in the development of bone substitutes. Microstructured HA are generally brittle with low tensile strength. The advances in nanotechnology have made possible an improvement in mechanical strength of nanostructured ceramics for load-bearing purposes. Nanostructured CaP-based scaffolds are a promising material for bone neoformation and vascularisation in the regenerative medicine and hard-tissue engineering fields, with satisfactory clinical outcomes [90–93]. Naturally, the nanosized grains in the ceramics also affect biological responses, such as cell morphology, adhesion and/or motility. The production of bone mineral *in vitro* by human MSCs was shown to be stimulated by nanostructured materials, even in the absence of osteogenic supplements [94]. This fact proves the osteoinductive characteristics of such materials. In addition, the stiffness of bioceramics is expected to be similar to precalcified bone (>30 kPa), creating mechanically tailored microenvironments for tissue conduction and modulating macrophage elasticity due to a Rac-1-mediated mechanosensory pathway mediation, actin polymerisation and rhoGTPase activity [95,96].

Still, Sr- and Zn-substituted ceramics have an effect on the production of cytokines and matrix metalloproteinases (MMPs), evincing the control of inflammatory processes by human monocytes [97–99]. An attractive approach for designing "immune-informed" bioceramics is creating ion-substituted or ion-doped CaPs, enabling the control of chemical cues, which influence bone development or regeneration.

9.3 CONCLUSIONS

Monocyte/macrophage responses to implanted biomaterials are important determinants of the inflammatory processes following the implantation. Here, we have reviewed the response of macrophages to three classes of biomaterials (polymers, metals and ceramics). Site- and application-specific design of biomaterials that takes into consideration the short- and long-term responses of macrophages is required for implantable systems that can establish a strong communication with the host immune system.

REFERENCES

1. Destouet, J. et al., Screening mammography in 350 women with breast implants: Prevalence and findings of implant complications. AJR. American *Journal of Roentgenology*, 1992. 159(5): p. 973–978.
2. Gorbet, M.B. and M.V. Sefton, Biomaterial-associated thrombosis: Roles of coagulation factors, complement, platelets and leukocytes. *Biomaterials*, 2004. 25(26): p. 5681–5703.
3. McGraw, J., G. Hiebert and J. Steeves, Modulating astrogliosis after neurotrauma. *Journal of Neuroscience Research*, 2001. 63(2): p. 109–115.

4. Sridharan, R. et al., Biomaterial based modulation of macrophage polarization: A review and suggested design principles. *Materials Today*, 2015. 18(6): p. 313–325.
5. Mokarram, N. and R.V. Bellamkonda, A perspective on immunomodulation and tissue repair. *Annals of Biomedical Engineering*, 2014. 42(2): p. 338–351.
6. Kzhyshkowska, J. et al., Macrophage responses to implants: Prospects for personalized medicine. *Journal of Leukocyte Biology*, 2015: p. 953–962.
7. Vishwakarma, A. et al., Engineering immunomodulatory biomaterials to tune the inflammatory response. *Trends in Biotechnology*, 2016. 34(6): p. 470–482.
8. Hanson, S., R.N. D'Souza and P. Hematti, Biomaterial–mesenchymal stem cell constructs for immunomodulation in composite tissue engineering. *Tissue Engineering Part A*, 2014. 20(15–16): p. 2162–2168.
9. Subbiahdoss, G. et al., Microbial biofilm growth vs. tissue integration: "The race for the surface" experimentally studied. *Acta Biomaterialia*, 2009. 5(5): p. 1399–1404.
10. Panilaitis, B. et al., Macrophage responses to silk. *Biomaterials*, 2003. 24(18): p. 3079–3085.
11. Boersema, G.S. et al., The effect of biomaterials used for tissue regeneration purposes on polarization of macrophages. *BioResearch Open Access*, 2016. 5(1): p. 6–14.
12. Bridges, A.W. et al., Chronic inflammatory responses to microgel-based implant coatings. *Journal of Biomedical Materials Research Part A*, 2010. 94(1): p. 252–258.
13. Hoffman, A.S. Hydrogels for biomedical applications. *Advanced Drug Delivery Reviews*, 2012. 64: p. 18–23.
14. El-Sherbiny, I.M. and M.H. Yacoub, Hydrogel scaffolds for tissue engineering: Progress and challenges. *Global Cardiology Science and Practice*, 2013: p. 38.
15. Oliveira, M.I. et al., Chitosan drives anti-inflammatory macrophage polarisation and pro-inflammatory dendritic cell stimulation. *European Cells & Materials*, 2012. 24: p. 136–152.
16. Ingram, J.H. et al., The influence of molecular weight, crosslinking and counterface roughness on TNF-alpha production by macrophages in response to ultra high molecular weight polyethylene particles. *Biomaterials*, 2004. 25(17): p. 3511–3522.
17. Rayahin, J.E. et al., High and low molecular weight hyaluronic acid differentially influence macrophage activation. *ACS Biomaterials Science & Engineering*, 2015. 1(7): p. 481–493.
18. Lewis, J.S., K. Roy, and B.G. Keselowsky, Materials that harness and modulate the immune system. *MRS Bulletin*, 2014. 39(01): p. 25–34.
19. Jones, J.A. et al., Proteomic analysis and quantification of cytokines and chemokines from biomaterial surface-adherent macrophages and foreign body giant cells. *Journal of Biomedical Materials Research Part A*, 2007. 83(3): p. 585–596.
20. Gao, G. et al., The biocompatibility and biofilm resistance of implant coatings based on hydrophilic polymer brushes conjugated with antimicrobial peptides. *Biomaterials*, 2011. 32(16): p. 3899–3909.
21. Rostam, H.M. et al., The impact of surface chemistry modification on macrophage polarisation. *Immunobiology*, 2016. 221(11): p. 1237–1246.
22. Hezi-Yamit, A. et al., Impact of polymer hydrophilicity on biocompatibility: Implication for DES polymer design. *Journal of Biomedical Materials Research Part A*, 2009. 90(1): p. 133–141.
23. Boehler, R.M., J.G. Graham, and L.D. Shea, Tissue engineering tools for modulation of the immune response. *Biotechniques*, 2011. 51(4): p. 239.
24. Bridges, A.W. and A.J. García, Anti-inflammatory polymeric coatings for implantable biomaterials and devices. *Journal of Diabetes Science and Technology*, 2008. 2(6): p. 984–994.
25. Franz, S. et al., Immune responses to implants–a review of the implications for the design of immunomodulatory biomaterials. *Biomaterials*, 2011. 32(28): p. 6692–6709.

26. Monchaux, E. and P. Vermette, Bioactive microarrays immobilized on low-fouling surfaces to study specific endothelial cell adhesion. *Biomacromolecules*, 2007. 8(11): p. 3668–3673.
27. Wang, D.-A. et al., In situ immobilization of proteins and RGD peptide on polyurethane surfaces via poly (ethylene oxide) coupling polymers for human endothelial cell growth. *Biomacromolecules*, 2002. 3(6): p. 1286–1295.
28. Duggal, S. et al., Phenotype and gene expression of human mesenchymal stem cells in alginate scaffolds. *Tissue Engineering Part A*, 2008. 15(7): p. 1763–1773.
29. Iwasaki, Y. et al., Platelet adhesion on the gradient surfaces grafted with phospholipid polymer. *Journal of Biomaterials Science*, Polymer Edition, 1998. 9(8): p. 801–816.
30. Goreish, H.H. et al., The effect of phosphorylcholine-coated materials on the inflammatory response and fibrous capsule formation: In vitro and in vivo observations. *Journal of Biomedical Materials Research Part A*, 2004. 68(1): p. 1–9.
31. Singh, N. et al., Covalent tethering of functional microgel films onto poly (ethylene terephthalate) surfaces. *Biomacromolecules*, 2007. 8(10): p. 3271–3275.
32. Wang, C. et al., Synthesis and performance of novel hydrogels coatings for implantable glucose sensors. *Biomacromolecules*, 2008. 9(2): p. 561–567.
33. Knopf-Marques, H. et al., Immunomodulation with self-crosslinked polyelectrolyte multilayers based coatings. *Biomacromolecules*, 2016. 17(6): p. 2189–2198.
34. Rostam, H. et al., Impact of surface chemistry and topography on the function of antigen presenting cells. *Biomaterials Science*, 2015. 3(3): p. 424–441.
35. Brown, B.N. et al., Macrophage polarization: An opportunity for improved outcomes in biomaterials and regenerative medicine. *Biomaterials*, 2012. 33(15): p. 3792–3802.
36. Bota, P. et al., Biomaterial topography alters healing in vivo and monocyte/macrophage activation in vitro. *Journal of Biomedical Materials Research Part A*, 2010. 95(2): p. 649–657.
37. Chen, S. et al., Characterization of topographical effects on macrophage behavior in a foreign body response model. *Biomaterials*, 2010. 31(13): p. 3479–3491.
38. Paul, N.E. et al., Topographical control of human macrophages by a regularly microstructured polyvinylidene fluoride surface. *Biomaterials*, 2008. 29(30): p. 4056–4064.
39. Garg, K. et al., Macrophage functional polarization (M1/M2) in response to varying fiber and pore dimensions of electrospun scaffolds. *Biomaterials*, 2013. 34(18): p. 4439–4451.
40. Madden, L.R. et al., Proangiogenic scaffolds as functional templates for cardiac tissue engineering. *Proceedings of the National Academy of Sciences*, 2010. 107(34): p. 15211–15216.
41. Cao, H. et al., The topographical effect of electrospun nanofibrous scaffolds on the in vivo and in vitro foreign body reaction. *Journal of Biomedical Materials Research Part A*, 2010. 93(3): p. 1151–1159.
42. Saino, E. et al., Effect of electrospun fiber diameter and alignment on macrophage activation and secretion of proinflammatory cytokines and chemokines. *Biomacromolecules*, 2011. 12(5): p. 1900–1911.
43. Smith, A.J. et al., Failure rates of stemmed metal-on-metal hip replacements: Analysis of data from the National Joint Registry of England and Wales. *The Lancet*, 2012. 379(9822): p. 1199–1204.
44. Campbell, P. et al., Histological features of pseudotumor-like tissues from metal-on-metal hips. *Clinical Orthopaedics and Related Research*, 2010. 468(9): p. 2321–2327.
45. Konttinen, Y.T. and J. Pajarinen, Surgery: Adverse reactions to metal-on-metal implants. *Nature Reviews Rheumatology*, 2013. 9(1): p. 5–6.
46. Vasconcelos, D.M. et al., The two faces of metal ions: From implants rejection to tissue repair/regeneration. *Biomaterials*, 2016. 84: p. 262–275.

47. Costain, D.J. et al., Perioperative mortality after hemiarthroplasty related to fixation method: A study based on the Australian Orthopaedic Association National Joint Replacement Registry. *Acta Orthopaedica*, 2011. 82(3): p. 275–281.
48. Germain, M. et al., Comparison of the cytotoxicity of clinically relevant cobalt–chromium and alumina ceramic wear particles in vitro. *Biomaterials*, 2003. 24(3): p. 469–479.
49. Champion, J.A., A. Walker and S. Mitragotri, Role of particle size in phagocytosis of polymeric microspheres. *Pharmaceutical Research*, 2008. 25(8): p. 1815–1821.
50. Langton, D. et al., Adverse reaction to metal debris following hip resurfacing. *Journal of Bone and Joint Surgery*, 2011. 93(2): p. 164–171.
51. Pandit, H. et al., Pseudotumours associated with metal-on-metal hip resurfacings. *Journal of Bone and Joint Surgery*, 2008. 90(7): p. 847–851.
52. Aroukatos, P. et al., Immunologic adverse reaction associated with low-carbide metal-on-metal bearings in total hip arthroplasty. *Clinical Orthopaedics and Related Research*, 2010. 468(8): p. 2135–2142.
53. Hasegawa, M. et al., Pseudotumor with dominant B-lymphocyte infiltration after metal-on-metal total hip arthroplasty with a modular cup. *Journal of Arthroplasty*, 2012. 27(3): p. 493.
54. Long, M. and H.J. Rack, Titanium alloys in total joint replacement—A materials science perspective. *Biomaterials*, 1998. 19(18): p. 1621–1639.
55. Wang, J.Y. et al., Titanium, chromium and cobalt ions modulate the release of bone-associated cytokines by human monocytes/macrophages in vitro. *Biomaterials*, 1996. 17(23): p. 2233–2240.
56. Cadosch, D. et al., Titanium uptake, induction of RANK-L expression, and enhanced proliferation of human T-lymphocytes. *Journal of Orthopaedic Research*, 2010. 28(3): p. 341–347.
57. St Pierre, C.A. et al., Periprosthetic osteolysis: Characterizing the innate immune response to titanium wear-particles. *Journal of Orthopaedic Research*, 2010. 28(11): p. 1418–1424.
58. Chiba, J. et al., The characterization of cytokines in the interface tissue obtained from failed cementless total hip arthroplasty with and without femoral osteolysis. *Clinical Orthopaedics and Related Research*, 1994. 300: p. 304–312.
59. Petković, A. et al., Proinflammatory cytokines (IL-1β and TNF-α) and chemokines (IL-8 and MIP-1α) as markers of peri-implant tissue condition. *International Journal of Oral & Maxillofacial Surgery*, 2010. 39(5): p. 478–485.
60. Olmedo, D. et al., Macrophages related to dental implant failure. *Implant Dentistry*, 2003. 12(1): p. 75–80.
61. Thomas, D.W., L. Clement, and E.M. Shevach, T lymphocyte stimulation by hapten-conjugated macrophages. *Immunological Review*, 1978. 40(1): p. 181–204.
62. Tomas, A. et al., "Peri-Implantitis": A complication of a foreign body or a man-made "disease". Facts and fiction. *Clinical Implant Dentistry and Related Research*, 2016.
63. Dorozhkin, S.V., Calcium orthophosphates: Occurrence, properties, biomineralization, pathological calcification and biomimetic applications. *Biomatter*, 2011. 1(2): p. 121–164.
64. Hench, L.L., N. Roki and M.B. Fenn, Bioactive glasses: Importance of structure and properties in bone regeneration. *Journal of Molecular Structure*, 2014. 1073: p. 24–30.
65. Velard, F. et al., Inflammatory cell response to calcium phosphate biomaterial particles: An overview. *Acta Biomaterialia*, 2013. 9(2): p. 4956–4963.
66. Laquerriere, P. et al., Importance of hydroxyapatite particles characteristics on cytokines production by human monocytes in vitro. *Biomaterials*, 2003. 24(16): p. 2739–2747.

67. Grandjean-Laquerriere, A. et al., The effect of the physical characteristics of hydroxyapatite particles on human monocytes IL-18 production in vitro. *Biomaterials*, 2004. 25(28): p. 5921–5927.
68. Grandjean-Laquerriere, A. et al., Importance of the surface area ratio on cytokines production by human monocytes in vitro induced by various hydroxyapatite particles. *Biomaterials*, 2005. 26(15): p. 2361–2369.
69. Nadra, I. et al., Effect of particle size on hydroxyapatite crystal-induced tumor necrosis factor alpha secretion by macrophages. *Atherosclerosis*, 2008. 196(1): p. 98–105.
70. Lange, T. et al., Size dependent induction of proinflammatory cytokines and cytotoxicity of particulate beta-tricalciumphosphate in vitro. *Biomaterials*, 2011. 32(17): p. 4067–4075.
71. Malard, O. et al., Influence of biphasic calcium phosphate granulometry on bone ingrowth, ceramic resorption, and inflammatory reactions: Preliminary in vitro and in vivo study. *Journal of Biomedical Materials Research*, 1999. 46(1): p. 103–111.
72. Mestres, G. et al., Inflammatory Response to Nano- and Microstructured Hydroxyapatite. *PLoS One*, 2015. 10(4): p. e0120381.
73. Albrecht, C. et al., Evaluation of cytotoxic effects and oxidative stress with hydroxyapatite dispersions of different physicochemical properties in rat NR8383 cells and primary macrophages. *Toxicology In Vitro*, 2009. 23(3): p. 520–530.
74. Rabolli, V. et al., The cytotoxic activity of amorphous silica nanoparticles is mainly influenced by surface area and not by aggregation. *Toxicology Letters*, 2011. 206(2): p. 197–203.
75. Muller, K.H. et al., The effect of particle agglomeration on the formation of a surface-connected compartment induced by hydroxyapatite nanoparticles in human monocyte-derived macrophages. *Biomaterials*, 2014. 35(3): p. 1074–1088.
76. Costantini, L.M., R.M. Gilberti, and D.A. Knecht, The phagocytosis and toxicity of amorphous silica. *PLoS One*, 2011. 6(2): p. e14647.
77. Zhou, T. et al., Switch regulation of interleukin-1 beta in downstream of inflammatory cytokines induced by two micro-sized silica particles on differentiated THP-1 macrophages. *Environmental Toxicology and Pharmacology*, 2015. 39(1): p. 457–466.
78. LeGeros, R.Z., Properties of osteoconductive biomaterials: Calcium phosphates. *Clinical Orthopaedics and Related Research*, 2002(395): p. 81–98.
79. Lange, T. et al., Proinflammatory and osteoclastogenic effects of beta-tricalciumphosphate and hydroxyapatite particles on human mononuclear cells in vitro. *Biomaterials*, 2009. 30(29): p. 5312–5318.
80. Lu, J. et al., The biodegradation mechanism of calcium phosphate biomaterials in bone. *Journal of Biomedicals Materials Research*, 2002. 63(4): p. 408–412.
81. Theiss, F. et al., Biocompatibility and resorption of a brushite calcium phosphate cement. *Biomaterials*, 2005. 26(21): p. 4383–4394.
82. Zhidao Xia and James, T.T., A review on macrophage responses to biomaterials. *Biomedical Materials*, 2006. 1(1): p. R1.
83. Hannink, G. and J.J. Arts, Bioresorbability, porosity and mechanical strength of bone substitutes: What is optimal for bone regeneration? *Injury*, 2011. 42 Suppl 2: p. S22–5.
84. Sheikh, Z. et al., Macrophages, foreign body giant cells and their response to implantable biomaterials. *Materials*, 2015. 8(9).
85. Anderson, J.M., A. Rodriguez and D.T. Chang, Foreign body reaction to biomaterials. *Seminars in Immunology*, 2008. 20(2): p. 86–100.
86. Jin, Q.M. et al., Effects of geometry of hydroxyapatite as a cell substratum in BMP-induced ectopic bone formation. *Journal of Biomedicals Materials Research*, 2000. 51(3): p. 491–499.

87. Watanabe, S. et al., Efficacy of honeycomb tcp-induced microenvironment on bone tissue regeneration in craniofacial area. *International Journal of Medical Sciences*, 2016. 13(6): p. 466–476.
88. Kuboki, Y. et al., Geometry of artificial ECM: Sizes of pores controlling phenotype expression in BMP-induced osteogenesis and chondrogenesis. *Connective Tissue Research*, 2002. 43(2–3): p. 529–534.
89. Chen, Z. et al., Osteoimmunomodulation for the development of advanced bone biomaterials. *Materials Today*, 2016. 19(6): p. 304–321.
90. LeGeros, R.Z., Biodegradation and bioresorption of calcium phosphate ceramics. *Clinical Materials*, 1993. 14(1): p. 65–88.
91. Kalita, S.J., A. Bhardwaj, and H.A. Bhatt, Nanocrystalline calcium phosphate ceramics in biomedical engineering. *Materials Science and Engineering: C*, 2007. 27(3): p. 441–449.
92. Zhou, H. and J. Lee, Nanoscale hydroxyapatite particles for bone tissue engineering. *Acta Biomaterialia*, 2011. 7(7): p. 2769–2781.
93. Dorozhkin, S.V., Calcium orthophosphate bioceramics. *Ceramics International*, 2015. 41(10, Part B): p. 13913–13966.
94. Dalby, M.J. et al., The control of human mesenchymal cell differentiation using nanoscale symmetry and disorder. *Nature Materials*, 2007. 6(12): p. 997–1003.
95. Rehfeldt, F. et al., Cell responses to the mechanochemical microenvironment—Implications for regenerative medicine and drug delivery. *Advanced Drug Delivery Reviews*, 2007. 59(13): p. 1329–1339.
96. Patel, N.R. et al., Cell elasticity determines macrophage function. *PLoS One*, 2012. 7(9): p. e41024.
97. Buache, E. et al., Effect of strontium-substituted biphasic calcium phosphate on inflammatory mediators production by human monocytes. *Acta Biomateriala*, 2012. 8(8): p. 3113–3119.
98. Renaudin, G. et al., Structural characterization of sol-gel derived Sr-substituted calcium phosphates with anti-osteoporotic and anti-inflammatory properties. *Journal of Materials Chemistry*, 2008. 18(30): p. 3593–3600.
99. Velard, F. et al., The effect of zinc on hydroxyapatite-mediated activation of human polymorphonuclear neutrophils and bone implant-associated acute inflammation. *Biomaterials*, 2010. 31(8): p. 2001–2009.

10 Biomaterials and Immune Response in Periodontics

Sivaraman Prakasam, Praveen Gajendrareddy, Christopher Louie, Clarence Lee and Luiz E. Bertassoni

CONTENTS

10.1 INTRODUCTION

Periodontics is a specialty of dentistry that deals with the prevention, diagnosis and treatment of periodontal diseases and peri-implant diseases. In addition, periodontists, the dental specialty practitioners of periodontics, perform other surgical procedures, examples of which include placement of dental implants and soft tissue surgical procedures, which enhance dental aesthetics and function. The term periodontium describes the supporting structures of a tooth. It includes the gingiva, cementum, periodontal ligament and alveolar bone.[1] The gingiva is the outermost soft tissue layer that surrounds a tooth. The cementum is a calcified hard tissue deposit on the tooth surface, which allows periodontal ligament fibre insertion. The periodontal ligament is a well-organised fibrous structure that anchors the teeth through the cementum to the underlying alveolar bone. The alveolar bone is the supporting bone that surrounds the teeth.[1] The periodontium, particularly the gingiva, protects the underlying tissues by acting as a barrier against the harsh external environment of the oral cavity. It not only acts as a physical barrier, but has a robust innate and adaptive immune mechanism that provides a dynamic biological barrier.

As described in the chapter on dental biofilms, one of the unique challenges the periodontium faces is the constant formation of dental biofilms at the tooth–periodontium interface. Dysbiosis of these dental biofilms initiates dysregulation of periodontal immune responses.[2] Dysregulation of the immune response results in activation of mechanisms that lead to progressive loss of periodontal tissues, resulting in periodontal diseases.[2] Untreated periodontal diseases eventually lead to loss of teeth. A recent estimate indicated that chronic periodontitis (CP), the most prevalent form of periodontal disease, affects an estimated 47% of the US adult population.[3,4] Severe forms of CP affect approximately 11% of the US and global global populations.[3,4] Thus, CP is a significant global health problem. The goal of periodontal treatment is to prevent, restore and reverse the tissue loss that happens with periodontal disease and ultimately the goal is to prevent tooth loss.

The primary therapeutic approach to restoration and reversion of tissue loss is a treatment modality called "guided tissue regeneration" (GTR).[5,6] A majority of biomaterials used in the field of periodontics are used towards GTR. GTR procedures overcome the disadvantage of slow proliferation of periodontal ligament fibroblasts and osteoblasts relative to the rapid proliferation and migration of epithelial cells. In an attempt to restore tissue integrity, epithelial cells proliferate and migrate into the defect areas created by tissue loss and prevent bone cells and periodontal ligament fibroblasts from migrating into the area.[7] The biomaterials used for GTR thus either inhibit epithelial migration by physically blocking them (cell exclusion) or by enhancing the proliferation and migration of periodontal ligament cells and alveolar bone osteoblasts (cell guidance), or combinations of both.[7] In addition, some biomaterials used for GTR provide a physical scaffold in defect areas for osteoblasts to migrate and form bone. An example of a GTR procedure is illustrated in Figure 10.1.

As discussed earlier, when periodontal disease is left untreated, it leads to tooth loss. While several options for rehabilitating the lost dentition exist, dental implants offer the best solution in achieving that. Reflecting this, dental implant placements have exponentially increased in the last few decades. One of the challenges in dental implant treatment is the loss of alveolar ridge dimensions subsequent to extraction of teeth. Similar to GTR, guided bone regeneration (GBR) strategies overcome this limitation by reconstructing the lost ridge dimensions.[6] The biomaterials used for these procedures are largely similar to biomaterials used for GTR and rely on either the exclusion of epithelial cells and gingival fibroblasts or the enhancement of proliferation and migration of alveolar osteoblasts, or combinations of both. An example of GBR procedure is illustrated in Figure 10.2. Once the availability of adequate ridge dimensions has been established, dental implants can be placed and restored with biocompatible materials like titanium alloys or zirconium-based ceramics.

While several biomaterials are used for other additional applications related to periodontics, this chapter will largely focus on materials used for GTR, GBR procedures and dental implant-related procedures.

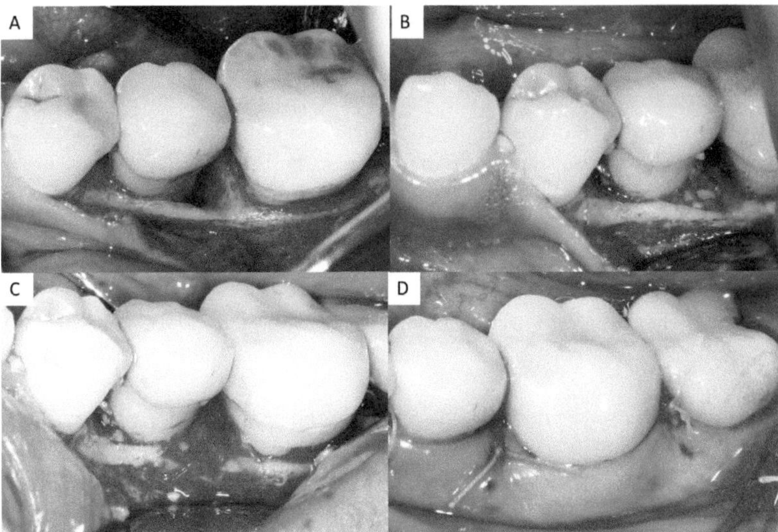

FIGURE 10.1 Guided tissue regeneration: (A) intraoperative image of a lower left second premolar immediately after flap elevation showing a three-walled defect on disto-buccal of the teeth. (B) Osseous defect filled with bone graft. (C) Placental membrane draped over bone graft. (D) Buccal view with sutures.

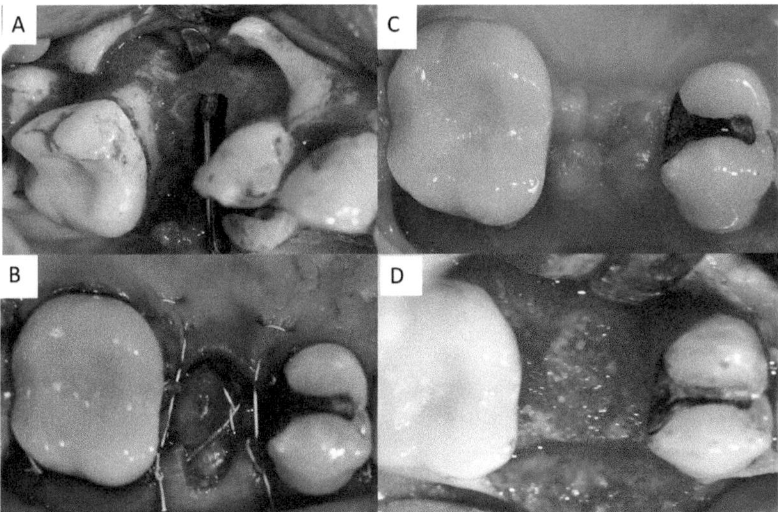

FIGURE 10.2 Alveolar ridge preservation: (A) extraction socket of maxillary right second premolar with a buccal fenestration. (B) Ridge preservation with bone graft and placental membrane. (C) Healing of edentulous area at three months post-operation. (D) Surgically exposed ridge at edentulous area after flap elevation for implant placement, 3.5 months after ridge preservation, showing successful bone regeneration.

10.2 MATERIALS USED FOR GUIDED TISSUE AND GUIDED BONE REGENERATION

Considering that both GTR and GBR procedures rely on principles of cell exclusion or cell guidance, the biomaterials used are largely similar. GTR and GBR procedures involve (1) the use of barrier membranes that exclude cells from migrating into the defect site while it is undergoing regeneration, (2) the use of scaffolds that maintain the defect space for allowing cell migration into the defect site and enhancing regeneration, (3) growth factors or chemotactic factors, collectively called "biologics," that enhance proliferation and/or migration of cells into defect space, thus enhancing regeneration or combinations of these biomaterials. Tables 10.1, 10.2 and 10.3 describe an overview of the materials that are available for GTR and GBR procedures.

Most commercially available biomaterials used for GTR and GBR procedures have been extensively tested for adverse effects prior to widespread clinical use. Consequently, a majority of materials are biocompatible and elicit minimal to no adverse immune responses. However, these biomaterials take advantage or are

TABLE 10.1
Barrier Membranes

Resorbable Membranes	Type	Immune Response
Platelet-rich fibrin	Autograft	No adverse immune responses, normal physiological turnover
Connective tissue	Autograft	No adverse immune responses, normal physiological turnover
Epithelial tissue	Autograft	No adverse immune responses, normal physiological turnover
Amnion chorion (human placenta)	Allograft	No adverse immune responses, bioactive molecules reduced inflammation and pain
Pericardium (human heart)	Allograft	No adverse immune responses, bioactive molecules may help regeneration
Collagen (from bovine, porcine or equine sources)	Xenograft	Minimal adverse immune response. Immune mechanisms help turn over the membrane
Poly glycolic acid	Synthetic/alloplast	Minimal adverse immune response. Immune mechanisms help turn over the membrane
Poly lactic acid,	Synthetic/alloplast	Minimal adverse immune response. Immune mechanisms help turn over the membrane
Non-Resorbable	**Type**	**Immune Response**
e-PTFE	Polytetrafluoroethylene	Adverse immune response in the presence of exposed membranes as a result of bacterial penetration
d-PTFE	Polytetrafluoroethylene	No adverse immune responses
Titanium mesh	Titanium	Adverse immune response in the presence of exposed membranes as a result of bacterial penetration

TABLE 10.2
Sources of Bone Graft Material

Type of Scaffold	Type	Bone-Forming Potential	Immune Response
Tuberosity or symphysis menti bone	Autograft	Osteogenic	No adverse immune responses, normal physiological turnover
Ileac crest bone marrow aspirate	Autograft	Osteogenic	No adverse immune responses, normal physiological turnover, may activate osteoclast and cause root resorption
Mesenchymal cell-laden bone matrices	Allograft	Osteogenic/ osteoinductive	Minimal adverse immune responses, normal physiological turnover
Demineralised human bone	Allograft	Osteoinductive	Minimal adverse immune response. Immune mechanisms help turn over the scaffold
Human bone	Allograft	Osteoconductive	Minimal adverse immune response. Immune mechanisms help turn over the scaffold
Bovine mineralised bone	Xenograft	Osteoconductive	Minimal adverse immune response. Immune mechanisms help turn over the scaffold
Beta – tri-calcium phosphate	Synthetics/ alloplasts	Osteoconductive	Minimal adverse immune response. Immune mechanisms help turn over the scaffold
Calcium sulfate	Synthetics/ alloplasts	Osteoconductive	Minimal adverse immune response. Immune mechanisms help turn over the scaffold

designed to take advantage of immune/inflammatory responses to enhance regenerative outcomes. Some biomaterials also have the capability to selectively activate/suppress certain immune mechanisms to further enhance regenerative outcomes. Nevertheless, select few biomaterials that are clinically used have been reported to have adverse immune responses. A comprehensive discussion of all biomaterials used for GTR or GBR is beyond the scope of the chapter. Hence the following sections will focus on (1) how the immune response enhances regenerative outcomes by using select examples of biomaterials and (2) select examples of biomaterials that have been reported to have adverse immune response.

10.2.1 Immune Response During Resorbable Barrier Membrane Turnover

As shown in Table 10.1, barrier membranes used in GTR/GBR procedures can be achieved with the use of resorbable and non-resorbable membranes with comparable outcomes.[8] These membranes have evolved substantially from the inert cell exclusive cellulose acetate (paper) laboratory filter[9,10] to biologically active, cell-guiding

TABLE 10.3
Growth Factors

Agent	Origin	Composition	MOA	Immune Resposne
rhPDGF-BB	Blood platelets	Protein	Chemotaxis and mitogenesis	No adverse immune response
FGF-2	Fibroblast growth factors family	Protein	Proliferation, migration and differentiation of PDL cells	No adverse immune response
PRP/PRF	Platelet alpha granules	PDGF, I-LGF, VEGF, TGF-β	Combination of MOAs of different growth factors	No adverse immune response
EMD	Hertwig's epithelial root sheath from porcine tooth buds	90% amelogenin	Precise MOA unknown	Occasional reports of adverse immune responses
BMP-2	Recombinant DNA using mammalian cells	Bone morphogenic protein-2	Increased proliferation, mineralisation and expression of alkaline phosphatase and osteocalcin	No adverse immune response when used as per manufacturer protocol
GDF-5	Recombinant DNA process using bacterial expression followed by *in vitro* refolding	Growth differential factor-5	Increased early differentiation and matrix production	No adverse immune response

growth factor laden devices.[11] Desirable design characteristics of membranes for periodontal/alveolar regeneration include (1) biocompatibility, (2) ability to provide cell exclusion, (3) the presence of bioactive molecules, (5) easy integration and (6) ease of use.[12]

The key difference between resorbable and non-resorbable membranes, as the name suggests, is that resorbable membranes resorb or turn over gradually and hence do not need to be removed from a surgical site. On the other hand, non resorbable materials require an additional surgical procedure, which poses potentials risks including patient discomfort, site morbidity and possibility of infection. This necessity for surgical re-entry and removal of the membrane thus makes the use of resorbable membranes over non-resorbable membranes attractive.

Resorbable membranes have been obtained from various sources, including[12] autologous sources, allogeneic sources, xenogeneic sources and synthetic materials.[13] The source from which the resorbable membrane is obtained determines the immunogenic potential. Autologous membranes, for example autologous palatal tissue, do not elicit any adverse immunological responses. Most allograft membranes, for example dermal allografts, are decellularised and have just the extracellular matrix, and they do not create any adverse reactions. Xenogeneic grafts, while having the theoretical potential of eliciting an immune response, generally do not elicit adverse immunological responses. This is primarily because, similar to allografts, these grafts are decellularised and, for the majority of these membranes, the collagen from the extracellular matrix is biochemically extracted and reconstituted as a membrane, thus significantly reducing immunogenicity. Alloplasts or synthetic membranes are designed with materials that are biocompatible and are selected for low immunogenicity. Thus, most resorbable membranes do not elicit a significant adverse immunological response. In fact, they take advantage of the inflammatory process for optimal function. Some membranes even possess the capability to reduce adverse inflammation by virtue of proteins embedded in their matrix.

With the progression of healing, the optimal tissues necessary for regeneration grow into the wound space and mature. As this occurs, the site's dependence on the barrier membrane to continue to function and hold its characteristics becomes less vital. Hence, resorbable barriers that contribute to regeneration during the early phases of healing and site maturation, and subsequently disintegrate, hold certain advantages over non-resorbable materials. Immuno-inflammation, a key characteristic of the healing process, also contributes to the degeneration of the resorbable barrier.

Collagen has been used widely as a resorbable barrier. The turnover of collagen membranes utilises the immune system similar to other resorbable membranes with perhaps minor differences. Consequently, in the following sections, we will use those turnover mechanisms as illustrative examples for most resorbable membranes. Apart from its low immunogenicity,[14] collagen has many favourable biological attributes that make it a popular choice as a resorbable barrier. Collagen, particularly type I collagen, is a predominant constituent in our body. It is found in tendon, bone and skin. Sixty per cent of gingival connective tissue and 90% of total protein in bone is collagen.[15] Collagen contributes to the healing process as a haemostatic agent and as an activator for neutrophils and fibroblasts.[16–18]

Collagen when implanted in the body, is primarily degraded by the enzymatic activity of infiltrating macrophages and neutrophils.[19] There are several ways in which collagen can be processed for various applications.[20,21] One of the most common ways of processing involves the the use of glutaraldehyde.[22] Glutaraldehyde processing of collagen has been shown to increase cross-linking of the collagen, resulting in decreased susceptibility to enzymatic degradation, increased tensile strength, decreased solubility, decreased water absorption, increased time to degradation.[23] This process has also been shown to result in a final product to be limited in tissue toxicity, even though glutaraldehyde alone has known toxicity.[19] This is particularly critical when the collagen is obtained from a xenogeneic source.

Once a biomaterial, such as collagen, is implanted in the body, it triggers multiple host reactions including clot formation, acute inflammation, provisional matrix formation, chronic inflammation, granulation tissue development, foreign body reaction and fibrous encapsulation. In the early phases of healing, the thrombin clot that forms and encapsulates the biomaterial also acts as the provisional matrix around it.[24–26] This blood protein deposition, described as provisional matrix formation, furnishes the structural and functional components that aid in healing around the biomaterial as well as the foreign body reaction that ensues.[27] The cytokines, growth factors, chemotactic and mitogenic agents derived from the provisional matrix provides the stimulatory or inhibitory responses that modulate macrophage activity and other cell populations necessary for healing and inflammatory responses.

As the inflammation and the foreign body response progress, macrophages are extravasated and migrate to the implanted site. This targeted migration is mediated by chemokines and other chemoattractants.[28] Platelets and the clot release chemoattractants such as transforming growth factor beta, platelet-derived growth factor, leukotriene and interleukin 1. These, along with mast cell degranulation products and factors released from macrophages recruited to the site, play a key role in recruiting more macrophages to the site of the implanted biomaterial.[29,30]

Upon adhesion to the biomaterial, the macrophage cytoskeleton changes allow for macrophages to spread over the material surface. This adhesion is facilitated by podosomes that form during the early stages of the adhesion process.[31–33] The adhered macrophages subsequently fuse to form foreign body giant cells.[34] Reflective of their origin, these foreign body giant cells display antigenic properties similar to monocytes and macrophages.[35]

The activation of these macrophages and the subsequent release of degrading agents result in the resorption and remodelling of regenerative biomaterials including collagen. Macrophages and foreign body giant cells release reactive oxygen species, degradative enzymes and acids into a privileged zone that exists between the cells and the biomaterial surface.[36–38] Thus, the surface of the biomaterial in the immediate vicinity of the inflammatory cells, macrophages and giant cells becomes susceptible to degradation. The rate and chemistry of this degradation depends on the chemistry of the biomaterial in use. At the minimum, the inflammatory response elicited by the material should not detrimentally affect the regenerative outcome intended for the use of the material.

An ideal membrane, in addition to not being detrimental, should also have components that would help reduce or direct the inflammatory response towards a favourable regenerative outcome. In fact, attempts are currently underway to engineer such membranes.[39] Existing synthetic and collagen-based devices that attempt incorporation of bioactive components[40] are limited in their ability to predictably incorporate bioactive molecules. Consequently, several naturally derived products have also been tested as devices for periodontal/alveolar regeneration, for example, duramater, oxidized cellulose mesh, cargille membranes[12] and fetal membranes. In the following sections, we will use a dehydrated human amnion-chorion allograft membrane (ACM) as an example of a bioactive resorbable membrane that favourably influences the immune system towards enhanced regenerative outcomes.

ACM is a human placenta-derived allograft that is constructed by laminating amnion and chorion membranes. Amnion and chorion layers are isolated from placenta and processed with proprietary cleansing process. The cleansed amnion and chorion layers are then laminated to form the composite graft, which is then dehydrated under controlled drying conditions.[41] The dehydrated graft retains bioactive proteins that can reduce inflammation and enhance regeneration. Koob et al. showed the presence of several growth factors, wound healing molecules and cytokines/chemokines that regulate inflammation[42,43] retained in ACM. Some key examples of molecules that are important GTR and GBR that are present in ACM include the following: PDGF-BB, TGF-beta1, bFGF, VEG and TIMP. They further demonstrated bioactivity of the molecules in ACM by demonstrating *in vitro* fibroblast proliferation, endothelial proliferation and migration of mesenchymal stem cells, in the presence of ACM.[42–44] In addition, ACM promotes *in vivo* mesenchymal progenitor cell recruitment in mice. Several preclinical and clinical studies have demonstrated the antibacterial properties of this membrane, which indirectly reduces immune responses during GTR/GBR procedures.[45–47] Amniotic membrane is also known to reduce pain,[46] as a consequence of its ability to reduce inflammation. In a recently concluded randomised clinical trial we noted a significant reduction in pain with the use of ACM (www.clinicaltrials.gov, registry ID number NCT02602223) compared to a control membrane (dense poly-tetrafluro-ethylene – dPTFE membrane).[48] In the above trial, we also noted significantly more new bone formation, as well as significant reduction of graft particles with the use of ACM over sockets grafted with freeze-dried bone allografts (FBDA) compared to a control membrane.[48] The placental barrier membranes used for the GTR and GBR procedures illustrated in Figures 10.1 and 10.2, respectively, are ACM membranes.

10.2.2 Immune Response to Non-Resorbable Barrier Membranes

Most non-resorbable membranes are inert, for example, dPTFE is completely inert and does not elucidate an immune response.[48] The older expanded PTFE, while being completely inert, was limited because of its larger pore size compared to the dPTFE. When flap dehiscence occurs and the ePTFE membranes were exposed they allowed bacterial infiltration and subsequent immune response.[49] Mesh membranes made from titanium are similarly inert and biocompatible, but when they are exposed prematurely due to flap dehiscence, the surgical site undergoes infection-related immune response reactions[50] similar to dPTFE. Table 10.1 compares the different commercially available non-resorbable membranes.

10.2.3 Immune Response During Scaffold Turnover

Bone-forming scaffolds used for GTR/GBR include autologous bone grafts, allogeneic bone grafts, xenogeneic bone grafts and synthetic bone substitutes. These scaffolds vary in their ability to promote regeneration based on their ability to be osteo-conductive, osteo-inductive or osteogenic (Table 10.2). The term osteo-conductive refers to the ability of a scaffold to passively allow cells to migrate into its matrix, while osteo-inductivity refers to the ability of a scaffold to actively induce cells to migrate into its matrix. Osteogenic refers to the potential of a scaffold to induce proliferation, migration and differentiation of cells into bone-forming cells from within the scaffold or from outside.

Bone autografts are obtained from different sites from the same host, for example, from the symphysis menti region, maxillary tuberosity, ramus or iliac crest. These grafts remodel using physiological mechanisms and do not elicit any immune response. Similarly, bone allografts and xenografts are decellularised and retain only the extracellular matrices, making them highly biocompatible and with negligible immunogenic potential. Synthetic bone substitutes are usually minerals that form part of the bone matrix, for example calcium sulfate particles, hydroxyapatite crystals or beta tri-calcium phosphates, and consequently are not highly immunogenic. However, like the resorbable barrier membranes, the bone scaffolds take advantage of the osteo-immunological mechanisms to enhance regenerative outcomes.

Amongst the most widely used for these purposes is the allograft, with over 200,000 cases involving the use of allografts each year in the USA.[51] Consequently, we will use them as an example of the osteo-immunological mechanisms that play a role in scaffold-mediated regeneration and compare them with autografts in the following section. Cancellous bone autografts, taken from the inner part of the bone, upon implantation, heal with the formation of a local haematoma that is rich in inflammatory cells and chemotactic mitogens that stimulate the further recruitment of mesenchymal stem cells. This is followed by the formation of fibrous granulation tissue,[51] recruitment of macrophages and neovascularisation.[52] Osteoblasts then line the periphery of the graft and start forming osteoid as the graft begins to be incorporated. The mineralisation of this osteoid results in new bone formation. Alternately, cortical autografts, which are primarily taken from the outer parts of bone, heal primarily through creeping substitution aided mostly by osteoclasts.[53,54] Unlike autografts, allografts are not as efficient in the promotion of healing, primarily as a result of the tissue preparation process, which also depletes the graft of many of the growth factors that are essential for osteo-induction. Cancellous allografts stimulate a more robust inflammatory response compared to autografts. This inflammatory response leads to the formation of a fibrous capsule around the graft particle, and the eventual deposition of osteoid, leading to the integration of the graft.[54] The incorporation of a cortical allograft is similar to a cancellous allograft in its nature to trigger a more robust inflammatory response and heals similar to the autogenic cortical graft through creeping substitution.[53] This happens by functional coupling of osteoblasts and osteoclasts. Osteoclasts formed from the fusion of mononuclear cells resorb the scaffold, while the osteoblasts lay down and mineralise in the areas of resorption (Figure 10.3).

Among allografts, the demineralised bone matrix is utilised in a significant number of grafting procedures. Demineralised bone has collagenous, non-collagenous structural components together with bone morphogenic proteins and those that stimulate growth. This makes the graft osteo-inductive and osteo-conductive. The osteo-inductive properties stimulate healing of the graft through growth factor-mediated recruitment and differentiation of mesenchymal stem cells into osteoblasts. As previously stated, the tissue processing depletes the graft of osteo-inductive properties and hence the mechanism of processing determines the osteo-inductive properties of the material. However, the capacity of the graft material for osteo-induction and conduction is greatly dependent on the method of processing of the graft. The different types of commercially available scaffolds and their bone-forming potential are listed in Table 10.2.

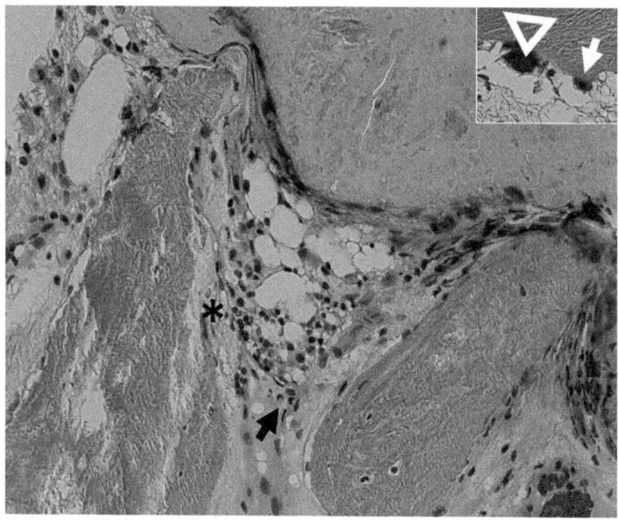

FIGURE 10.3 Goldner's trichrome staining of a bone core obtained after GBR mediated alveolar regeneration. Bone is stained in green and bone marrow cells in pink showing neutrophils (black arrow), mononuclear cells (*). Inset shows a higher magnification of multinuclear osteoclasts (white arrowhead) right next to osteoblasts (white arrow), demonstrating active remodelling of the graft particles.

10.3 IMMUNE RESPONSE TO BIOLOGICS

Biologic agents accelerate regeneration by introducing either recombinant human growth factors or biomolecules to wound sites and upregulating healing mechanisms. Current products that are used in GTR/GBR include recombinant human platelet-derived growth factor-BB (rhPDGF-BB), enamel matrix derivative (EMD), platelet-rich plasma/platelet-rich fibrin (PRP/PRF), fibroblast growth factor (FGF), bone morphogenic protein (BMP) and growth differential factor (GDF).[55] Given that many of the biologic agents are naturally present molecules that play critical roles in human physiology, albeit in a highly concentrated purified or recombinant form, its unsurprising that there are very few reports on adverse immunological events related to these agents. Of the biologic agents, the commonly used EMD is the only commercially available product that is of xenogeneic source. It is obtained from porcine tooth buds. This, and the fact that the precise mechanism of action of EMD is unknown, has led to extensive investigation into how EMD interacts with host immune cells. Here, we use EMD as an illustrative example of how biologic agents modulate the immune response and enable enhanced regenerative outcomes for GTR/GBR procedures.

10.3.1 EMD – CD4+ T-Helper Cells

EMD affects CD4+ lymphocyte migration. CD4+ plays a critical role in the immune response that takes place in the periodontium. In addition, EMD also enhances the expression of CD25 receptors by 2–12%. CD25 receptors are important regulators of activation-induced cell death. 100 mg of EMD/ml induces upregulation of T-lymphocyte apoptosis by about 32.4%, which likely explains the increased healing observed when EMD is used for periodontal regeneration.[56,57]

10.3.2 EMD – Macrophages and Monocytes

In a rat experimental periodontitis model, EMD gel was applied to the furcation area of the first molar region and monitored for changes in expression of macrophage cytokines and growth factors. Fourteen days after EMD treatment, periodontal tissue regeneration and new bone formation occurred. Compared to the no-treatment group, there was a significant decrease in inflammatory infiltrate near the bone surface, expression of IL-1β and TGF-β1 was absent and BMP-2 and BMP-4 were associated with polylayer-arranged osteoblasts near the dentin. These results suggest that EMD may play a role in the conversion of inflammatory macrophages to wound-healing macrophages, thus facilitating faster regeneration.[58]

Another study demonstrated that when monocytes were stimulated with lipopolysaccharide (LPS) and treated with varying concentrations of EMD (0, 50, 100, 200 μg/ml), TNF-α and IL-1β production became detectable under ELISA. The concentration of these cytokines was not influenced by EMD concentration, suggesting that EMD does not promote inflammation or resorption. Another assay measured increased monocyte phagocytic activity after three days in the presence of EMD. The results indicate that EMD may activate monocytes to clear a higher volume of foreign bodies, expediting the resolution of inflammation.[59]

Whole blood from healthy donors was incubated with different concentrations of EMD (1, 10, 100, 300 μg/ml) or 8-CPT-cAMP (10, 25, 50, 100 μM) and challenged with bacterial LPS (10 ng/ml) or peptidoglycan (10 μg/ml). Significant EMD dose-dependent reductions of LPS and peptidoglycan-induced cytokine release were observed with TNF-α and IL-8, but not IL-10. A similar dose-dependent decrease was observed with cAMP, which was decreased five and ten minutes after EMD exposure. Since macrophage-mediated cytokine burst is downregulated by cAMP formation, these findings prove that EMD may limit the release of pro-inflammatory cytokines induced by LPS or peptidoglycan via a secondary cAMP pathway.[60]

10.3.3 EMD – Tissue Inhibitors of Metalloproteinases

In a randomised clinical trial, 36 infrabony defects were randomly assigned to be treated by either flap surgery plus EMD or flap surgery plus placebo. GCF was sampled at baseline and 2, 4 and 12 weeks after surgery. Levels of tissue inhibitors of metalloproteinase-1 (TIMP-1), MMP-1 and MMP-8 were measured. At two weeks, the concentration of MMP-1 was significantly lower in the EMD compared to the placebo group. At four weeks, the concentration of TIMP-1, MMP-1 and MMP-8 was significantly lower in the EMD group compared to the placebo group. At 12 weeks the concentration of MMP-1 and MMP-8 was significantly lower in the EMD group compared to the placebo group. When calculating the TIMP-1/MMP-1+MMP-8 ratio, there was a significant increase at 2 weeks when compared to baseline, but a significant decrease at 4 and 12 weeks when compared to 2 weeks. These data conclude that EMD may assist with the early stages of remodelling in soft tissue and allow for quicker return to baseline pre-surgical conditions.[61]

10.3.4 EMD – Polymorphonuclear Leukocytes

PMN response to EMD was tested in the presence of fMLP (N-formyl-methionyl-leucyl-phenylalanine), a bacterially derived chemotactic factor, and OZ (serum-opsonized zymosan), a trigger molecule for MMP-8. When treated with EMD (200 μg/ml) and fMLP (1 μM), PMNs were observed to promote earlier and more sustained superoxide production and increased chemotaxis compared to those not treated with EMD (200 μg/ml). Both of these mechanisms are important for wound healing and bacterial clearance. Additionally, the combination of EMD (200 μg/ml) + fMLP (1 μM) and EMD (200 μg/ml) + OZ (2.5 mg/ml) resulted in significant decreases of MMP-8 release compared to fMLP (1 μM) and OZ alone (2.5 mg/ml). This result illustrates that EMD may also play a role in the suppression of tissue damage and degradation by MMP-8.[62]

The effect of EMD on cellular proliferation was studied by stimulating sub-confluent cultures of gingival and periodontal ligament fibroblasts with varying concentrations of EMD (10, 50, 100, 150 μg/ml). As negative and positive controls, 0.2% and 10% fetal calf serum (FCS) were used, respectively. At concentrations of 50 μg/ml or greater, EMD had a positive stimulatory effect on [3H] thymidine incorporation of gingival and periodontal ligament fibroblast DNA. Fibroblast wound healing and cellular proliferation was tested in the presence of EMD (20 μg/ml). After 16 days, EMD-treated fibroblasts all showed significantly greater wound reduction compared to 0.2% FCS controls, but less than 10% FCS controls. There were also significant increases in gingival and dermal fibroblasts proliferation, but not in periodontal ligament fibroblasts. These data indicate that EMD may aid in the rapid closure of wounds via fibroblast proliferation and migration.[63]

10.4 DENTAL IMPLANTS

Dental implants have become a large part of the practice of dentistry and dental implant placement, maintenance and treatment of peri-implant diseases has become a large part of the practice of periodontics. Approximately three million US adults have dental implants, with a predicted annual growth of 500,000.[64] A variety of materials and alloys have been evaluated in the search of a durable and biocompatible dental implant. Metals such as nickel, gold, lead, iridium, stainless steel, cobalt/chromium alloys and polymers such as polyurethane, polyethylene, polyamide, polytetrafluroethylene and polymethylmethacrylate have all been used as materials or alloyed for the fabrication of dental implants.[65] However, many of these materials do not meet the functional and mechanical requirements necessary for dental implants or have been limited due to their ability to cause adverse immunologic reactions.

An illustrative example is the use of metals alloyed with nickel. Nickel alloys have been shown to cause severe immunologic responses and cytotoxicity and thus fell out of favour for use as dental implants. When placing nickel implants into rats and analysing the soft tissues using X-ray scanning analytical microscopy (XSAM), severe inflammatory responses were observed. Histologically, the concentration of nickel dispersed within the soft tissue correlated with the observed inflammatory area and degree of tissue damage.[66] Nickel ions in solution were shown through biochemical analyses of lactate dehydrogenase (LDH), superoxide anion, TNF-α and scanning electron microscopy to destroy the cell membranes of neutrophils.[67] The non-toxic concentrations and cytotoxic nickel concentrations were later investigated and quantified in human dermal fibroblasts. It was determined that nickel may have a modulating effect on the cytotoxicity of hexavalent chromium, another possible alloy of dental implants. Over a 24-hour period of exposure to nickel and chromium with a nickel concentration of 250 μM, massive necrosis with enhanced oxidative stress was observed, decreasing the viability and increasing the stress response of primary human dermal fibroblasts. A nickel concentration of 25 μM was determined to be non-cytotoxic, suppressing chromium-induced stress signaling and inhibiting apoptosis of human dermal fibroblasts.[68]

Most dental implants currently used with significant success are made of titanium and its alloys. This mirrors the widespread use of titanium in the field of orthopedics. The advent of use of titanium for dental implants occurred in the early 1940s. Titanium is widely accepted due to its excellent biocompatibility via the rapid formation of a stable oxide film and its relative resistance to corrosion. Through a 12-month longitudinal study and utilising cytokine microarrays, mean volumes of cytokine levels were measured in the peri-implant crevicular fluid (PICF) and gingival crevicular fluid (GCF). It was demonstrated that the levels of IL-4, -6, -10 and -12p70, tumor necrosis factor-α and interferon-γ in the GCF and PICF over a 12-month period were not significantly different. No immune response was noted, and the response was concluded to be similar in respects to the cytokine levels examined in the GCF and PICF.[69]

However, an examination of the potential risk and detrimental effects of titanium ions, titanium corrosion and the corrosive titanium alloy byproducts on the surrounding peri-implant tissues is of great clinical importance. Studies within the field of orthopaedics have reviewed and noted a number of allergic reactions to titanium.[70] Symptoms and immune responses to titanium included urticaria, eczema, edema, redness and pruritus of the skin or mucosa, atopic dermatitis, impaired healing of fractures, necrosis and weakening of orthopaedic implants, and non-keratinised, edematous, proliferative hyperplastic tissue.[71–79] Chronic immune responses with infiltrating macrophages, fibroblasts and CD4 and CD8 positive lymphocytes, suggesting a delayed-type hypersensitivity reaction to titanium, have been examined in tissues adjacent to titanium orthopaedic fracture plates.[80] In addition, a comparison of the tissue response using light microscopy between asymptomatic and symptomatic patients with titanium orthopaedic bone plates noted a chronic granulomatous inflammatory reaction in the tissues of the symptomatic patients with persistent pain.

Significantly more lymphocytes and macrophages were noted in the soft tissue covering the titanium plates and there was localised tissue discolouration adjacent to the fixation screws and titanium was identified in this area by atomic absorption analysis.[81] Understanding how titanium ions and other metal debris becomes embedded into the surrounding soft tissue can be explained by the effects of metal-on-metal (MOM) wear on the host immune system and infection in hip arthroplasty. It was suggested that MOM wear products influenced the risk of infection by hampering the immune system.[82,83] MOM bearings produce nanometer- to submicrometer-sized metal particles.[84] Furthermore, recent research has suggested that particulate debris of any composition promotes bacterial growth by providing a scaffold for bacterial adhesion and biofilm growth.[85]

This understanding and examination of the effects of titanium ions in the rehabilitation of long bone fractures and arthroplasty in orthopaedics can be compared to the immunological responses to titanium of the dental implant. There is a suspected association of allergic reactions to titanium dental implants occurring in rare circumstances for some patients.[86] Allergic contact stomatitis caused by titanium nitride-coated implant abutments clearly dictates the incidence of a titanium allergy.[87] There have also been reports of a strong temporal relation between titanium dental implants and the onset of exfolliative cheilitis.[88]

Given that a large section of the population is being treated with dental implants, the advent of peri-implant diseases is becoming a public health concern. Peri-implant diseases include peri-implant mucositis and peri-implantitis. Both are inflammatory processes around dental implants. Peri-implantitis is distinguished from peri-mucositis by the presence of peri-implant bone loss with the former disease. The etiology of peri-implantitis is not truly understood but a possible cause and contributing factor can be associated with the exposure of the peri-implant tissues to titanium particulate debris eliciting a host immune response. In a study comparing the submucosal plaque of implants with peri-implantitis and implants determined to be healthy, the results showed significantly higher mean levels of dissolved titanium, after adjusting for the amount of plaque collected per site, in the submucosal plaque of implants with peri-implantitis versus the submucosal plaque of healthy implants. This demonstrated an association between titanium particles and the development of peri-implantitis.[89] When comparing epithelial cells and macrophages in cytologic smears of peri-implant mucosa between patients with or without peri-implantitis, metal-like particles were observed inside and outside these cells, whereas no metal particles were found in the control samples where implants were not placed. The concentration of titanium was higher in the peri-implantitis group compared to the healthy implant group and no traces of titanium were observed in the controls.[90]

Pro-inflammatory cytokines, infiltration of immune cells and activation of osteoclasts are stimulated in peri-implant tissues in the presence of metal particles and ions. It was suggested that the degradation of dental implants and the debris that is then released has cytotoxic and genotoxic potential for the peri-implant tissues demonstrated by the degenerative changes reported in macrophages and neutrophils that phagocytised titanium particles in human cells cultured in medium containing titanium-based nanoparticles.[91] Examining the cellular responses of gingival epithelial-like cells (GE-1) to varying concentrations of titanium ions demonstrated that at high concentrations of titanium ions, induction of necrosis occurred in GE-1 cells. Titanium ion concentrations of more than 13 ppm significantly decreased the viability of GE-1 cells and the mRNA expression levels of TLR-4 and ICAM-1 in GE-1 cells were significantly enhanced at a concentration of 9 ppm. It has been suggested that Ti ions are cytotoxic, elevate the sensitivity of the gingival epithelial cells to microorganisms and elicit monocyte infiltration and induce inflammation at the interfaces of dental implants and gingival tissues.[92,93] As the titanium levels of tissue samples obtained in the vicinity of the titanium implants increased to higher levels (≥40 μm) human macrophages *in vitro* were stimulated and secretion of IL-1B occurred.[94] Additionally, the size of the titanium particles plays a key role in cytotoxicity. Titanium particles of 1–3 μm size are phagocytised by phagocytic cells (which are approximately 5 μm) and an immunological response was not elicited.[67]

Factors triggering titanium dissolution into the peri-implant tissues, as well as the role of titanium corrosion in the peri-implant inflammatory process, are unclear and a number of suggestions have been made to elucidate such triggering factors. Titanium particles could be released upon implant placement as a result of the friction between bone and dental implants at high insertion torque values. Free titanium particles are then capable of eliciting the activation of the DNA damage response via DDR pathway in oral epithelial cells, disrupting its genomic stability, and leaving the peri-implant tissues more prone to infiltration and destruction by foreign bodies.[95] Fluoride, a common additive to many toothpastes and oral hygiene products, has shown to cause corrosion of the implant surface and more titanium ions were detected around the peri-implant tissues following sodium fluoride treatment. Corrosion of the titanium dental implant does not only compromise its structural integrity, but can also cause an immunogenic effect, amplifying the host inflammatory response and increasing bone loss by means of an increased release of pro-inflammatory cytokines such as TNF-alpha, IL-1B and RANKL by host cells.[96]

For the most part, dentistry has been successful in creating a fairly biocompatible dental implant utilising titanium. However, it is undeniable that with recent findings, a body of literature is developing and demonstrating some form of an elicitation of an immunological response when the peri-implant tissues are exposed to titanium ions, debris or corrosive byproducts. These immunological effects and response elicited by these foreign particles in the oral cavity are still being investigated and additional research is needed to fully understand this multi-factorial and complex host response.

10.4.1 Luting Agents

Luting agents are cements that provide a link between the prepared tooth/dental implant and the restoration, bonding them together through mechanical, chemical or combined properties.[97] While dental implants can be restored with screw-retained restorations, a large number of practitioners use cement-retained restorations with equal success. Excess cement at the dental implant to abutment interface and flowing towards the bone has been shown as one of the main etiological factors for peri-implantitis in dental implants that are restored with cement-retained restorations.[98]

Luting agents can be classified into two types: conventional and resin-based. Conventional luting agents are zinc phosphate, zinc oxide eugenol, polycarboxylate, glass ionomer cement (GIC) and resin-modified GIC. Resin-based agents contain the matrix, inorganic fillings and monomers, such as methyl methacrylate, aromatic dimethacrylate-based resin (bisfenol-glycidylmethacrylate - Bis-GMA), triethylene glycol dimethacrylate (TEGDMA), 4-methacryloxyethyl trimellitate (4-META) and urethane dimethacrylate (UDMA).[97,99,100]

Adverse reactions towards luting cements have long been described,[101–108] but prevalence among patients is difficult to ascertain due to the scarcity of clinical trials and because the reporting of adverse effects concerning dental materials is voluntary for most countries.[109]

The luting agents that have mostly been associated with adverse reactions are eugenol and polymer-based materials. Glass ionomer cements and zinc oxide allergies are extremely rare, but eugenol may act as a contact irritant and induces anaphylactic symptoms[101,102] and type IV hypersensitivity.[110] Even though resinous agents are considered safe, and most of the unreacted methacrylate groups are not capable of being leached into aqueous environments, a significant amount of unreacted monomer can be released[111] and cause allergic contact stomatitis in susceptible patients.[112] Oral contact allergic reactions may manifest as redness, swelling, mucosal erosion or lichenoid reactions near restoration. The patient may complain of itching or pain.[113,114]

10.4.2 Ceramics for Crowns and Implants

Ceramic structures composed of zirconium dioxide have been used as a metal replacement for implant abutments and crown and bridge work.[115] They are biocompatible, showing similar levels of pro-inflammatory cytokines in peri-implant tissue similar to those found in contralateral teeth or titanium implants.[116] In fact, there are case reports indicating the use of ceramic implants and ceramic veneering as substitutes for titanium for patients with sensitisation to metals.[117,118] Dental ceramics are basically composed of metal oxides and half-metals. The most frequently used oxides for crowns are silicium dioxide, Al_2O_3, K2O3, MgO, CaO and B_2O_3, which are all highly biocompatible with no related immune reactions.[114]

10.4.3 Metal Alloys

Periodontal or implant procedures for oral rehabilitation may involve the use of metal-based alloys such as dental crowns, casts, metal frameworks, temporisation materials and metal-ceramic restorations. Commonly these alloys present a combination of nickel (Ni), cobalt (Co), chromium (Cr), palladium (Pd) or gold (Au), which are considered of little risk because of their very low dissolution rate.[119,120] However, the oral cavity is an adverse environment owing to the presence of mechanical stress, electrolyte-rich saliva and complex microflora, which may increase the metal corrosion process, metal ion dissolution and the onset of adverse reactions.[105,121]

Patients' sensitisation to metal alloys is quite common. Patch test clinical studies to detect metal sensitivity in large populations indicate sensitisation rates from 8[122] to 25%[123] – women being more affected than men.[109] Yet, it is unusual for patients to present adverse reactions against dental alloys. When the patient shows symptoms of dental metal alloy immunoreactivity, this is mainly related to palladium chloride,[123–126] gold sodium thiosulfate[105] and nickel alloys.[105,127] Patients generally complain of pain, taste disturbances, burning sensation, dry mouth, associated with objective findings such as ulcerations, vesicles, lichenoid reaction, non-plaque-related gingivitis, stomatitis, recurrent aphtosis, cheilitis, hand/face dermatitis, eczema and/or atopy.[105,109,125]

The mechanism of immune activation by dental alloys is still under investigation. Metal ions and proteins possibly form stable bonds, becoming haptens with immunogenic potential. Au-Pd alloys seem to be a weaker allergen than Ni, Cr or Co in other alloys, and individuals who are sensitive to Ni are likely to be allergic to Pd.[128] *In vitro* studies suggest that human peripheral blood mononuclear cell (PBMC) sensitisation to Co, Cr, Pd and Au may result in a Th1- and Th2-type mixed cellular immune response.[129] PBMC can increase the levels of interleukin synthesis (IL) in accordance to the type of metal. Contact with Co increases IL-2 and 13, Pd raises IL-2 and IL-4, Au promotes IL-13 and interferon gamma (IFN- γ release), and Ni is related to high levels of IL-2, IL-4, IL-13, IFN- γ.[129] Patients with oral nickel exposure may present increased levels of cytokines such as IL-4, IFN- γ, IL-5 and IL-10, which are related to type I hypersensitivity and type V immune reaction.[127] Dental cast alloys can activate human monocyte-derived dendritic cells by inducing IL-8 production.[130] Also, it has been described that Ni, Co and Pd directly bind to the toll-like receptor 4 (TLR4)[131,132] and Au binds to TLR3 commencing the maturation of antigen-presenting cells.[133]

Taken together, these studies show that dental appliances may represent an active source of metals in the body, especially Pd and Ni, and this can favour the clinical setting of hypersensitivity in a subgroup of susceptible patients.

10.5 MOUTHWASHES

One of the key aspects of the practice of periodontics is helping the patient maintain adequate oral hygiene practices for health as well as disease control. Periodontists often prescribe mouth rinses containing chlorhexidine (CHX) for routine post-operative care, but CHX mouthwashes have been used since the 1970s to control plaque and gingivitis[134–136] due to their antimicrobial properties and substantivity. Other healthcare professionals use chlorhexidine-containing products as topical antimicrobial agents. However, there is growing evidence that CHX is capable of inducing hypersensitivity reaction in adults and children.[137–142] Enger et al. (2009) described severe and life-threatening reactions towards CHX in 104 men during operative procedures of either urological or cardiothoracic surgery. Noteworthy from the diverse sources of CHX sensitisation is the fact that three men from this series related previous exposure to CHX only from mouthwash formulations.[143]

CHX can cause allergic contact stomatitis (type VI hypersensitivity),[144] type I allergy and anaphylactic symptoms.[40,145] Recently, the Food and Drug Administration launched a warning that CHX used as a skin antiseptic can cause rare but serious allergic reactions. Thus, healthcare professionals should always ask patients about previous CHX reactions, advise patients about the possibility of having an unexpected adverse symptom and consider using alternative antiseptics in case of suspicion of CHX allergy.[146]

10.6 SUMMARY AND CONCLUDING REMARKS

The biomaterials currently used in the practice of periodontics are largely biocompatible and elicit minimal immune responses. On the other hand, the turnover of graft materials and biomembranes are critically dependent on an active immune system. The increasing use of immune modulatory drugs, for example, monoclonal antibodies that target specific cytokines and anti-resorptive drugs, is already impacting periodontal and dental implant-related procedures.[147] In addition, several of the materials discussed here for regeneration have several limitations that make predictable outcomes a challenge. The size and shape of defects are critical factors in determining outcomes. While three-walled narrow intrabony defects and class two mandibular buccal furcations are predictable sites to regenerate,[7] any exponential increase in complexity of defect size or morphology reduces the predictability. Thus, the next challenge that needs to be addressed in GTR/GBR procedures is towards treating medically complex patients as well as predictably regenerating larger/complex defects. This would need bioengineering strategies like (1) pre-vascularisation of large grafts,[148] (2) 3D printing of graft materials to match defect shape size and morphology,[148] (3) incorporation of progenitor cells,[149] and (4) incorporation of biologics into engineered scaffolds that allow their sustained or controlled release.[149] In terms of dental implants, the prevention of peri-implantitis in osseo-integrated implants is an emerging and critical area of clinical relevance.

REFERENCES

1. Bannister, S. R. *Glossary of Periodontal Terms*, https://members.perio.org/libraries/glossary?_ga=2.253816268.538891445.1512266559-235718969.1507236679&ssopc=1 (2017).
2. Hajishengallis, G. Periodontitis: From microbial immune subversion to systemic inflammation. *Nat Rev Immunol* 15, 30–44 (2015).
3. Eke, P. I. et al. Update on prevalence of periodontitis in adults in the United States: NHANES 2009 to 2012. *J Periodontol* 86, 611–622 (2015).
4. Services, U. S. D. o. H. a. H. Vol. 2016–1232 (ed. Health and Human Services) (DHHS, 2015).
5. Hammerle, C. H., Giannobile, W. V. & Working Group 1 of the European Workshop on, P. Biology of soft tissue wound healing and regeneration—Consensus report of Group 1 of the 10th European Workshop on Periodontology. *J Clin Periodont* 41 Suppl 15, S1–5, doi:10.1111/jcpe.12221 (2014).
6. Ramseier, C. A., Rasperini, G., Batia, S. & Giannobile, W. V. Advanced reconstructive technologies for periodontal tissue repair. *J Periodontol* 2000 59, 185–202, doi:10.1111/j.1600-0757.2011.00432.x (2012).

7. Sculean, A. et al. Biomaterials for promoting periodontal regeneration in human intrabony defects: A systematic review. *J Periodontol* 2000 68, 182–216, doi:10.1111/prd.12086 (2015).
8. Moses, O. et al. Biodegradation of three different collagen membranes in the rat calvarium: A comparative study. *J Periodontol* 79, 905–911, doi:10.1902/jop.2008.070361 (2008).
9. Nyman, S., Gottlow, J., Karring, T. & Lindhe, J. The regenerative potential of the periodontal ligament. *J Clin Periodontol* 9, 257–265 (1982).
10. Nyman, S., Lindhe, J., Karring, T. & Rylander, H. New attachment following surgical treatment of human periodontal disease. *J Clin Periodontol* 9, 290–296 (1982).
11. Freitas, R. M. et al. Alveolar ridge and maxillary sinus augmentation using rhBMP-2: A systematic review. *Clin Implant Dent Relat Res* 17, e192–e201 (2015).
12. Tatakis, D. N., Promsudthi, A. & Wikesjö, U. M. Devices for periodontal regeneration. *J Periodontol* 2000 19, 59–73 (1999).
13. Lim, R. Concise review: Fetal membranes in regenerative medicine: New tricks from an old dog? *Stem Cells Transl Med* 6, 1767–1776, doi:10.1002/sctm.16-0447 (2017).
14. Soo, C., Rahbar, G. & Moy, R. L. The immunogenicity of bovine collagen implants. *J Dermatol Surg Oncol* 19, 431–434 (1993).
15. Schroeder, H. E., Munzel-Pedrazzoli, S. & Page, R. Correlated morphometric and biochemical analysis of gingival tissue in early chronic gingivitis in man. *Arch Oral Bio* 18, 899–923 (1973).
16. Chang, C. & Houck, J. C. Demonstration of the chemotactic properties of collagen. *Proc Soc Exp Biol Med* 134, 22–26 (1970).
17. Postlethwaite, A. E., Seyer, J. M. & Kang, A. H. Chemotactic attraction of human fibroblasts to type I, II, and III collagens and collagen-derived peptides. *Proc Natl Acad Sci USA* 75, 871–875 (1978).
18. Wang, C. L., Miyata, T., Weksler, B., Rubin, A. L. & Stenzel, K. H. Collagen-induced platelet aggregation and release. II Critical size and structural requirements of collagen. *Biochim Biophys Acta* 544, 568–577 (1978).
19. M, C. in *Fundamental aspects of biocompatibility* (eds Williams & DE), 87–104 (CRC Press, 1981).
20. Khor, E. Methods for the treatment of collagenous tissues for bioprostheses. *Biomaterials* 18, 95–105 (1997).
21. ST, L. in *The biomedical engineering handbook* (ed. Bronzino, J. D.) 627–647 (CRC Press, 1995).
22. Petite, H., Frei, V., Huc, A. & Herbage, D. Use of diphenylphosphorylazide for crosslinking collagen-based biomaterials. *J Biomed Mater Res* 28, 159–165, doi:10.1002/jbm.820280204 (1994).
23. Pachence, J. M. Collagen-based devices for soft tissue repair. *J Biomed Mater Res* 33, 35–40, doi:10.1002/(SICI)1097-4636(199621)33:1<35::AID-JBM6>3.0.CO;2-N (1996).
24. Anderson, J. M. Multinucleated giant cells. *Curr Opin Hematol* 7, 40–47 (2000).
25. Gretzer, C., Emanuelsson, L., Liljensten, E. & Thomsen, P. The inflammatory cell influx and cytokines changes during transition from acute inflammation to fibrous repair around implanted materials. *J Biomater Sci Polym Ed* 17, 669–687 (2006).
26. Luttikhuizen, D. T., Harmsen, M. C. & Van Luyn, M. J. Cellular and molecular dynamics in the foreign body reaction. *Tissue Eng* 12, 1955–1970, doi:10.1089/ten.2006.12.1955 (2006).
27. Horbett, T. in *Biomaterials Science: An Introduction to Biomaterials in Medicine* (eds B. Ratner et al.), 237–246 (ElsevierAcademic Press, 2004).
28. Esche, C., Stellato, C. & Beck, L. A. Chemokines: Key players in innate and adaptive immunity. *J Invest Dermatol* 125, 615–628, doi:10.1111/j.0022-202X.2005.23841.x (2005).

29. Tang, L., Jennings, T. A. & Eaton, J. W. Mast cells mediate acute inflammatory responses to implanted biomaterials. *Proc Natl Acad Sci USA* 95, 8841–8846 (1998).
30. Broughton, G., 2nd, Janis, J. E. & Attinger, C. E. The basic science of wound healing. *Plast Reconstr Surg* 117, 12S–34S, doi:10.1097/01.prs.0000225430.42531.c2 (2006).
31. Giancotti, F. G. & Ruoslahti, E. Integrin signaling. *Science* 285, 1028–1032 (1999).
32. Marx, J. Cell biology. Podosomes and invadopodia help mobile cells step lively. *Science* 312, 1868–1869, doi:10.1126/science.312.5782.1868 (2006).
33. Rose, D. M., Alon, R. & Ginsberg, M. H. Integrin modulation and signaling in leukocyte adhesion and migration. *Immunol Rev* 218, 126–134, doi:10.1111/j.1600-065X.2007.00536.x (2007).
34. Chen, E. H., Grote, E., Mohler, W. & Vignery, A. Cell-cell fusion. *FEBS Lett* 581, 2181–2193, doi:10.1016/j.febslet.2007.03.033 (2007).
35. Athanasou, N. A. & Quinn, J. Immunophenotypic differences between osteoclasts and macrophage polykaryons: Immunohistological distinction and implications for osteoclast ontogeny and function. *J Clin Pathol* 43, 997–1003 (1990).
36. Henson, P. M. The immunologic release of constituents from neutrophil leukocytes. I. The role of antibody and complement on nonphagocytosable surfaces or phagocytosable particles. *J Immunol* 107, 1535–1546 (1971).
37. Henson, P. M. The immunologic release of constituents from neutrophil leukocytes. II. Mechanisms of release during phagocytosis, and adherence to nonphagocytosable surfaces. *J Immunol* 107, 1547–1557 (1971).
38. Haas, A. The phagosome: Compartment with a license to kill. *Traffic* 8, 311–330, doi:10.1111/j.1600-0854.2006.00531.x (2007).
39. Bottino, M. C., Thomas, V. & Janowski, G. M. A novel spatially designed and functionally graded electrospun membrane for periodontal regeneration. *Acta Biomaterialia* 7, 216–224 (2011).
40. Rose, L. & Rosenberg, E. Bone grafts and growth and differentiation factors for regenerative therapy: A review. *Practical procedures & aesthetic dentistry: PPAD* 13, 725 (2001).
41. Davis, J. S. Skin transplantation. *Johns Hopkins Hospital Reports* 15, 307–396 (1910).
42. Koob, T. J. et al. Biological properties of dehydrated human amnion/chorion composite graft: Implications for chronic wound healing. *Int Wound J* 10, 493–500 (2013).
43. Koob, T. J., Lim, J. J., Massee, M., Zabek, N. & Denoziere, G. Properties of dehydrated human amnion/chorion composite grafts: Implications for wound repair and soft tissue regeneration. *J Biomed Mater Res B: Applied Biomaterials* 102, 1353–1362 (2014).
44. Koob, T. J. et al. Angiogenic properties of dehydrated human amnion/chorion allografts: Therapeutic potential for soft tissue repair and regeneration. *Vasc Cell* 6 (2014).
45. Gurinsky, B. A novel dehydrated amnion allograft for use in the treatment of gingival recession: An observational case series. *J Implant Adv Clin Dentistry* 1, 65–73 (2009).
46. Velez, I., Parker, W. B., Siegel, M. A. & Hernandez, M. Cryopreserved amniotic membrane for modulation of periodontal soft tissue healing: A pilot study. *J Periodontol* 81, 1797–1804 (2010).
47. Wallace, S. Radiographic and histomorphometric analysis of amniotic allograft tissue in ridge preservation: A case report. *J Imp Adv Clin Dent* 2, 49–55 (2010).
48. Hassan, M., Prakasam, S., Bain, C., Ghoneima, A. & Liu, S. S.-Y. A randomized split-mouth clinical trial on effectiveness of amnion-chorion membranes in alveolar ridge preservation: A clinical, radiologic, and morphometric study. *Int J Oral Maxillofac Implants* 32 (2017).
49. Ling, L. J., Hung, S. L., Lee, C. F., Chen, Y. T. & Wu, K. M. The influence of membrane exposure on the outcomes of guided tissue regeneration: Clinical and microbiological aspects. *J Periodontol Res* 38, 57–63 (2003).

50. Torres, J. et al. Platelet-rich plasma may prevent titanium-mesh exposure in alveolar ridge augmentation with anorganic bovine bone. *J Clin Periodontol* 37, 943–951 (2010).
51. Russell A. T., T. C., Lavelle, D. G. in *Fractures in Adults* Vol. 3 (eds Heckman J. D., Bucholz R. W., Court- & Brown, C. M.) 1915– 1982 (Rockwood and Green, 1991).
52. Oakes, D. A. & Cabanela, M. E. Impaction bone grafting for revision hip arthroplasty: Biology and clinical applications. *J Am Acad Orthop Surg* 14, 620–628 (2006).
53. Khan, S. N. et al. The biology of bone grafting. *J Am Acad Orthop Surg* 13, 77–86 (2005).
54. JM, F. Fracture repair and bone grafting. *OKU 10: Orthopaedic Knowledge Update. Rosemont, IL; American Academy of Orthopaedic Surgeons*, 11–21 (2011).
55. Suarez-Lopez Del Amo, F., Monje, A., Padial-Molina, M., Tang, Z. & Wang, H. L. Biologic agents for periodontal regeneration and implant site development. *Biomed Res Int* 2015, 957518, doi:10.1155/2015/957518 (2015).
56. Gassmann, G., Schwenk, B., Entschladen, F. & Grimm, W. D. Influence of enamel matrix derivative on primary CD4+ T-helper lymphocyte migration, CD25 activation, and apoptosis. *J Periodontol* 80, 1524–1533, doi:10.1902/jop.2009.080612 (2009).
57. Petinaki, E., Nikolopoulos, S. & Castanas, E. Low stimulation of peripheral lymphocytes, following in vitro application of Emdogain. *J Clin Periodontol* 25, 715–720 (1998).
58. Fujishiro, N., Anan, H., Hamachi, T. & Maeda, K. The role of macrophages in the periodontal regeneration using Emdogain gel. *J Periodontal Res* 43, 143–155, doi:10.1111/j.1600-0765.2007.01004.x (2008).
59. Khedmat, S., Hadjati, J., Iravani, A. & Nourizadeh, M. Effects of enamel matrix derivative on the viability, cytokine secretion, and phagocytic activity of human monocytes. *J Endod* 36, 1000–1003, doi:10.1016/j.joen.2010.02.032 (2010).
60. Myhre, A. E. et al. Anti-inflammatory properties of enamel matrix derivative in human blood. *J Periodontal Res* 41, 208–213, doi:10.1111/j.1600-0765.2005.00863.x (2006).
61. Okuda, K. et al. Levels of tissue inhibitor of metalloproteinases-1 and matrix metalloproteinases-1 and -8 in gingival crevicular fluid following treatment with enamel matrix derivative (EMDOGAIN). *J Periodontal Res* 36, 309–316 (2001).
62. Karima, M. M. & Van Dyke, T. E. Enamel matrix derivative promotes superoxide production and chemotaxis but reduces matrix metalloproteinase-8 expression by polymorphonuclear leukocytes. *J Periodontol* 83, 780–786, doi:10.1902/jop.2011.110397 (2012).
63. Rincon, J. C., Haase, H. R. & Bartold, P. M. Effect of Emdogain on human periodontal fibroblasts in an in vitro wound-healing model. *J Periodontal Res* 38, 290–295 (2003).
64. Prakasam, S. Create a Safety Culture. *Dimens Dent Hyg* 13, 67–70 (2015).
65. Saini, M., Singh, Y., Arora, P., Arora, V. & Jain, K. Implant biomaterials: A comprehensive review. *World J Clin Cases* 3, 52–57, doi:10.12998/wjcc.v3.i1.52 (2015).
66. Uo, M., Watari, F., Yokoyama, A., Matsuno, H. & Kawasaki, T. Dissolution of nickel and tissue response observed by X-ray scanning analytical microscopy. *Biomaterials* 20, 747–755 (1999).
67. Kumazawa, R. et al. Effects of Ti ions and particles on neutrophil function and morphology. *Biomaterials* 23, 3757–3764 (2002).
68. Rudolf, E. & Cervinka, M. Nickel modifies the cytotoxicity of hexavalent chromium in human dermal fibroblasts. *Toxicol Lett* 197, 143–150, doi:10.1016/j.toxlet.2010.05.011 (2010).
69. Nogueira-Filho, G. et al. Longitudinal comparison of cytokines in peri-implant fluid and gingival crevicular fluid in healthy mouths. *J Periodontol* 85, 1582–1588, doi:10.1902/jop.2014.130642 (2014).

70. Goutam, M., Giriyapura, C., Mishra, S. K. & Gupta, S. Titanium allergy: A literature review. *Indian J Dermatol* 59, 630, doi:10.4103/0019-5154.143526 (2014).
71. Bircher, A. J. & Stern, W. B. Allergic contact dermatitis from “titanium” spectacle frames. *Contact Dermatitis* 45, 244–245 (2001).
72. Haug, R. H. Retention of asymptomatic bone plates used for orthognathic surgery and facial fractures. *J Oral Maxillofac Surg* 54, 611–617 (1996).
73. Hensten-Pettersen, A. Casting alloys: Side-effects. *Adv Dent Res* 6, 38–43, doi:10.1177/08959374920060011401 (1992).
74. Lhotka, C. G. et al. Are allergic reactions to skin clips associated with delayed wound healing? *Am J Surg* 176, 320–323 (1998).
75. Matthew, I. & Frame, J. W. Allergic responses to titanium. *J Oral Maxillofac Surg* 56, 1466–1467 (1998).
76. Mitchell, D. L., Synnott, S. A. & VanDercreek, J. A. Tissue reaction involving an intraoral skin graft and CP titanium abutments: A clinical report. *Int J Oral Maxillofac Implants* 5, 79–84 (1990).
77. Tamai, K. et al. A case of allergic reaction to surgical metal clips inserted for postoperative boost irradiation in a patient undergoing breast-conserving therapy. *Breast Cancer* 8, 90–92 (2001).
78. Thomas, P., Bandl, W. D., Maier, S., Summer, B. & Przybilla, B. Hypersensitivity to titanium osteosynthesis with impaired fracture healing, eczema, and T-cell hyperresponsiveness in vitro: Case report and review of the literature. *Contact Dermatitis* 55, 199–202, doi:10.1111/j.1600-0536.2006.00931.x (2006).
79. Valentine-Thon, E. & Schiwara, H. W. Validity of MELISA for metal sensitivity testing. *Neuro Endocrinol Lett* 24, 57–64 (2003).
80. Hunt, J. A., Williams, D. F., Ungersböck, A. & Perrin, S. The effect of titanium debris on soft tissue response. *J Mater Sci Mater Med* 5, 381–383, doi:10.1007/bf00058968 (1994).
81. Ungersboeck, A., Geret, V., Pohler, O., Schuetz, M. & Wuest, W. Tissue reaction to bone plates made of pure titanium: A prospective, quantitative clinical study. *Journal of Materials Science: Materials in Medicine* 6, 223–229, doi:10.1007/bf00146860 (1995).
82. Hosman, A. H., van der Mei, H. C., Bulstra, S. K., Busscher, H. J. & Neut, D. Metal-on-metal bearings in total hip arthroplasties: Influence of cobalt and chromium ions on bacterial growth and biofilm formation. *J Biomed Mater Res A* 88, 711–716, doi:10.1002/jbm.a.31922 (2009).
83. Hosman, A. H., van der Mei, H. C., Bulstra, S. K., Busscher, H. J. & Neut, D. Effects of metal-on-metal wear on the host immune system and infection in hip arthroplasty. *Acta Orthop* 81, 526–534, doi:10.3109/17453674.2010.519169 (2010).
84. Campbell, P., Doorn, P., Dorey, F. & Amstutz, H. C. Wear and morphology of ultra-high molecular weight polyethylene wear particles from total hip replacements. *Proc Inst Mech Eng H* 210, 167–174, doi:10.1243/PIME_PROC_1996_210_409_02 (1996).
85. Anwar, H. A., Aldam, C. H., Visuvanathan, S. & Hart, A. J. The effect of metal ions in solution on bacterial growth compared with wear particles from hip replacements. *J Bone Joint Surg Br* 89, 1655–1659, doi:10.1302/0301-620X.89B12.19714 (2007).
86. Egusa, H., Ko, N., Shimazu, T. & Yatani, H. Suspected association of an allergic reaction with titanium dental implants: A clinical report. *J Prosthet Dent* 100, 344–347, doi:10.1016/S0022-3913(08)60233-4 (2008).
87. Lim, H. P., Lee, K. M., Koh, Y. I. & Park, S. W. Allergic contact stomatitis caused by a titanium nitride-coated implant abutment: A clinical report. *J Prosthet Dent* 108, 209–213, doi:10.1016/S0022-3913(12)60163-2 (2012).
88. Pigatto, P. D., Berti, E., Spadari, F., Bombeccari, G. P. & Guzzi, G. Photoletter to the editor: Exfoliative cheilitis associated with titanium dental implants and mercury amalgam. *J Dermatol Case Rep* 5, 89–90, doi:10.3315/jdcr.2011.1084 (2011).

89. Safioti, L. M., Kotsakis, G. A., Pozhitkov, A. E., Chung, W. O. & Daubert, D. M. Increased levels of dissolved titanium are associated with peri-implantitis – a cross-sectional study. *J Periodontol* 88, 436–442, doi:10.1902/jop.2016.160524 (2017).
90. Olmedo, D. G., Nalli, G., Verdu, S., Paparella, M. L. & Cabrini, R. L. Exfoliative cytology and titanium dental implants: A pilot study. *J Periodontol* 84, 78–83, doi:10.1902/jop.2012.110757 (2013).
91. Noronha Oliveira, M. et al. Can degradation products released from dental implants affect peri-implant tissues? *J Periodont Res*, n/a-n/a, doi:10.1111/jre.12479.
92. Makihira, S. et al. Titanium ion induces necrosis and sensitivity to lipopolysaccharide in gingival epithelial-like cells. *Toxicol In Vitro* 24, 1905–1910, doi:10.1016/j.tiv.2010.07.023 (2010).
93. Wachi, T., Shuto, T., Shinohara, Y., Matono, Y. & Makihira, S. Release of titanium ions from an implant surface and their effect on cytokine production related to alveolar bone resorption. *Toxicology* 327, 1–9, doi:10.1016/j.tox.2014.10.016 (2015).
94. Pettersson, M. et al. Titanium ions form particles that activate and execute interleukin-1beta release from lipopolysaccharide-primed macrophages. *J Periodontal Res* 52, 21–32, doi:10.1111/jre.12364 (2017).
95. Suarez-Lopez Del Amo, F. et al. Titanium activates the DNA damage response pathway in oral epithelial cells: A pilot study. *Int J Oral Maxillofac Implants* 32, 1413–1420, doi:10.11607/jomi.6077 (2017).
96. Nishimura, K. et al. Influence of titanium ions on cytokine levels of murine splenocytes stimulated with periodontopathic bacterial lipopolysaccharide. *Int J Oral Maxillofac Implants* 29, 472–477, doi:10.11607/jomi.3434 (2014).
97. Ladha, K. & Verma, M. Conventional and contemporary luting cements: An overview. *J Indian Prosthodont Soc* 10, 79–88, doi:10.1007/s13191-010-0022-0 (2010).
98. Korsch, M., Obst, U. & Walther, W. Cement-associated peri-implantitis: A retrospective clinical observational study of fixed implant-supported restorations using a methacrylate cement. *Clin Oral Implants Res* 25, 797–802 (2014).
99. Jivraj, S. A., Kim, T. H. & Donovan, T. E. Selection of luting agents, part 1. *J Calif Dent Assoc* 34, 149–160 (2006).
100. Kim, T. H., Jivraj, S. A. & Donovan, T. E. Selection of luting agents: Part 2. *J Calif Dent Assoc* 34, 161–166 (2006).
101. Tammannavar, P., Pushpalatha, C., Jain, S. & Sowmya, S. V. An unexpected positive hypersensitive reaction to eugenol. *BMJ Case Rep* 2013, doi:10.1136/bcr-2013-009464 (2013).
102. Sarrami, N., Pemberton, M. N., Thornhill, M. H. & Theaker, E. D. Adverse reactions associated with the use of eugenol in dentistry. *Br Dent J* 193, 257–259, doi:10.1038/sj.bdj.4801539 (2002).
103. Evrard, L. & Parent, D. Oral allergies to dental materials. *Bull Group Int Rech Sci Stomatol Odontol* 49, 14–18 (2010).
104. Gall, H. [Allergies to dental materials and dental pharmacologic agents]. *Hautarzt* 34, 326–331 (1983).
105. Raap, U., Stiesch, M., Reh, H., Kapp, A. & Werfel, T. Investigation of contact allergy to dental metals in 206 patients. *Contact Dermatitis* 60, 339–343, doi:10.1111/j.1600-0536.2009.01524.x (2009).
106. Ratz, K. H. & Heise, H. Allergies of the oral cavity caused by dental materials and dental pharmaceuticals. *Z Arztl Fortbild (Jena)* 80, 1033–1036 (1986).
107. Szepesi, M., Radics, T., Vitalyos, G. & Hegedus, C. Allergies to dental materials and effectiveness of treatment in the north-eastern region of Hungary. *Fogorv Sz* 107, 135–139 (2014).
108. Wiltshire, W. A., Ferreira, M. R. & Ligthelm, A. J. Allergies to dental materials. *Quintessence Int* 27, 513–520 (1996).

109. Schedle, A., Ortengren, U., Eidler, N., Gabauer, M. & Hensten, A. Do adverse effects of dental materials exist? What are the consequences, and how can they be diagnosed and treated? *Clin Oral Implants Res* 18 Suppl 3, 232–256, doi:10.1111/j.1600-0501.2007.01481.x (2007).
110. Silvestre, J. F., Albares, M. P., Blanes, M., Pascual, J. C. & Pastor, N. Allergic contact gingivitis due to eugenol present in a restorative dental material. *Contact Dermatitis* 52, 341, doi:10.1111/j.0105-1873.2005.0612c.x (2005).
111. Ferracane, J. L. Hygroscopic and hydrolytic effects in dental polymer networks. *Dent Mater* 22, 211–222, doi:10.1016/j.dental.2005.05.005 (2006).
112. Johns, D. A., Hemaraj, S. & Varoli, R. K. Allergic contact stomatitis from bisphenol-a-glycidyl dimethacrylate during application of composite restorations: A case report. *Indian J Dent Res* 25, 266–268, doi:10.4103/0970-9290.135941 (2014).
113. Lygre, G. B., Gjerdet, N. R., Gronningsaeter, A. G. & Bjorkman, L. Reporting on adverse reactions to dental materials—Intraoral observations at a clinical follow-up. *Community Dent Oral Epidemiol* 31, 200–206 (2003).
114. Lygre, H. Prosthodontic biomaterials and adverse reactions: A critical review of the clinical and research literature. *Acta Odontol Scand* 60, 1–9 (2002).
115. Hashim, D., Cionca, N., Courvoisier, D. S. & Mombelli, A. A systematic review of the clinical survival of zirconia implants. *Clin Oral Investig* 20, 1403–1417, doi:10.1007/s00784-016-1853-9 (2016).
116. Cionca, N., Hashim, D., Cancela, J., Giannopoulou, C. & Mombelli, A. Pro-inflammatory cytokines at zirconia implants and teeth. A cross-sectional assessment. *Clin Oral Investig* 20, 2285–2291, doi:10.1007/s00784-016-1729-z (2016).
117. Oliva, X., Oliva, J. & Oliva, J. D. Full-mouth oral rehabilitation in a titanium allergy patient using zirconium oxide dental implants and zirconium oxide restorations. A case report from an ongoing clinical study. *Eur J Esthet Dent* 5, 190–203 (2010).
118. Cionca, N., Hashim, D. & Mombelli, A. Zirconia dental implants: Where are we now, and where are we heading? *Periodontology 2000* 73, 241–258, doi:10.1111/prd.12180 (2017).
119. Gil, F. J., Sanchez, L. A., Espias, A. & Planell, J. A. In vitro corrosion behaviour and metallic ion release of different prosthodontic alloys. *Int Dent J* 49, 361–367 (1999).
120. Wu, M. K. et al. Corrosion behaviours of the dental magnetic keeper complexes made by different alloys and methods. *Int J Oral Sci* 8, 155–163, doi:10.1038/ijos.2016.21 (2016).
121. Milheiro, A., Muris, J., Kleverlaan, C. J. & Feilzer, A. J. Influence of shape and finishing on the corrosion of palladium-based dental alloys. *J Adv Prosthodont* 7, 56–61, doi:10.4047/jap.2015.7.1.56 (2015).
122. Kranke, B. & Aberer, W. Multiple sensitivities to metals. *Contact Dermatitis* 34, 225 (1996).
123. Muris, J. et al. Sensitization to palladium and nickel in Europe and the relationship with oral disease and dental alloys. *Contact Dermatitis* 72, 286–296, doi:10.1111/cod.12327 (2015).
124. Muris, J. et al. Sensitization to palladium in Europe. *Contact Dermatitis* 72, 11–19, doi:10.1111/cod.12295 (2015).
125. Muris, J. et al. Palladium-based dental alloys are associated with oral disease and palladium-induced immune responses. *Contact Dermatitis* 71, 82–91, doi:10.1111/cod.12238 (2014).
126. Cristaudo, A. et al. Release of palladium from biomechanical prostheses in body fluids can induce or support PD-specific IFNgamma T cell responses and the clinical setting of a palladium hypersensitivity. *Int J Immunopathol Pharmacol* 22, 605–614, doi:10.1177/039463200902200306 (2009).
127. Buyukozturk, S. et al. Oral nickel exposure may induce Type I hypersensitivity reaction in nickel-sensitized subjects. *Int Immunopharmacol* 26, 92–96, doi:10.1016/j.intimp.2015.03.012 (2015).

128. Budinger, L. & Hertl, M. Immunologic mechanisms in hypersensitivity reactions to metal ions: An overview. *Allergy* 55, 108–115 (2000).
129. Minang, J. T., Arestrom, I., Troye-Blomberg, M., Lundeberg, L. & Ahlborg, N. Nickel, cobalt, chromium, palladium and gold induce a mixed Th1- and Th2-type cytokine response in vitro in subjects with contact allergy to the respective metals. *Clin Exp Immunol* 146, 417–426, doi:10.1111/j.1365-2249.2006.03226.x (2006).
130. Rachmawati, D., von Blomberg, B. M. E., Kleverlaan, C. J., Scheper, R. J. & van Hoogstraten, I. M. W. Immunostimulatory capacity of dental casting alloys on endotoxin responsiveness. *J Prosthet Dent* 117, 677–684, doi:10.1016/j.prosdent.2016.08.013 (2017).
131. Raghavan, B., Martin, S. F., Esser, P. R., Goebeler, M. & Schmidt, M. Metal allergens nickel and cobalt facilitate TLR4 homodimerization independently of MD2. *EMBO Rep* 13, 1109–1115, doi:10.1038/embor.2012.155 (2012).
132. Schmidt, M. et al. Crucial role for human Toll-like receptor 4 in the development of contact allergy to nickel. *Nat Immunol* 11, 814–819, doi:10.1038/ni.1919 (2010).
133. Barry, R. J. et al. Association analysis of TGFBR3 gene with Behcet's disease and idiopathic intermediate uveitis in a Caucasian population. *Br J Ophthalmol* 99, 696–699, doi:10.1136/bjophthalmol-2014-306198 (2015).
134. Loe, H. & Schiott, C. R. The effect of mouthrinses and topical application of chlorhexidine on the development of dental plaque and gingivitis in man. *J Periodontal Res* 5, 79–83 (1970).
135. Loe, H., Schiott, C. R., Karring, G. & Karring, T. Two years oral use of chlorhexidine in man. I. General design and clinical effects. *J Periodontal Res* 11, 135–144 (1976).
136. Schiott, C. R. et al. The effect of chlorhexidine mouthrinses on the human oral flora. *J Periodontal Res* 5, 84–89 (1970).
137. Cogne, Y. et al. Chlorhexidine-induced IgE-mediated allergy in a 6-year-old child. *J Allergy Clin Immunol Pract* 5, 837–838, doi:10.1016/j.jaip.2016.11.019 (2017).
138. Faber, M. et al. Allergy to chlorhexidine: Beware of the central venous catheter. *Acta Anaesthesiol Belg* 63, 191–194 (2012).
139. Garvey, L. H. et al. IgE-mediated allergy to chlorhexidine. *J Allergy Clin Immunol* 120, 409–415, doi:10.1016/j.jaci.2007.04.029 (2007).
140. Garvey, L. H., Roed-Petersen, J. & Husum, B. Anaphylactic reactions in anaesthetised patients – four cases of chlorhexidine allergy. *Acta Anaesthesiol Scand* 45, 1290–1294 (2001).
141. Koch, A. & Wollina, U. Chlorhexidine allergy. *Allergo J Int* 23, 84–86, doi:10.1007/s40629-014-0012-6 (2014).
142. Pemberton, M. N. Allergy to Chlorhexidine. *Dent Update* 43, 272–274 (2016).
143. Egner, W. et al. Chlorhexidine allergy in four specialist allergy centres in the United Kingdom, 2009-13: Clinical features and diagnostic tests. *Clin Exp Immunol* 188, 380–386, doi:10.1111/cei.12944 (2017).
144. Liippo, J., Kousa, P. & Lammintausta, K. The relevance of chlorhexidine contact allergy. *Contact Dermatitis* 64, 229–234, doi:10.1111/j.1600-0536.2010.01851.x (2011).
145. Thune, P. Two patients with chlorhexidine allergy—Anaphylactic reactions and eczema. *Tidsskr Nor Laegeforen* 118, 3295–3296 (1998).
146. FDA. *FDA warns about rare but serious allergic reactions with the skin antiseptic chlorhexidine gluconate*, www.fda.gov/downloads/Drugs/DrugSafety/UCM539059.pdf (2017).
147. Otomo-Corgel, J., Pucher, J. J., Rethman, M. P. & Reynolds, M. A. State of the science: Chronic periodontitis and systemic health. *J Evid Based Dent Pract* 12, 20–28 (2012).
148. Bertassoni, L. E. et al. Hydrogel bioprinted microchannel networks for vascularization of tissue engineering constructs. *Lab on a Chip* 14, 2202–2211 (2014).
149. Thrivikraman, G., Athirasala, A., Twohig, C., Boda, S. K. & Bertassoni, L. E. Biomaterials for craniofacial bone regeneration. *Dental Clinics* 61, 835–856 (2017).

Index

Page numbers followed by f and t indicate figures and tables, respectively.

B

D

E

F

G

H

K

L

M

N

O

P

W

X

Y

Z